Health Now

HEALTH

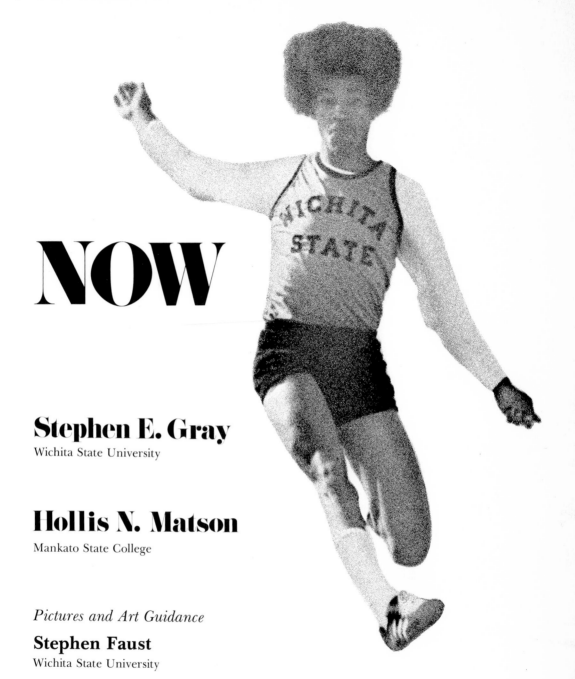

NOW

Stephen E. Gray
Wichita State University

Hollis N. Matson
Mankato State College

Pictures and Art Guidance
Stephen Faust
Wichita State University

Macmillan Publishing Co., Inc.
New York

Collier Macmillan Publishers
London

Macmillan Publishing Co., Inc.
866 Third Avenue, New York, New York 10022

Collier Macmillan Canada, Ltd.

Library of Congress Cataloging in Publication Data

Gray, Stephen E
  Health now.

  Includes index.
  1. Hygiene. 2. Hygiene, Public. I. Matson,
Hollis N., joint author. II. Title.
[DNLM: 1. Health. WB120 G782h]
RA776.G788   613   75-4929
ISBN 0-02-346140-3

Printing: 1 2 3 4 5 6 7 8   Year: 6 7 8 9 0 1

To Babs

She did more than type; she wrote.
She did more than suggest; she researched.
She did more than criticize; she encouraged.

Preface

This is a book to be read. All books are, of course. But some are meant to be studied more than read, analyzed more than discussed, memorized more than thought about. This isn't a book that lends itself to that kind of approach. This is the day when health relates to dirty sewers, pot smoking, euthanasia, pregnancy out of wedlock, national health insurance, and group marriage. These are the 1970s, a time of affluent depression, ecstatic guilt, confused organization. Health now has little to do with platitudes, pedantics, instructions on brushing teeth and moving bowels. This is the time for looking at ourselves as we are, the world as it is.

There are five parts to *Health Now,* plus an introductory chapter that deals with the meaning of health, its history, its present and future. Why should a young person study health? Surely he knows he should take an occasional bath, that smoking and drinking can be hazardous, that a speeding automobile can be hazardous. Is this a "preachy" subject, the same old approach to some worn-out data? We hope not.

Part One, titled "Social Health," answers questions like the following: Do girls who weren't virgins at marriage have a greater chance of becoming divorcees, carping mothers, unhappy companions? Do Blacks have a stronger sex urge than Whites? How about newlyweds—can the honeymoon euphoria last? And don't forget the mother-in-law and Mother and Dad. Part One deals with mental health, even though no one really knows what that is. Everyone wants it, though, and conducts his own special search for an emotional Holy Grail. Some seek it in love, work, and faith. Others feel it's contained in sports, relaxation, good books, good food. Some get so frustrated in their efforts to find it that their sense of well being and their rationality leave them. They can end up in institutions.

Part Two, "Health Escapes," deals with drugs, alcohol and tobacco, and quacks. What can be said about these things that hasn't already been said? They're dangerous, they're frightening, they lead to cancer, schizophrenia, delirium tremens, and bankruptcy? They're for people with no sense of responsibility toward society and loved ones, no pride in themselves, no common sense? No. This has been said before, probably too often, and it's probably not quite true. There are some very intelligent people who visit quacks, some responsible people who take illegal drugs, some healthy people who drink and smoke. Besides, this book isn't supposed to preach. It should present several sides of the issues, though, and it does. The reader can choose the side he likes.

Part Three deals with "Physical Health." Human anatomy and physiology are covered, of course. Each system of the body is described according to structure and function. And diet is covered. Fads are rejected, whether they're "natural food" fads or quick reducing schemes. The only known way to have that lean and hungry look is to be hungry. It should be "balanced hunger," though. There should be sufficient vitamins, proteins, minerals, fats, and carbohydrates in any diet to meet bodily needs. Fads involving body building are rejected, too. Isometrics really won't change basic body build. And nothing will turn a 140-pounder into a guard for Green Bay. There are kinds of exercise that are worthwhile, though. They improve circulation, strengthen the heart, and make life a lot more enjoyable.

Part Four discusses "Health Impairments." There's coverage of illnesses currently known to plague man. What man has done about them, is doing about them, and possibly will do about them gets emphasis. What man should be doing about safety and accident prevention gets emphasis, too. Accidents kill and maim more young people than any germ, any fever, any virus. They also wreak havoc with Mom and Dad and Granddad.

Part Five covers "Community Health." This outlines the American system, or "nonsystem," of health care delivery. Certainly American hospitals, doctors, nurses, health insurance plans, and drug companies aren't the envy of the world—despite propaganda from special interest groups saying otherwise. We don't have a health care system that happily enriches itself from sickness, ignorance, and poverty, either. You can get excellent care in this country, but you have to understand the system, know where to look. The final chapter, "Man's Crisis: His Environment," deals with pollution of all forms, various ways of dealing with it, and the progress we seem to be making. It's a dirty world, one that seems to be getting dirtier, one that needs a lot of thought and leadership to keep man from destroying himself along with birds, fish, and aardvarks.

Man has become such a complex actor that only the sincere can understand him. Society has become so self-righteous, so bureaucratic, so conformist oriented that only the easygoing can tolerate it. And man and society are what health is about. Sincerity, readability, and easygoing pleasure are what this book is meant to be about—that and current health facts. Put them together, and the reader has something to think about and, we hope, remember and apply.

We can't thank everyone who has helped us with this book. There are hundreds who have given suggestions, encouragement, criticism. And all of it has been used—sensibly, we hope. There are some, though, whose help was essential to turning out the kind of product we hope you approve of. They are Henry Gurney, Bridgewater State College, Bridgewater, Massachusetts; John Tansley, Glendale College, Glendale, California; Karen King, University of Tulsa, Tulsa, Oklahoma; Bryan E. M. Cooke, University of Northern Colorado, Greeley, Colorado; Helen Thomas, Wichita State University, Wichita, Kansas; and, above all, Lloyd Chilton, Executive Editor, College Department, Macmillan.

S. E. G.

H. N. M.

Contents

Contents

Part Three
Physical Health

Part Four
Health Impairments

Part Five
Community Health

1 The Health Scene

It can be a bore. You've had a health course before, maybe a couple of them. Certainly, you know you should brush your teeth regularly, take a bath every so often, and eat a balanced diet. You've heard the latest on drugs. You know that driving mixed with martinis can lead to serious health problems; martinis without driving can lead to some health problems, too. Or maybe you've never had a course in health, but certainly you know the basics of healthy living. So why a course in something your mother has stressed since kindergarten, Dad backed her up on, and your girlfriend alludes to from time to time?

You could ask just about the same questions on courses in sociology, psychology, American history, civics, philosophy, and ethics. Any discussion can be trite; any topic can be nontopical; any teaching can be pedantic and preachy. Teaching can be stimulating; discussions can be thought-provoking; subject matter can be current, too. Health can be a boring course, just as trigonometry, accounting, and business law can be boring. Or it can be a vital course, a creative one—one that gives you an idea of who you are, how to approach being the kind of person you want to be, how to appreciate the kinds of people other people are and the kinds of things that make up the universe.

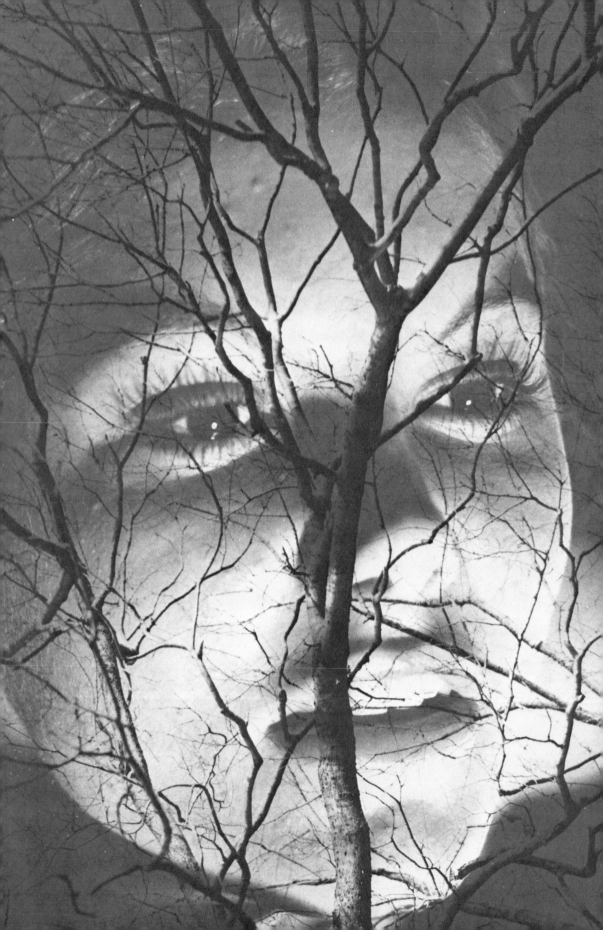

Definition of Health

What is health? That feeling you have when you're 18 and don't have when you're 48? The way you feel when you don't have a cold, when you've had a good night's sleep, when you don't have a toothache or athlete's foot? There's more to it than that, according to the World Health Organization. Health is a "state of complete physical, mental, and social well-being and not merely the absence of disease or infirmity."[1] Fifty-four nations agreed on this definition at the World Health Assembly, so there has to be something said for it. It's not a perfect definition, however. Health, like love, passion, and understanding, is such a broad concept that you can't really define it in absolutes, can't tie it down. There has to be a little sickness in health, a touch of insanity, a smattering of poverty for it to be a realistic ideal. Even the most wild-eyed zealot at WHO doesn't believe that all men or any man can have a complete sense of physical well-being. Certainly, there'd be a canker sore, dim eyesight, a touch of asthma, or old age to make this healthy person human, not a god. And it's yogis, fakirs, and mystics, not health practitioners, who believe in complete mental well-being. As to social well-being, breathes there a soul so optimistic as to believe we can eliminate hate, greed, poverty, crime, and war? Isn't an ideal so euphoric more closely related to nirvana than health?

"Health is a quality of life involving dynamic interaction and interdependence among the individual's physical well-being, his mental and emotional reactions, and the social complex in which he exists."[2] The School Health Education Study said this and expressed it well. Health really is an interaction among physical, mental, and social status. And this interaction is dynamic. But this definition is so broad that it could apply to the Christian Church, the Boy Scouts, or a political party. "Health is the soul that animates all the enjoyments of life, which fade and are tasteless without it." Sir William Temple wrote this. And, although it's true, it doesn't define what health is. The same is true of the statement by Aristotle's grandson, Herophylus, in 300 B.C.: "To lose one's health renders science null, art inglorious, strength unavailing, wealth useless, and eloquence powerless." An old Arabian proverb in the same context stated, "He who has health has hope, and he who has hope has everything." There are hundreds, thousands of sayings about this precious state, yet none really explains what it's about—and with good reason.

Health, like personality, is pretty much of an individual thing. A "good personality" is one that fits in well with the people and circumstances around it. How good it is varies from time to time, from place to place. General Patton's personality was great for leading the Third Army. It wouldn't have worked out too well in a monastery or a university, or at an insurance convention. The same applies to health. "Good health" to an 18-year-old is a different concept from "good health" to an 88-year-old. Good health to a track star is different from good health to a businessman or a bartender. And if

FIGURE 1-1. *Health—a quality of life.*

we're talking about the total concept of health, which involves the mental and social aspects, the variables become unlimited.

No one is quite sure about what mental health is, but most agree that it's not a fixed definition. It varies between men and women, young and old, athlete and spectator, corporation president and scientist, certainly professor and student. There's more than one who's a little "strange" who's a great artist, a first-class writer, an effective psychiatrist, a top teacher, a successful entrepreneur. Social well-being is more variable yet. There really are those who don't care about money, status, friends, family, fame. And there are those who get sick trying to acquire one or more of these things. Of money, status, and fame, some can never have enough. To others, friends and family make their lives complete, whether they're living in a boxcar or a penthouse. Social well-being, like the other aspects of health, varies with who's describing it and who's listening.

But health, no matter how you view it, is dynamic. It's not the same today as it was a week ago. It won't be the same a month from now. This applies to the mental and social aspects of it as well as the physical, applies to any person or any group. It's an ever-changing scale, varying between the death point of zero and optimum degrees beyond the description of numbers. It's an ecological type of concept, involving not just man himself, but myriad interactions with his environment.[3] What kind of medical and

FIGURE 1-2. *Feeling good!*

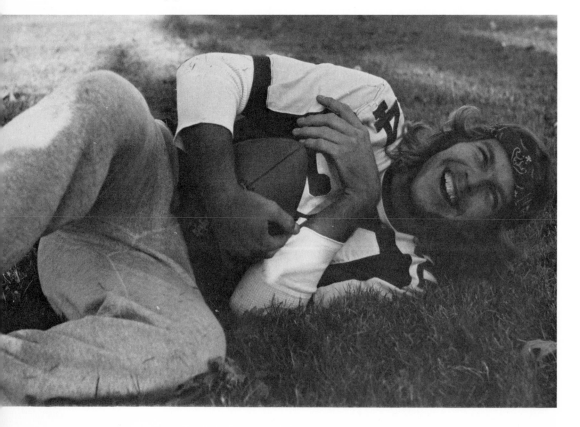

dental care is he getting? How about his food, his exercise, and his feelings about his job, his school, his church? What kind of thoughts does he have about the past? Has it been a good life, the kind he wants to share and build on? There's sexual adjustment. This involves others, not just the individual. There's the aesthetic feelings he gets from nature, from music, paintings, and books. There are challenges, adventures, spiritual faith, and ideals. There's this feeling about ourselves, partly good, partly bad, partly something we dream up, partly something the world gives us.

Health is really as complex as life itself, as infinite as the universe. Good health is really the good life. And though it may seem elusive, fortuitous, infinite, it's within the grasp of most of us. After all, if health is infinite, so is man's mind. There are few problems we can't solve or few situations we can't improve with a positive attitude and a little knowledge.

Heredity's Role in Health

Men may be created equal spiritually, but certainly not physically and mentally. There's the 7-foot-4-inch basketball center, the girl with the Miss America body, the 270-pound middle linebacker, the mongoloid, the mathematical genius, the girl with buck teeth. Heredity can play hateful tricks, funny tricks, provide bounties that Howard Hughes or John Paul Getty couldn't touch.

Most of us pick pretty good ancestors. We've got reasonable heads and reasonable bodies and average senses. If we're a little below average, that's no problem. Social standards are pretty loose. If we happen to have a minor gift, we're lucky. But be we fortunate or unfortunate, there's not a lot we can do about what Mother Nature gave us. Despite the advertisements in the centerfold of comic books, you really can't turn a 98-pound weakling into a Mr. World. You can't give someone a speed reading course and improve his IQ by 30 or 40 points, either. And there's no way to cure epilepsy, Huntington's chorea, mongolism, congenital dislocation of the hip, or club feet with good thoughts. We inherit certain kinds of health problems, tendencies toward certain kinds of health problems, and we have to learn to adjust to our limitations. The likelihood of being afflicted with schizophrenia, coronary artery disease, intestinal cancer, asthma, and most other ills, including premature death, is probably influenced, and sometimes caused, by genes—DNA, RNA, or whatever predetermines that we'll have blue eyes, red hair, bowed legs.[4] Heredity places limitations on health for all of us. Sometimes they're restrictive limitations, but usually they're not. Most of us have all that we need for the good life. Mother Nature really isn't to blame if we don't get it.

Environment's Role in Health

There used to be some bitter battles between people who claimed that heredity was a greater force in shaping what we become than environment and people who looked at it from the other angle. But, despite the bickering and the tomes of material supporting both sides, the matter has never been resolved and probably never will be. Certainly, you might inherit weaker lungs than your neighbor in the next county. But he'll have a better chance of coming down with emphysema than you will if he smokes and you don't. The same, of course, applies to the liver, cirrhosis, and alcohol; to the mind, hallucinations, and LSD. What's done to us and what we do to ourselves after we're born has a big influence on how long and how well we live. And environment, unlike heredity, is something we have a little control over. You can select the life style you follow, the girl you marry, the friends you hang out with, your job, your church, your political party; select the television programs you watch, the books you read, where you live. All of these things influence your health in one way or another. And they influence who you are, which is what health is really about.

There are different types of environment that act on us in different ways. There's "physical environment," which takes in heat and light and food and pollution and traffic and microorganisms. These determine not just how well we live, but whether we live at all. There are "psychological environment" and "social environment," which affect our personalities, our attitudes, our philosophies of life. This is where the habits of winning or losing, living in a ghetto or suburbia, get formed. And there is a category called "personal environment," which is probably the most important. This refers to your surroundings at the moment, your immediate friends, your immediate habits such as smoking or driving a motorcycle, your immediate sicknesses, your immediate successes, fears, goals, faith.[5]

Decision Making

There are our physical selves, the world around us, and decisions to make about this world. Put them all together, and you've got the unique human being. No two people have exactly the same environment. No two people respond to environment exactly the same way. Part of this response is based on our physical makeup—our nerves, our muscles. Part comes from the uniqueness of stimuli and reactions to stimuli we've experienced in the past. Some claim there's no such thing as a decision-making process. We're just reacting to a complex set of stimuli in a complex but predetermined way. We're intricate computers that breathe, eat, and get programmed. According to this philosophy, there really is no difference between environment and decision making. But most people don't carry this line of reasoning to the ultimate. Human behavior is so complex that there almost has to be a mind, a thought process, or free will to explain it.[6] Someone really does have the choice of whether to engage in sexual intercourse, take "speed," drink bourbon, have an abortion, drive at 90 miles per hour. These decisions definitely affect health, express health in the way that they're made.

A Healthy Person

Because health is an individual thing, an expression of a life style, a philosophy, an art, how can you say that there's such a thing as a healthy person? In the strictest sense, you can't. But, in the strictest sense, you can't say someone

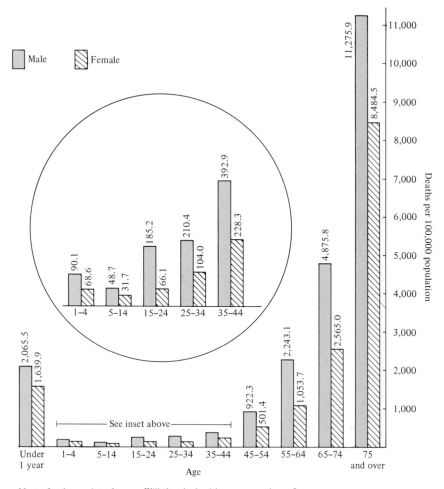

Most of us have a lot of years. Will they be healthy ones, good ones?

SOURCE: Public Health Service, National Center for Health Statistics, unpublished data.

FIGURE 1-3. *Death rates by age and sex, 1971.*

is beautiful, honest, intelligent, or strong. Society does make judgments, though, about health practices. It considers some worthwhile, and most people who follow them live longer and spend less time in hospitals and doctors' offices than ones who don't. A healthy person, according to society,

1. Stays in good physical condition. This includes a program of rest, sleep, and recreation, as well as exercise.
2. Eats a balanced diet of proteins, carbohydrates, minerals, vitamins, and fats. He eats his share of calories, but not many more or fewer than his body burns.
3. Decides wisely about the use of alcohol, tobacco, and drugs. There's a lot of argument about what "wise decisions" in this area are. And they're the kinds of decisions that no one can make for another person. But "wisdom" is something most of us get when we think a little.

4. Has a healthy philosophy of life. Even churches and psychiatrists can't agree on what this means. It's a broad area that includes responsibility, consideration of others, love, self-confidence, sincerity, hard work— sometimes. Sometimes it includes a little hate and self-pity. A lot depends on the circumstances, at times on who's involved. But there are philosophies that help us adjust to a trying and disappointing world, and there are philosophies that put us in mental institutions, on welfare, in penitentiaries. The former philosophies are worth seeking, even though no one is quite sure what they are. Probably you'll find them if you look. Surely you won't if you don't.
5. Visits a dentist twice a year to have plaque removed, teeth polished, and a checkup for caries and periodontal disease. And he practices good oral hygiene habits like brushing his teeth twice a day and using dental floss.
6. Has good safety habits, particularly when he drives. He's considerate and alert; he knows the highway regulations and follows them.
7. Has a physical checkup periodically and keeps his immunizations up to date.
8. Stays reasonably clean, preferably by bathing and changing undergarments daily. Some refined people aren't quite this fastidious, but it's probably better to err on the side of too much soap than too little.
9. Makes intelligent decisions about his sex role and his sex life. Obviously this is double talk. Sex is much more physical and emotional than it is intellectual. Intelligent decisions in this area come hard, but they seem to come to most who work at being honest with themselves.
10. Is aware of the medical services available to him and his family and has an effective medical care plan.
11. Knows the difference between the quack and the legitimate health care practitioner and avoids the former, no matter how disappointed he becomes with the latter. Also, if he's sure he's run into a quack, he reports it to the Food and Drug Administration or the Better Business Bureau.[7]

Health in an Earlier Day

Disease is a lot older than man is. Geologists have found fossils of microorganisms that existed 500 million years ago. So man who lived in the caves, fought sabertoothed tigers and carried clubs, suffered from stomachaches, diarrhea, bad teeth, boils, and athlete's foot.[8] Primitive man blamed these problems on the gods. After all, there were lots of them; they had unlimited power; and they were amenable to flattery. Speak to them nicely, give them a sacrifice or two, and they might cure your headache, fallen arches, even old age. Spiritualism and medicine were one and the same. Demons and evil spirits were coronary thrombosis, glaucoma, stomach ulcers, phlebitis, and otitis media. And there were the wonder drugs of spells, prayers, omens, chants, and dancing. Then along came the civilizations of Egypt and Mesopotamia, and man began to get the idea that there was more to health care than carrying the right amulet. Homer considered the Egyptian physicians the finest of his day. And Herodotus wrote of Egyptians as the healthiest of all people. King Hammurabi of Mesopotamia published a code around 2250 B.C. outlining community health procedures, health practices that individuals and families should follow, and recommended medical fees and punishments for malpractice. "An eye for an eye and a tooth for a tooth" in the Old Testament probably came from Hammurabi's thoughts on the subject.

Around 1490 B.C. the Israelites received the Mosaic Code. Probably based on Egyptian theories, the code stressed cleanliness, safety, obstetrics, disease prevention and control, sewage disposal, first aid, quarantine, and sterilization of surgical instruments. During this same time there were Indians in Mexico who used hundreds of medicinal plants to treat disease and had an excellent knowledge of narcotics and their effects. They practiced dieting, bathing, bloodletting, even surgery and suturing. And the Hindus of India developed surgery to a fine art. Successful amputations weren't uncommon; neither was the removal of skin cancers, cysts, and tumors.

Greek and Roman Health

But the belief that divine power reigned supreme persisted until about 500 B.C., when the Greeks and their philosophies began spreading throughout the civilized world. Hippocrates crystallized a new health care viewpoint, claiming that man's physical ills sprang from natural, not supernatural causes. This "father of scientific medicine" established principles of medical observation and treatment still in use today. Today's physicians still subscribe to the Oath of Hippocrates.

Personal hygiene was at the heart of the Greek health care philosophy. Cleanliness was stressed; so were exercise, diet, and disease control. The Romans, though, were more interested in community health. Attempting to improve the health of their general population, they built sewage systems, aqueducts, and public baths, and paved their streets. They even established medical societies, arranged for physicians to work for the state, and set up health insurance. Some of their administrative and engineering accomplishments in this field haven't been bettered to this day.

The Middle Ages

But then came the barbarians and the powerful church of the Middle, or "Dark," Ages. Herb doctors, witchcraft, alchemy, and astrological cures took over completely. If you needed an operation, you could see your surgeon-barber. Treatment by an educated physician was almost out of the question; manual labor was beneath him. The vile human body was studied in philosophical terms only. These were the days of the great plagues, and death was as common a visitor as rainfall and the evening wind. Smallpox, leprosy, influenza, typhoid fever, and diphtheria controlled destiny far more than kings and armies. However, the practice of quarantine became well developed during this period. People felt, and sometimes rightly so, that close association with the sick would make them sick. So lepers had to wear bells or blow horns to warn people of their presence. And massive hospitals were built, where the sick were placed five or six in a bed to die.

FIGURE 1-4. *One of the true kings of the Dark Ages. This fellow shaped more lives and ended more lives than the strongest of popes, the most terrifying of generals, the cleverest of prime ministers.*

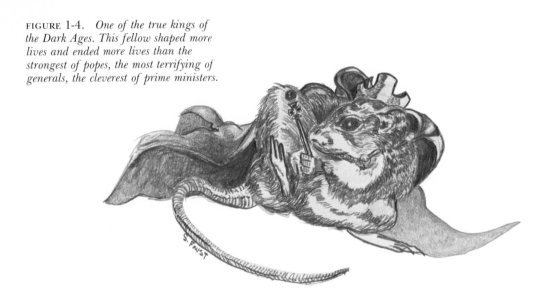

But at least some men insisted on using their heads. Superstition had its place in old women's parlors, hermits' hideaways, and monasteries. But there was a real world to be faced, to be described, tested, and thought about. Leonardo da Vinci conducted physiological experiments and did dissections. Paracelsus conducted thousands of rudimentary chemical experiments and is looked on as the father of modern chemotherapy. Andreas Vesalius founded the science of anatomy by cutting corpses apart. An Englishman, William Harvey, discovered that blood circulates. And another Englishman, Thomas Sydenham, established the study of internal medicine. These Renaissance men may not have made the Dark Ages bright, but they did start a flame that began to glow.

And then came 1675. Man suddenly had a method and a tool to examine a universe he never knew existed. Anton van Leeuwenhoek, a Dutch brewmaster, invented the microscope. Bacteria and protozoa now came under human scrutiny. Drops of water, human hair, bits of skin, bits of anything looked quite different under magnification than they did with the unaided human eye. Modern biological science was about to be created; modern thought about disease and illness was being formed.

The Eighteenth Century

Knowledge came so rapidly in the eighteenth century that it had to be consolidated into basic disciplines to give it form. There were chemistry, physics, physiology, bacteriology, biology, and anatomy. And there were men who saw these disciplines as weapons against suffering. Giovanni Battista Morgagni formulated modern disease theories by correlating symptoms with autopsy findings. James Lind, an English naval surgeon, found that citrus fruits could cure scurvy. John Hunter founded modern surgery, and René Laennec developed the stethoscope to refine the physical diagnosis process originated by Leopold Auenbrugger.

Probably the most exciting eighteenth-century discovery came as the 1700s were about to end. Edward Jenner, an English country doctor, discovered how to vaccinate against smallpox—opening up the health miracle of immunology. Thomas Malthus, another Englishman, pioneered studies in population problems. And Philippe Pinel, of France, pioneered treatment for the mentally ill, originating modern psychiatry.

The Nineteenth Century

The nineteenth century was a race for progress. With modern tools and knowledge to work with, scientists anticipated earthshaking results. And got them. Ignaz Semmelweis showed how infant and maternal mortality could be almost eliminated when people delivering babies washed their hands. William Morton, an obscure dentist, discovered that ether could be used as an anesthetic, making surgery something other than a petrifying horror. Gregor Mendel, an Austrian monk, explained heredity in terms of genetics. And there was Louis Pasteur, possibly the greatest scientist of all time. He originated the "germ theory" of disease and refined the sciences of bacteriology and immunology, along with Robert Koch, a German. On the female side of the ledger, there was Florence Nightingale, the "Lady of the Lamp." Modern nursing and much of hospital administration are based on her work during the Crimean War. Joseph Lister perfected antiseptic surgery. And Wilhelm Roentgen discovered the X-ray. And no list of nineteenth-century health leaders would be complete without Sigmund Freud. Freud's writings on psychoanalysis and treatment of the emotionally disturbed are classics.

The Twentieth Century

Then came the 1900s and so many dramatic achievements that no one is quite sure which are the most important. Carl Ehrlich developed salvarsan, an effective treatment for syphilis. Walter Reed proved that mosquitoes transmit yellow fever. Best and Banting, from Canada, showed that insulin could control diabetes mellitus. Gerhard Domagh isolated the sulfa drugs. Alexander Fleming discovered penicillin. But these were just a few of the twentieth-century health care miracles. A few others:

1. Major advances were made in the uses of sulfa drugs and antibiotics and other forms of chemotherapy.
2. Major vaccination programs were mounted against smallpox, poliomyelitis, tetanus, and diphtheria.
3. The electrocardiograph and electroencephalograph were invented. These instruments, absolute essentials for modern diagnosis, gave doctors the tools to study outputs of the heart and brain.
4. Pesticides and insecticides were used to control disease on a broad scale.
5. Comprehensive methods of treating mental illness were developed. And, though the problem hasn't been conquered, there are many in today's society leading vigorous and well-adjusted lives who would have been in straightjackets or behind barred windows in yesterday's society. There are drug therapy, individual and group therapy, electric shock and insulin shock, surgery, occupational therapy, and other treatments.

6. Although the X-ray had been discovered in the prior century, it wasn't until the 1900s that its therapeutic and diagnostic uses were perfected.
7. Advances were made in surgical procedures, particularly around the brain and chest. Even organ transplantation came into being. And, to some extent, there was substitution of artificial body parts for the real things.
8. Scurvy, beriberi, pellagra, rickets, and other diseases associated with nutritional deficiency were pretty well eliminated, at least in Western countries.
9. There was a tremendous advance in drug research. Tranquilizers were discovered, antihistamines were found to control allergies, and a host of pills were developed to deal with a host of ills.
10. Biophysics entered the medical care scene. Isotopes and trace elements were used for diagnosis and treatment of cancer, neurological disorders, and circulatory problems.
11. The vitamin came into its own. So did carbohydrates and minerals and other components of foods. Nutrition became a science and a highly popular public pastime.
12. Yellow fever, hookworm, tuberculosis, and malaria were attacked on an international scale, were pretty well eliminated in industrialized countries, significantly reduced in countries not so industrialized.
13. Cortisone and ACTH and other drugs controlling hormone functions were used in the new field of endocrinology.

There are a host of other problems twentieth-century science is working on and, to some degree, solving. There are arthritis and rheumatism, alcoholism, suicide, drug addiction and dependency, cerebral palsy, and muscular dystrophy. There's cardiovascular disease, of course. And there are cancer and kidney disorders, and allergies, and some bacterial and viral infections that haven't been cleared up already.

And there are social and preventive measures scientists are looking into. Slums and poverty probably cause more sickness and death than any specific disease or accident. So there are slum clearance projects and urban renewal projects. And there are water fluoridation projects to prevent cavities in the young. There are vaccination programs, maternal and infant care programs, anti-VD campaigns, antismoking posters and campaigns.[9]

American Sickness

Naturally, these campaigns, whatever form they take, aren't completely effective. And, naturally, there are a lot of problems in America's health care picture that need more attention. Here are a few:

1. Seventeen per cent of our population have some type of mental disorder, the type that calls for professional treatment and help.
2. By the time he's 40, the average U.S. citizen has lost half of his teeth. This is a shame, as the loss, in most cases, is needless.
3. The alcoholics of the 1970s number about 9.6 million. Ten years ago,

TABLE 1-1
Days of Disability, by Type and Sex of Patient: 1960–1971

(In millions, except as indicated. 1960 and 1965, for years ending June 30; thereafter, calendar years. Data refer to civilian non-institutional population. Based on sample and subject to sampling variability.)

Item	1960 Total Days	1960 Days per Person	1965 Total Days	1965 Days per Person	1970 Total Days	1970 Days per Person	1971 Total Days	1971 Days per Person
Restricted-activity days*	2,830.1	16.2	3,086.1	16.4	2,913.1	14.6	3,275.6	15.7
Male	1,214.8	14.3	2,339.1	14.7	1,272.7	13.2	2,390.4	14.2
Female	1,615.3	18.0	1,747.0	18.0	1,640.4	15.8	1,785.2	17.0
Bed-disability days†	1,054.8	6.0	1,160.2	6.2	1,222.3	6.1	2,238.9	6.1
Male	454.3	5.3	483.7	5.3	502.6	5.2	525.8	5.4
Female	600.5	6.7	676.5	7.0	719.8	6.9	713.1	6.8
Work-loss days‡	369.9	5.6	399.5	5.7	417.2	5.4	396.2	5.1
Male	244.4	5.5	260.9	5.7	242.6	5.0	236.0	4.9
Female	125.5	5.6	138.6	5.6	174.6	5.9	160.2	5.5
School-loss days§	195.5	5.3	214.0	5.2	221.5	4.9	249.6	5.5
Male	93.3	4.9	103.3	4.9	107.9	4.7	119.6	5.2
Female	102.2	5.6	110.7	5.4	113.6	5.1	130.0	5.9

* A day when a person cut down on his usual activities for the whole day because of illness or injury. Includes bed-disability, work-loss, and school-loss days.
† A day when a person was kept in bed either all or most of the day because of illness or injury. Includes those work-loss and school-loss days actually spent in bed.
‡ A day when a person lost the entire work day because of illness or injury. Computed for persons 17 years of age and over in the currently employed population, defined as those who were working or had a job or business from which they were not on layoff during the 2-week period preceding the week of interview.
§ Child's loss of entire school day because of illness or injury. Computed for children 6–16 years of age.

Source: Health Statistics from the U.S. National Health Survey: *Vital and Health Statistics*, series 10, Nos. 72 and 79 (Washington, D.C.: U.S. National Center for Health Statistics).

there were about 5 million alcoholics in the United States. Now there are almost that many alcoholic women.

4. There are 70 million of us with one or more chronic conditions, and there are a million so seriously afflicted that they're confined to their homes.
5. Fifty per cent of all U.S. dwellings are overcrowded, lack heat, lack effective bathing facilities, have open gas burners, or have other basic deficiencies that make living in them unsanitary and unsafe.
6. We spend an average of 6 days in bed each year and average 16 days of restricted activity because of sickness, injuries, and impairments.
7. Three million of us have serious visual problems, 1 million of whom can't even read a newspaper, no matter how strong the corrective lenses are. And there are 6 million with hearing impairments.[10]

American Death

And these are just statistics on sickness. What about death? Is the American mortality picture depressing? In a way, no. The leading cause of death in the United States is heart disease; the second is cancer; the third is stroke; and fourth is accidents. This is a big contrast to the turn of the century listing, which placed tuberculosis in first place, pneumonia and influenza in second, and gastritis in third. Five communicable diseases were among the top ten killers in 1900. Today only two are in this position. There has been a lot of progress in infectious disease prevention and control. Diagnosis is more accurate, detection faster, immunization more widespread. And though this is a health care blessing in one sense, it has paved the way for new health care problems in another. Also, Americans aren't as long-lived as they might be. The life span of the average American woman ranks eleventh compared to that of female citizens of other countries. For American men, the ranking is seventeenth.[11]

Health of America's Youth

American youth have a few health care problems of their own. If you're in your teens, you certainly don't think of death. Arthritis, coronaries, stroke, and cancer couldn't be more remote. But VD isn't remote; accidents aren't remote; neither is mental illness. Consider the numbers:

1. Twenty-two per cent of all infectious VD cases occur in the under-20-years-old group.
2. More than half of all deaths of people between 15 and 24 years old come from accidents. Accidents continue to be the leading cause of death for people under 35.
3. People between 16 and 29 comprise 16 per cent of all new admissions to state mental hospitals.
4. Some consider juvenile delinquency an illness. If it is, then this illness statistic has been rising steadily since 1948.

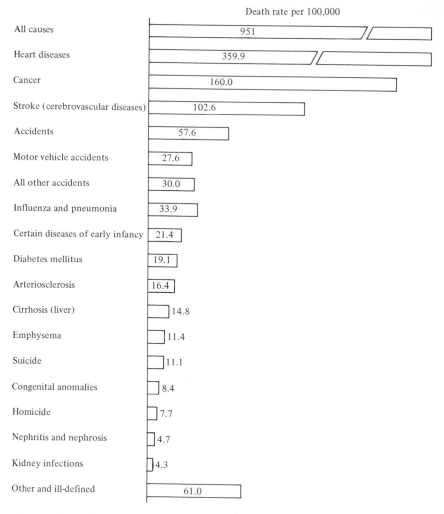

Death rate per 100,000

All causes	951
Heart diseases	359.9
Cancer	160.0
Stroke (cerebrovascular diseases)	102.6
Accidents	57.6
Motor vehicle accidents	27.6
All other accidents	30.0
Influenza and pneumonia	33.9
Certain diseases of early infancy	21.4
Diabetes mellitus	19.1
Arteriosclerosis	16.4
Cirrhosis (liver)	14.8
Emphysema	11.4
Suicide	11.1
Congenital anomalies	8.4
Homicide	7.7
Nephritis and nephrosis	4.7
Kidney infections	4.3
Other and ill-defined	61.0

SOURCE: *Monthly Vital Statistics Report,* Department of Health, Education, and Welfare (Jan. 1973).

FIGURE 1-5. *Leading causes of death in the United States, 1972.*

5. Ten per cent of all students in school have speech defects.
6. A quarter of all people under 21 have vision problems.
7. Three of the four leading causes of mortality among the 15- to 24-years-old group have some kind of psychogenic connection.

As mentioned before, accidents are the greatest killer, then comes homicide, then cancer, then suicide.[12] Apparently, youth is a time for excitement, thrills, fun, almost unbearable pleasure. Apparently, there are some unbearable pain and unhappiness, too.

Health Dilemma

Laser beams pulverize tumors, seal broken blood vessels, coagulate tissue over torn retinas. Hearts from dead people force blood through veins and arteries of the living; kidneys get transplanted; lungs get transplanted; so do livers. There are drugs to make us calm, drugs to make us sleep, drugs to

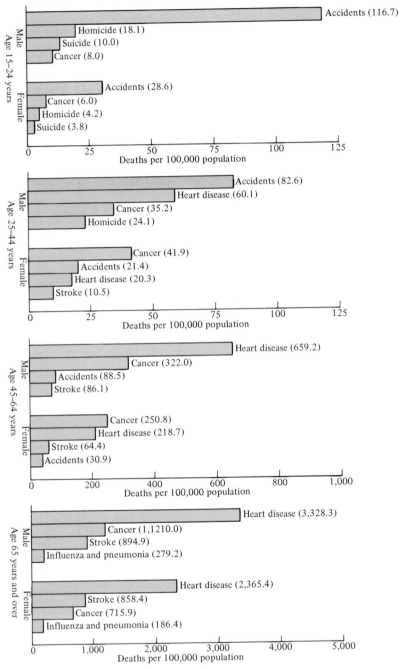

Note the leading role that psychogenic-related problems play in death of the young.

SOURCE: Public Health Service, National Center for Health Statistics, unpublished data.

FIGURE 1-6. *Death rates ranked for four leading causes, by age and sex, 1969.*

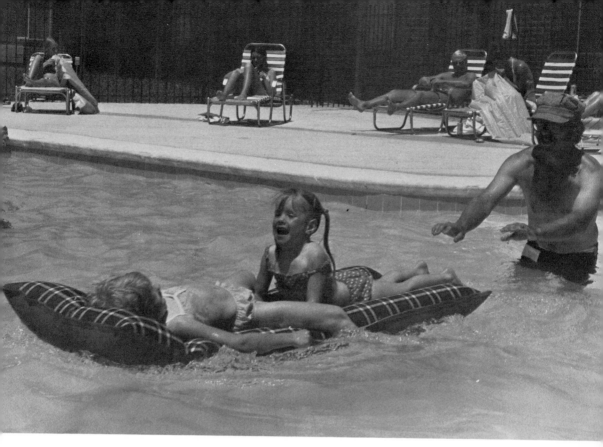

FIGURE 1-7. *In the swim of life.*

build our memories and improve our ability to learn. If your heart can't keep up the rhythm, get a cardiac pacemaker. There's kidney dialysis if you're having trouble in that area. There are heart-lung machines, there are cryosurgery, diagnostic computers, tissue banks, and spectrum analysis for disease detection. Truly, we live in a world of medical-technical miracles. Research, in the last 10 years, has produced an effective vaccination against German measles, an enzyme treatment for leukemia, L-dopa to treat parkinsonism, transplantation of the first human heart.[13]

But then there are space travel, urbanization, routine travel faster than the speed of sound, computers whose memories are limitless, whose speed is infinite. Somehow, mental illness, divorce, alcoholism, drug dependency, juvenile deliquency have taken a prominent place in American culture. These are the days of stress, the days of dissatisfaction of the young, uncertainty of the old, confusion of the middle-aged. These are the days when governments crumble, philosophies change, religions try to adjust. People want solutions—in the health care field as well as others. Technology has produced some wondrous answers. It has produced some shocking problems, too. Possibly technology itself will solve them. Possibly the problems will just get bigger and more terrifying.

How about euthanasia? Should someone live when life no longer means dignity, rationality, self-sufficiency? How about someone who suffers unbearable pain, humiliation, someone who's costing his loved ones money

17

they can't afford, heartbreak they can afford but shouldn't have to bear. Who's to make the decision on whether this person should die? And can you extend decisions of this type to the mentally ill, epileptics, sexual deviates, criminals, people society doesn't approve of at the moment? Technology can extend life, sometimes make it more tolerable. But it won't define what life is about, what makes the mystery worthwhile.

Another technological problem is living together without first visiting the priest, rabbi, preacher, or justice of the peace. Granted, this involves technology in an indirect way only. But it wouldn't have happened in the day of the plantation economy, horse-drawn transportation, and the hand-made dress. At least, it wouldn't have happened on the scale it occurs on many college campuses. The affluent and secure life created by the indus-trial revolution has contributed to this phenomenon. No longer does the young man shake with terror at the displeasure of irascible Dad. So what if he gets thrown off the farm, barred from the house, scorned by his family. He can go to work for Montgomery Ward, IBM, General Motors, the fed-eral government. There are thousands of paternalistic-type organizations willing to take Dad's place as provider, counselor, and dispenser of prestige. And the young lady, be her infraction slovenliness, poor grades, poor atti-tude, or pregnancy out of wedlock, doesn't tremble at the wrath of Mom, either. Technology will provide for her, just as it does for the young man she might want to room with. Oil, steam, and machines are bringing on problems Eli Whitney never dreamed of. There are sex-gender clinics and people who get their sexes changed. There are communes, millions of broken homes, swingers, and X-rated movies. Who's got solutions? Or are these really problems? No scientist or computer in the world would ven-ture an answer.

The Fountains of Youth and Eternity

The average Greek had a life span of less than 20 years, the average Roman about the same. Mister Average American, when our country was formed, lived around 32 years—by the turn of the century, around 48. But now our average citizen lives around three score years and ten.[14] And, considering the infectious diseases, rotten teeth, malnutrition, and poor hearing and eyesight his ancestors had to bear, he lives quite well. But where will it end? Will citizens of the 1980s or 1990s have life spans into the hundreds? By the year 2000, will 80-year-olds look like teenagers, scream at rock concerts, play pro football, and reproduce a new generation? Unfortunately, probably not. Ponce de Leon had a great dream four centuries ago. But the Fountain of Youth will probably be a dream a few more centuries down the road.[15] We can have good lives, though, vigorous, free of too many worries, filled with our share of fun, love, and accomplishment—even though the lives will end, and youth will end, and dreams will change. Life, as we currently know it, is a dynamic process, one where we fight for emotional, intellectual, and ethical growth. It's certainly not some static state of euphoria. That would be

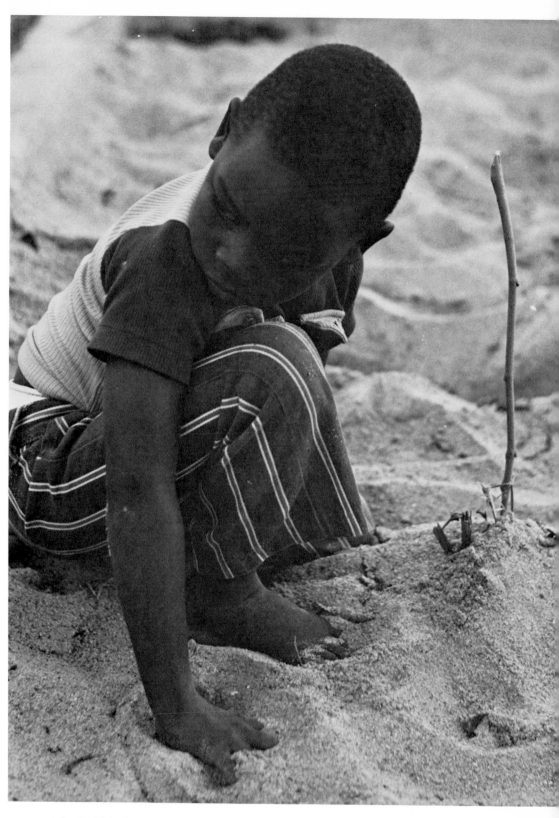

FIGURE 1-8. *Faith in tomorrow.*

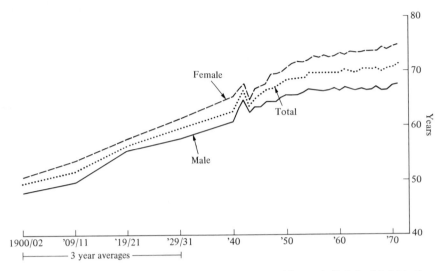

SOURCE: *Social Indicators 1973* (Washington, D.C.: The Social and Economic Statistics Administration, U.S. Department of Commerce), p. 2.

FIGURE 1-9. *Life expectancy at birth, by sex, 1901–1971.*

paradise. And paradise, probably, will never come to the Kingdom of Earth. Making the most of what you have, working for more, praying for the ideal, cultivating faith it will come—that's health. It may not be perfection, but it's worth having.

Notes

1. Constitution of the World Health Organization, p. 3, *Chronicle of the World Health Organization*, 1 (1947), 29–43.
2. *Health Education: A Conceptual Approach to Curriculum*, School Health Education Study (St. Paul, Minn.: 3M Company, 1967), p. 10.
3. Howard S. Hoyman, "Our Modern Concept of Health," *Journal of School Health*, Vol. 32 (September 1962), 253.
4. Alan E. H. Emery, *Heredity, Disease, and Man* (Berkeley: University of California Press, 1968), pp. 148–177.
5. Stephen Maltz, *Critical Issues for College Health* (Dubuque, Ia.: William C. Brown Co., 1968), pp. 411–421.
6. Caleb Ticknor, *Philosophy of Living* (New York: Arno Press, 1972), pp. 13–21.
7. Herman E. Hilleboe and Granville W. Larimore, eds., *Preventive Medicine* (Philadelphia: Saunders, 1965).
8. Erwin H. Ackerknecht, *A Short History of Medicine* (New York: Ronald Press, 1955), p. 4.
9. Frederick F. Cartwright, *Disease and History* (New York: Crowell, 1972).
10. Stephen Lewin, *The Nation's Health* (New York: H. W. Wilson Co., 1971).
11. U.S. Department of Health, Education, and Welfare, National Vital Statistics Division, National Center for Health Statistics, Public Health Service, 1969.

12. U.S. Department of Health, Education, and Welfare, National Vital Statistics Division, National Center for Health Statistics, Public Health Service, 1970.
13. Monroe Lerner and Odin W. Anderson, *Health Progress in the United States* (Chicago: University of Chicago Press, 1963).
14. Alvin Toffler, *Future Shock* (New York: Random House, 1970).
15. Rene Dubos, *Mirage of Health—Utopias, Progress, and Biological Change* (New York: Harper and Row, 1959), pp. 235–236.

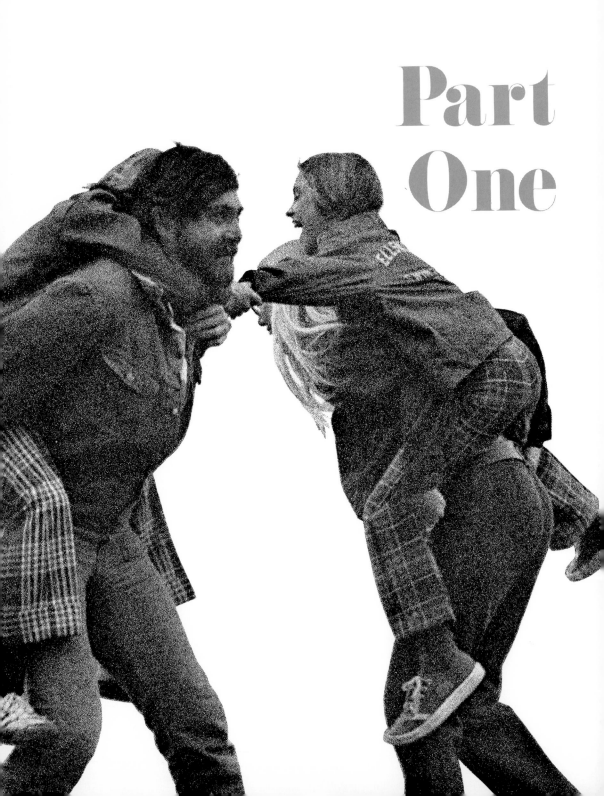

Part
One

Social Health

2 Human Sexuality

It's a revolution. There are no political parties involved, though. There are no economic theories or class struggles, either. There have been no public demonstrations, no street riots, no governments to be overthrown. Leaders for this revolution? They really don't exist. Nor are there heroes, bureaucrats, or intellectuals. The revolution has taken place without plan, without organization, and with questionable coverage by the press, radio, and television. But it's been an all-pervasive revolution. It's touched every family in the modern world, affected each individual. The soldiers of this revolution have been both male and female. The battleground has been the bedroom.[1]

The sex revolution is here. But not all agree that it's a true revolution. Some feel that "revolution" implies a promiscuous sexual code, a widespread breakdown of American morality. This just isn't what's happening. What is happening is that young people have assumed more responsibility for their own sexual behavior. The parents, the church, the schools have had less and less influence in this area. Many think that there has been a growing tendency for couples to engage in premarital intercourse. But even if this were true—and it isn't—is this revolution? Is it revolution to talk about sex in something other than whispers, let unwed mothers adjust to society, teach and preach family planning, acknowledge variant sexual behavior rather than ignore it? Perhaps not. Maybe it's just a change that's taken place in our

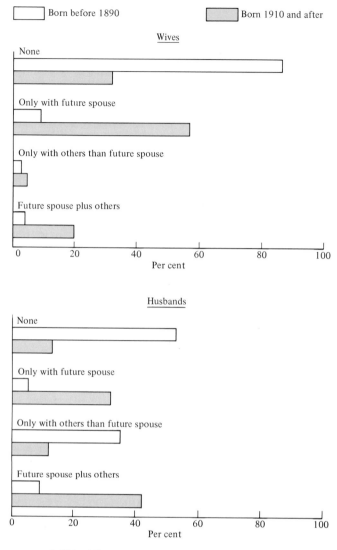

Born before 1890   Born 1910 and after

Wives

SOURCE: J. Richard Udry, *The Social Context of Marriage* (Philadelphia:
J. B. Lippincott, 1971), p. 139.

FIGURE 2-1.   *Incidence of premarital intercourse.*

cultural styles similar to changes that have taken place in our work habits,
prestige, and spending.

It's a common belief that the percentage of nonvirgins has been on the
rise for the last 10 or 20 years. Not so. There was a big change in the female
nonvirginity situation around the turn of the century. In the 1920s there was
another major increase in "bad girls." But since that time the curve has
leveled off. Why, then, the widespread belief in the growth of premarital intercourse? Visibility has a lot to do with the situation. Today there are over
200 million Americans. Fifty years ago there were only half that number. So

when there are more people doing a given thing we get the idea that something phenomenal is taking place. Also, there's a lot more willingness to talk about sexual relations than there was in past generations. Talk increases public interest and awareness.

And there has been a change in attitude about premarital sex. Although the same percentage of females may be participating in coitus, more of them accept this behavior without the feelings of guilt their mothers and older sisters did. This has been a bold attack on the puritanical philosophy of abstinence and has created a lot of public anxiety. It seems to be what the "sex revolution" is all about. There are a lot of people doing a lot of talking about something that has been going on for a long time.[2]

Sexual Sensations

Sexual intercourse is pleasurable, of course. It wouldn't be such a popular act if it weren't. It involves inserting the male sex organ, the penis, into the female's vagina. The male will probably ejaculate. The female may experience orgasm. But neither of these is necessary to constitute intercourse. Ejaculation and orgasm aren't necessary for pregnancy to occur, either. And even intercourse isn't necessary for a sexual response.

The human body sexually responds to hundreds of different stimuli. There are sights, sounds, and odors that stimulate us constantly. And the sexual response of our genital structures doesn't have to be brought about by a person of the opposite sex. Homosexual stimulation and autosexual stimulation (masturbation) can produce a similar reaction. And the type of response we experience varies with our state of physical health, our feeling of fatigue, pregnancy, a given stage in the menstrual cycle, or intoxication from alcohol or drugs, and will definitely vary according to our attitudes and background experience relating to the sexual act.[3]

Human Anatomy and Physiology

There's an area between a woman's legs called the vulva that encompasses her external sexual parts. The parts of the vulva covered with hair are called the labia majora. There are also the labia minora, which are the tissue folds protruding around the vulva opening. The head of skin at the uppermost part of the labia minora covers the female counterpart of the male penis. This is the clitoris, which can be as small as a pea or as large as a marshmallow. Just underneath the clitoris is the urethra, a small opening that connects with the urinary bladder.

About a half inch from the outer edge of the vulva is the hymen. This is tissue about a sixteenth of an inch thick. It separates the vagina from the vulva. It contains many small blood vessels and often bleeds the first time a woman has intercourse.

The vagina, the area behind the hymen, is quite flexible. Usually its walls touch each other. But these walls can adjust to the shape of a tampon, a

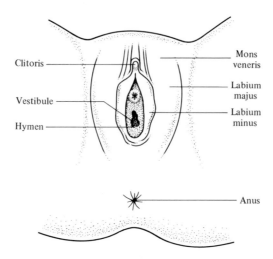

FIGURE 2-2. *Female external genital organs.*

penis, a baby. The vagina, as well as the vulva, contains nerves, blood vessels, and muscular tissue that respond to stimulation.

The cervix is at the top of the vagina. This is the neck of the uterus, the part that extends into the vagina from the abdominal cavity. The uterus, sometimes called the womb, contains glands and blood vessels contributing to the menstrual flow.[4]

Fallopian tubes extend from both corners of the uterus and carry an

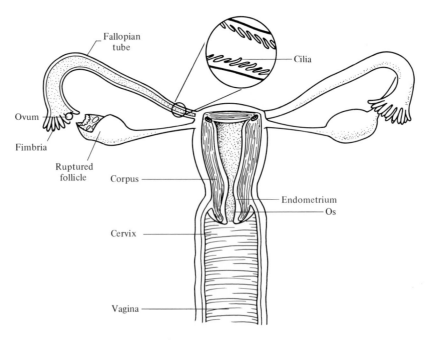

FIGURE 2-3. *Uterus and related organs (front view).*

egg from the ovaries each month. Fertilization takes place in these tubes, the sperm traveling from the penis to the vagina through the cervix and into the fallopian tubes. When conception takes place, the egg takes about 6 days to pass through the cervix and then begins growing in what is called the endometrial lining. If pregnancy doesn't occur, the egg passes to the uterus and then becomes discarded.

The eggs the ovaries produce are smaller than grains of sand. Usually one per month is released. But it is not uncommon for a month to go by when a woman doesn't produce an egg. And sometimes more than one egg is released, which is one of the contributing factors to the conception of twins and triplets. The ovaries produce the hormones estrogen and progesterone, which play a primary role in the female menstrual cycle. When menstrual flow begins, the hormones are at their lowest level. But soon the estrogen level increases, causing changes in the lining of the uterus. Progesterone is produced immediately after the egg is released, and then the ovaries continue to produce both hormones until about 5 days before the woman's next period. Production then stops, the bodily levels decrease, and the female cycle starts again.

Estrogen and progesterone have quite an influence on the woman's emotional and physical state. Breasts enlarge when these hormones are produced. Estrogen helps her skin to clear. But a high progesterone level can contribute to acne. Progesterone can also cause women to retain fluid, can lead to bloating of the stomach, changes in bowel habits, and sensitivity around the breasts. A low estrogen level, which usually occurs just prior to menstruation, can cause mild to severe depression.

The time between menstrual periods varies from woman to woman. Also, emotional upset, diet, and travel can affect the cycle. The girl who has a period every 28 days, no matter what the circumstances, is a rarity. The normal range is from 21 to 35 days, but even this isn't a firm figure. Skipping a period every so often doesn't necessarily indicate sickness or pregnancy. But it's a good idea to check problems of this type with a doctor.[5]

The penis and testicles are external sexual organs of the male. The penis, usually soft, becomes erect when the man is sexually aroused. There's a canal running through the center of the penis that can carry either sperm or urine, but can't carry the two at the same time. The testicles, the counterpart of the female ovaries, rest in a sac of skin underneath the penis called the scrotum. There is an epididymis at the top of each testicle leading to an ejaculatory duct. This duct empties into the urethra, the canal running through the center of the penis.

Testicles manufacture sperm, which can unite with the female's eggs to cause conception. There are glands next to the ejaculatory duct that produce secretions to carry the sperm from the epididymis to the urethra. These glands are called the prostate, the Cowper's glands, and the seminal vesicles. The fluid containing the sperm leaves the genital tract by ejaculation, and there are about 500 million sperm released when this happens. Ejaculation doesn't take place only during intercourse, of course. It can be brought on by masturbation or petting, or even take place spontaneously during sleep.

In addition to sperm, the testicles produce male hormones called androgens. These aren't produced on a cyclical basis the way female hormones

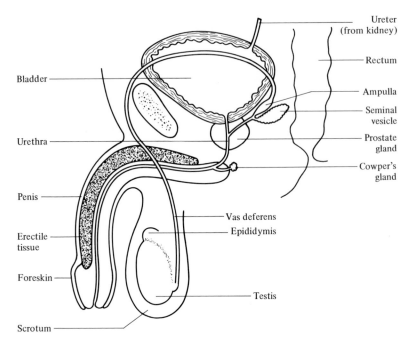

FIGURE 2-4. *The male reproductive organs.*

are. And there is no male version of the female's menstrual flow. One of the more prominent androgens is testosterone. This contributes to the growth of facial hair, hair on the chest, and male characteristics such as a deep voice.[6]

Sexual Response

Obviously, males and females are built differently. And their sexual responses are different as well. These have been categorized in several ways by different authorities, who usually break the sex act down in various phases. Here's how one recent team of researchers has done it:

1. There is the excitement phase. This is the initial part of the sexual act, when the partners become physically aroused. The male's penis becomes erect. The female's vagina becomes lubricated. Pulse rate increases in both the man and the woman. Blood pressure rises, and there are contractions of both voluntary and involuntary muscles. A rash that looks a little like measles appears on the skin. This is called the "sex flush."
2. Next is the plateau phase, which is really a continuation of the excitement phase. The erection of the male's penis becomes complete, and the female exhibits what is called the "orgasmic platform." Her vagina swells and reduces the vaginal area by almost 50 per cent.
3. Then comes the orgasmic phase, the climax of the sexual experience. This is characterized by a rhythmic series of muscular contractions in the outer third of the female's vagina. And there are similar contractions in

30

the male's penis. These contractions take place at intervals of approximately $\frac{4}{5}$ second when the orgasm is at its peak. Muscular tension is released in a series of spasms throughout the entire body. The partner is usually grasped forcefully as the orgasmic phase ends.

4. The final phase, the resolution phase, begins as the male loses his erection. Blood pressure in both partners returns to normal. So do pulse rate and levels of respiration. This phase lasts for around $\frac{3}{4}$ hour for the female, as she remains sexually aroused after orgasm and could experience subsequent orgasms if she were effectively stimulated. During this time the male experiences what is called a "refractory period." This is when he cannot become sexually aroused. It may last for just a few minutes, sometimes a few hours.[7]

These phases shouldn't be looked on as a description of a perfect or even a typical sexual experience. We're individuals. We respond, act, think, and create in individual ways. We express this individuality in the sexual act as we do in the rest of life. Each sexual encounter has characteristics of its own, expressing the individual feelings, backgrounds, and physiological endowments of participants. Sexual intercourse is too meaningful and enjoyable an experience to be looked on as "good," "bad," "typical," "normal," or an "ideal" to live up to.

Sex Before Marriage?

Of course, learning about intercourse, experimenting with it, learning to give and get the greatest pleasure from it is often an easier path to follow when you're married than when you're single. Some single people have no problem at all in this regard. They feel that intercourse should take place only within marriage and won't face the problem until the wedding bells have sounded. But there are others, often engaged or having found someone special, who struggle with the decision on whether to wait. They have their religious beliefs to contend with, the attitudes of their families. They're afraid of pregnancy, sometimes of a bad reputation. Sometimes they're haunted by past emotional experiences. And then there are decisions made in moments of passion. "Yes" seems to be the only conclusion that makes sense at these times.

A lot of the old guidelines in this area are gone. Dorm regulations have vanished on many campuses. On others they've become so permissive and loosely enforced that no one pays much attention to them. Peer morality or worrying about what a roommate might think? Hardly! This is the day when there can be a certain amount of pressure to have relations. Students often wonder what's wrong with friends or themselves if they're still virgins. Professors and administrators aren't the terrifying symbols of righteousness they once were. And parents and preachers have lost a lot of their awesomeness. The decision on whether to participate in the sexual act is largely up to the individual. And this decision can be frightening.

The first years in college are often confusing. Values you've had since birth are challenged. Sometimes families are far away. Sometimes people who seem nice, intelligent, and helpful claim that premarital sex is fine. No problem about pregnancy, of course. Contraceptives are readily available. And you should show that you don't have hang-ups, that you're sexually "normal," that you can win and keep an attractive girlfriend or boyfriend. And there's talk about repression of "instincts." Everyone knows that's bad. It's hard not to give way to this kind of pressure.

Sex is a broader concept than intercourse, of course. Some couples feel that they can have a satisfying, deeply sexual relationship without copulation. Kissing can be a tender and intimate act. Combine this with sincerity, mutual respect, and genuine enjoyment in being together, and you have a complete expression of the love relationship. Others feel that more is required. This is a decision that each person has to make on his own.[8]

Sexual Standards

There are still "nice girls," of course. And there are still men who won't take the marriage vows with girls who aren't virgins. There are some pretty diverse sexual standards throughout the United States, and they've been categorized in several ways. One of the more popular categories identifies four basic sexual concepts that Americans of all backgrounds embrace.

1. There is the double standard. Here the men can have all the premarital intercourse they want. In fact, they're encouraged to carry on this activity. But no such encouragement is given to women. They must be chaste and even be shocked at the suggestion they give up their virginity prior to the wedding bells.
2. Another standard involves permissiveness without affection. None of this double-standard business. Premarital intercourse is good for men, right? It's good for women, too. Does affection have to be present? It certainly does not. Sex is as normal as eating, as natural as breathing, as relaxing as sleeping, and much more fun. Why fight it? Accept it as a fact of life, and go from there.
3. The third standard is permissiveness with affection. Again, the double standard is rejected. There's no reason why women can't enjoy premarital sex without being scorned and humiliated. But neither men nor women should participate in this act unless there's a strong bond of affection between them. Promiscuity, under this standard, is condemned.
4. The fourth standard is abstinence for both sexes. Sex without marriage is a sin. The church says so, mother says so, and it's so. It's not just a sin for girls, either. It's a sin for men as well. Both must be chaste before the wedding.

Which is the best of these four standards? It's entirely up to the individual and couple concerned. The abstinence standard is still accepted by many young ladies and some young men. The double standard, despite women's lib, is still quite popular. The concept of permissiveness without affection really isn't popular and probably never will be. Our society is just too deeply imbued with conservative philosophies of life to treat sex in such a light fash-

FIGURE 2-5. *Tenderness.*

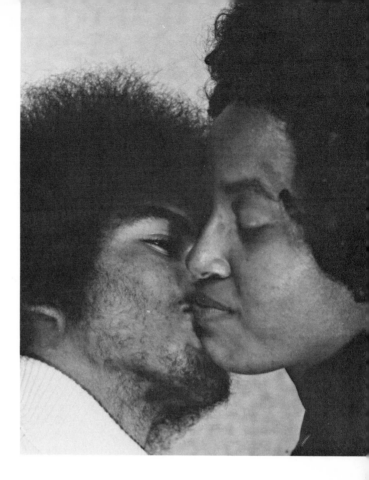

ion. Western culture may tolerate body-centered relationships, but the culture implies that these relationships should lead to marriage or some other type of stable union. Permissiveness with affection has become quite popular—particularly among college students. Sexual intercourse, according to this code, isn't an end in itself. It's an expression of the partners' feelings for each other. The female isn't overly censured for participating in the sexual act, as she's participating in an act of love. Besides, she and the young man have a good chance of getting married and raising a family.[9]

Sexual Myths and Fallacies

Which sexual standard a couple decides to follow should be based on a lot of thought and realistic information. Unfortunately, young people often don't know as much as they should about sex. And those who talk about it a lot are often feigning more knowledge than they really have. Here are some of the more common sexual myths and fallacies that abound on many college campuses.

1. *A girl can become pregnant if she hasn't had coitus.*

   Some say this a myth or fallacy. But there have been pregnant girls who swore they were still virgins. It seems possible that if a man ejaculated near a girl's vulva during sex play, semen could make its way into the vagina and

33

then into the uterus. So maybe this isn't a myth. But it's a near-myth. The odds of a virgin birth are darn thin.

2. *Masturbation can interfere with being an effective partner in heterosexual relations.*

This fortunately isn't true, as an overwhelming number of male students masturbate, and about 50 per cent of female students do. And the practice doesn't lead to emotional illness, either. If it did, the mental health of America's college population would be in serious crisis. It doesn't affect the ability of the male or the female to respond during intercourse. It doesn't prevent the male from controlling ejaculation effectively. It doesn't prevent women from reaching climax. Most females don't attain orgasm during the first few months of intercourse, but masturbation has nothing to do with this problem. It should be pointed out, though, that masturbation isn't a necessary part of the sexual growth cycle. Many women and some men who have never masturbated enjoy complete sexual maturity.

3. *Promiscuity is common on college campuses.*

This is a myth, if "promiscuity" implies that students usually copulate with several partners during a short period of time. The incidence of premarital campus intercourse is high in terms to puritanical ideals. But, for the most part, females have been having relations with one partner only. True, recent research has indicated that more than 46 per cent of American females lose their virginity by age 20. But, despite the number of nonvirgins, young people aren't all that active sexually. Over 40 per cent of the girls questioned had not participated in coitus at all during the month prior to the survey. Seventy per cent had done so only once or twice during the month. About 60 per cent of the girls had never had more than one partner, half of whom were men they intended to marry. Most women find it hard to maintain fulfilling emotional and sexual relationships with several people. And many men have the same attitude. Others take quite a pride in the number of partners with whom they've "made out." But, by and large, even for college men, promiscuity is not widespread.

4. *Young men will go almost crazy if they don't have intercourse.*

No! It's not pleasant to wait, of course. But waiting can be done without serious impairment to the male's mental and physical health. Catholic priests have been following the celibacy pattern for centuries and have managed just fine.

5. *A girl can't get pregnant if her boyfriend doesn't reach orgasm.*

No, no, no! This is a fallacy that has created a lot of false security, shock, and heartache. If intercourse is prolonged, the male's penis can emit several drops of fluid, not semen, which contains some sperm cells. So even if intercourse is interrupted prior to ejaculation, the girl can become impregnated.

6. *Drugs can lift you to new heights during intercourse.*

No one knows that this is true. But, to be fair, no one knows that it's not true. Some feel that marijuana, peyote, hashish, and heroin increase male sexual response during the excitement and plateau phases of intercourse, but make the attainment of orgasm difficult. Some say that LSD makes individuals so sensitive to external stimuli that sexual intercourse is difficult to tolerate. But these are opinions of only a few people about a few people. And there's extreme variation in individual response.

7. *A girl who doesn't attain orgasm easily is frigid.*

This is ridiculous. The orgasm idea has become a tyranny on American culture. Multiple orgasms and simultaneous orgasms have been looked on as absolute musts for satisfactory sexual relationships. This just isn't so. Women can have completely happy and satisfying relations without reaching orgasm, even though the attainment of it may be desirable.

8. *A girl can't get pregnant during her menstrual period.*

She can, she can! She can get pregnant if she doesn't reach orgasm, also. Incidentally, there is no physical reason why copulation can't take place at any time. But some couples prefer not to do it during the female's menstrual cycle because of the "mess."

9. *A girl who has lost her hymen is definitely not a virgin.*

Not so. It's true that hymenal tissue is usually ruptured during the first act of sexual intercourse—assuming that it was present in the first place. Some girls are born without this tissue. Some are born with a very small amount of it. And even a normal hymen can be ruptured during sports or a severe fall. Sometimes this tissue is so tough that a doctor must rupture it. Otherwise, the menstrual flow couldn't escape, and the girl would never be able to participate in coitus.

10. *A man with a large penis can satisfy women's sexual gratification better than a man with a small penis.*

Nope. Penal size has practically no relationship to a male's prowess in the bedroom. In extreme cases, the penis can be so large it causes the woman pain. And sometimes it's so small that penetration and pelvic contact can't be maintained. But this is highly unusual. Most men have no worries in this regard.

11. *Blacks have a greater sex drive than Whites.*

This myth may have had its origin in bigotry or envy. But it just isn't so. Fortunately or unfortunately, there's no scientific evidence to support one race's being more sexually active than another.

12. *A girl who urinates after coitus or who has intercourse in a standing position can't get pregnant.*

Some couples have relied on these "methods of contraception" and have found them as reliable as placing a lizard's ear in the left nostril or french kissing a water moccasin. A woman's bladder doesn't empty through her vagina, so urine couldn't possibly wash out sperm that entered her vaginal canal. And coitus, whether it takes place in a lying, standing, or sitting position, can cause sperm to be deposited at or near the cervix. Almost immediately the sperm start moving toward the uterus. A standing position, definitely, doesn't make these sperm pour out of the vagina.

13. *Frigid women aren't as likely to conceive as women with normal sexual response.*

Fortunately, conception doesn't have a thing to do with whether a woman enjoys sexual activity. If it did, the human race just might become extinct. If a woman holds herself back from orgasm in order to prevent conception, she's frustrated herself and possibly her partner for no good reason. A passive and indifferent girl during coitus can get just as pregnant as one who enjoys it thoroughly.[10]

Sexual Attitudes

Not everyone enjoys sex. Most people do, of course, in varying degrees. This degree is related a lot more closely to attitude than to inherent physical characteristics. We have a tendency to think of sexual satisfaction in physical terms only. But sex is a much broader concept, involving a total relationship between the participants. Each sexual act is an experience encompassing the feelings, the thoughts, the backgrounds of the partners. The act can be one of love and devotion, an almost spiritual sensation of sharing and needing. The act can be a completely sensual one. In this case, anything other than the fulfillment of bodily desires is totally unimportant. It may be a casual experience, an act of simple acceptance or even indifference. And there can be times when intercourse releases pent-up tension, bringing on a state of complete relaxation and quietness. Or it can be just something to do to pass time. A couple doesn't feel like playing bridge or going to the movies—so what else? And intercourse, certainly, can be just plain fun. It's time to experiment with the other's body, to look for new and varied heights of emotional excitement. These are some of the positive expressions of sex—actions and attitudes that build harmonious relationships and loving ones.

But sexual attitudes don't always contribute to growth or express love. The sex act can express hostility, disdain, complete selfishness. It can reflect a struggle for dominance between male and female. It can force compliance and create humiliation. Maybe one of the partners has a flair for the dramatic, enjoys going through histrionic and patronizing recitations as to why intercourse should be avoided. There can be the passive partner, the hateful partner, the childish partner. It's important that the couple realize the sex act matures like any other human relationship—by eliminating or cutting short bad experiences and emphasizing the good ones.[11]

Positive Sexual Attitudes

There are attitudes that usually accompany a healthy relationship and are worth cultivating. Probably the most important is mutual acceptance and respect. This is a must if love is to exist in any form. It lets each partner understand the other's needs and emotions and make allowances for ones he doesn't like. It keeps us from expecting perfection, feeling sorry for ourselves, or treating the other person as something to be manipulated. It allows for differences in philosophy, background, and religion, differences in momentary desire. It builds understanding if these desires aren't satisfied.[12]

Gentle and sensitive communicativeness is an attitude the couple should cultivate. An attitude? Love can be and should be expressed verbally, of course, but there's an emotion behind the words that makes them significant. We express these same emotions through gesture, dress, posture, expression, touch. Some feel that men have a stronger reaction to physical expressions than women do and that women's main response runs in the verbal area. But this is more of an individual reaction than it is a sexually related one. All of us respond to communication cues in different ways, and all of us should learn which cues carry the greatest significance for loved ones.[13]

Sexual responsiveness is a form of communication. It's a form of personal enjoyment as well, of course. And a lot of couples don't get much enjoyment during the initial months of a relationship. This can create real disappointment and feelings of inadequacy. Why shouldn't there be instantaneous and complete success? After all, isn't sexual responsiveness instinctive? No, it's not, if we're referring to the higher and more gratifying forms of responsiveness. These have to be learned, just as any other creative and self-fulfilling act has to be learned. There's instinct involved in painting, writing, throwing a baseball. But to get proficient in these fields, you have to keep trying and know that you're going to succeed.[14]

Negative Sexual Attitudes

There are some feelings we ought to avoid as well as cultivate. Naturally, a list like this could go on for volumes. But there are a few thought traps worth discussing.

One involves inappropriate comparisons. Sex is an individual thing. No two people perform the act the same way, just as no two people swing a baseball bat or do a tap dance the same way, either. But we have a tendency to compare ourselves with others. This can be helpful, but it can be overdone and create problems. How often we have intercourse, the types of sex play we enjoy, the positions we use, and where and when we have our sexual experiences are going to be different from those of other couples. Sometimes there's a girl or boy we share personal secrets with, or there's a book that describes the sex act in the most ecstatic of terms. We hear or read that intercourse takes place on a daily basis or more often. Heights are reached beyond the pinnacle of Mount Everest. Tales of this type usually have no resemblance to reality. And even if there are a few that are true, they ought to be looked on as unique experiences only. After all, we're looking for a sense of well-being and self-fulfillment. This is too individual and creative a goal to benefit from daydreams.

Another common trap involves hopeless expectations. This is natural. After all, most of us thought about the sex act for years before we experienced it. There was a new world it would create for us—wonderment, thrill, release. Colored lights would flash, bells would ring, pulses would thunder. Then comes reality. Some people are so bitterly disappointed at their first sexual experiences that they resent their partners. Sometimes they feel a deep sense of personal guilt that can seriously interfere with the growth of a fulfilling relationship.

The final trap involves rigidity of pattern. People get so concerned with carrying on intercourse "properly" that they have a tendency to turn it into a regimen. Perfume, soft music, certain routines to be followed, definite days, definite times, and definite places for the act are a must. Who likes to do things the same way all the time? Even Marine sergeants can get bored and lose enthusiasm. There's got to be a naturalness, a spontaneity to the sex act, like there is to any act we anticipate. Maybe a little mystery, a little experimentation wouldn't hurt, either.[15]

Premarital Pregnancy

There are a certain number of college coeds who become pregnant each year. No one knows exactly how many, as some of these pregnancies are terminated by abortion. In several cases the girls get married, so there is no longer unmarried pregnancy. Then there are cases where the girls decide to "go home" or "visit a relative" for a while and return to college the following year. So statistics on unmarried college pregnancies aren't exact. But authorities have estimated that the rate for the country runs from 6 to 15 per cent.[16] Why?

In some cases, ignorance is the problem. Pregnant girls have claimed that they didn't know what contraception was all about—didn't even know what intercourse meant. "Is that what we did? I thought there was more to it than that." This might be a little hard to believe in the 1970s. But it's not hard to believe that young couples won't face the responsibilities of their relationships. Youth means that nothing really bad can happen to you. Every battle you enter you win. Complete happiness and freedom from worry is the natural state of affairs. The overwhelming majority of pregnant, unmarried girls have reported that neither they nor their partners used any type of contraceptive precaution. They just couldn't believe that "this" was happening to them.

Many pregnancies have resulted from a spur-of-the-moment decision to have intercourse. Both the girl and the boy were aware of contraceptive techniques, but emotions got in the way of caution. And there are girls who look on pregnancy as a way to "beat the system." Living at home, going to classes, and holding a part-time job have their unpleasant side effects. Get pregnant—maybe get married—and problems like these disappear. Approximately half of all teenage brides are pregnant, so this philosophy must have a certain amount of support. Unfortunately, 80 per cent of these marriages end in divorce. Escape doesn't always go according to plan.

There are girls who have an emotional need to punish themselves for having intercourse. These become pregnant due to "contraceptive failure." Then there are girls who are rebelling against their parents. Getting pregnant represents a new sense of independence or a way of punishing parents for lack of affection, mistreatment, or being too strict. There are boys who like to get their girls pregnant to show that they're "real men." There are members of minority groups who look on the use of contraceptives as racial genocide fostered by the White majority. A few girls look on pregnancy as the ultimate expression of femininity. Abstinence in this case isn't old-fashioned—it's unthinkable. Guilt and fear are replaced by anticipation. Contraception is laughed at or ignored.[17]

Contraceptive Techniques

But most couples, married or single, who participate in coitus use some type of contraceptive technique. There are condoms, vaginal spermicides, the pill, the diaphragm and jelly, intrauterine devices, the rhythm method, the cervical cap, douching, and coitus interruptus. The pill is probably the safest and most effective of these methods. A female takes them for 20 or 21 days each month, beginning on the fifth day of her menstrual cycle. The pills have to be prescribed by a physician, and there are minor side effects in some cases. Some women with histories of diabetes, liver malfunction, heart disease, migraine headaches, and high blood pressure shouldn't take them. But other than abstinence and sterilization the pill is the most effective method of birth control known.

The diaphragm, intrauterine devices, and the cervical cap can be messy. With intrauterine devices, there are often pain, bleeding, and expulsion without the girl's knowing it. Condoms, used by the male, interfere with sensation to some extent. And occasionally the condom breaks or leaks. Vaginal spermicides, which can be purchased without prescription in most drugstores, have the disadvantage of having to be used $\frac{3}{4}$ of an hour prior to intercourse. And spermicides, like the diaphragm, can be messy.

The rhythm method, the one contraceptive method currently approved by the Catholic Church, is only moderately effective. It calls for abstinence from sexual intercourse during the female's fertile period. But it's impossible to determine with complete assurance just when this fertile period occurs. Douching is almost totally ineffective. And coitus interruptus, withdrawal of the penis from the vagina immediately prior to ejaculation, is completely unsatisfactory. It demands extreme self-control on the part of the male, requiring him to give up a highly pleasurable part of the sexual act. And it usually limits the sexual satisfaction of the woman as well, as withdrawal often takes place before she can attain orgasm. And, even if the male does perform this act as planned, there is no guarantee that the woman will not become impregnated by a few premature drops of fluid containing sperm cells.

There is a recently developed technique that is growing in acceptance involving use of the "morning-after pill." It requires that the girl see her doctor within 3 to 5 days after having engaged in intercourse and explain that she might be pregnant. The doctor, if he has no bias against this procedure, may prescribe estrogen to terminate the possible conception. There can be some unpleasant side effects, and the morning-after pill shouldn't be prescribed for women with certain types of illnesses. It is a highly effective technique, though. But because of its expense, inconvenience, and possible physical harm, it should be used only as a backup method of contraception.

There is also surgical sterilization, which is completely effective. Sterilization can be performed on either the female or the male, and most proce-

TABLE 2-1
Methods of Contraception

Methods	The Pill	Intrauterine Device (IUD)	Diaphragm with Jelly or Cream	Foam, Jelly, or Cream
How does it work	Prevents egg's release from woman's ovaries	It is not known exactly how the IUD prevents conception	Blocks and prevents sperm from reaching egg.	Prevents sperm from reaching egg.
How reliable is it?	More effective than any method other than sterilization.	Highly effective. Protects about 97% of users a year.	Highly effective. Protects 95% of users per year if used consistently and properly.	Foam: medium effectiveness. Creams and jellies: low effectiveness.
Are there problems with it?	Must be taken only when prescribed by a doctor. Some women should not take the pill. All women should have a medical exam before.	Cannot be used by all women. Sometimes the body "pushes" it out.	Must be fitted by doctor. Some women find it inconvenient.	Must be used just before intercourse. Some find it messy and inconvenient.
Side effects?	May cause clotting, weight gain, or internal bleeding. If this occurs, see a doctor.	May cause cramps or bleeding, spotting. If this occurs, see a doctor.	No.	Causes some irritation in rare cases.
Advantages?	Convenient, reliable, and not messy. Does not interfere with sex act.	Always there when needed, yet not felt by either partner.	Not felt by either partner.	Can be purchased at drugstore.
Prescription needed?	Yes.	Yes.	Yes.	No.

Source: DHEW Publication No. (HSM) 73-16002 (Washington, D.C.: U.S. Department Health, Education, and Welfare, 1973).

Condom (Rubber)	Condom and Foam Used Together	Rhythm	Sterilization
Prevents sperm from reaching egg.	Blocks and destroys sperm.	Intercourse only during "safe time" of woman.	Closing of tubes in male prevents sperm reaching egg; closing of tubes in female prevents egg from reaching sperm.
Highly effective, particularly if used during foreplay and when removed with care to prevent spilling the fluid in the woman's vagina.	Highly effective.	Low effectiveness. 25% of women become pregnant each year.	Highest effectiveness. No one should have the operation unless he or she is sure no more children are desired.
Objectionable to some. Condom may break or tear.		Difficult to be sure of the safe time if menstrual cycle is irregular.	All surgery has some risk, but new procedures make these operations simple and safe.
No.	Causes some irritation in rare cases.	No.	No. There is no loss of sexual desire or ability.
Condoms offer excellent protection against venereal disease and can be purchased at drugstore.		Little if any religious objection to this method.	Many feel that removing fear of pregnancy improves sexual relations.
No.	No.	No.	Yes.

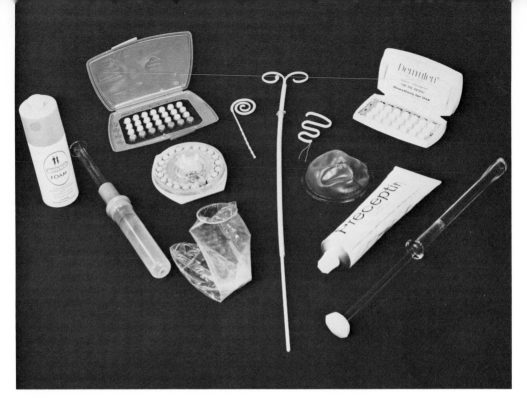

FIGURE 2-6. *Some of the more common contraceptive devices.*

dures in no way interfere with the sexual response of the individual concerned. This has never been a popular procedure, though, because the effects often are permanent. But, for people who no longer want to bear children, voluntary sterilization is almost the ideal contraceptive technique. It eliminates worry, mess, side effects.

For the male, sterilization can be performed in a doctor's office in a matter of hours. There is no hospitalization, and total recovery takes place in about a week. The procedure is called a vasectomy and consists of tying the vas deferens. The operation on the female is called tubal ligation. This is a major abdominal procedure, consisting of tying off the fallopian tubes. It requires hospitalization, it is more costly than the type performed on the male, and the recovery time is longer. A new female sterilization technique, done by laparoscopy, consists of dividing the tubes with an electrode. This requires only a small incision in the abdomen, but it does call for 48 hours of hospitalization.[18]

Abortion and Adoption

Despite the existence of sterilization, contraception, and the rhythm method, unmarried girls do become pregnant. What to do? The first step, of course, is to assure that pregnancy does exist. A late period isn't an absolute sign that the egg has been fertilized. See a doctor; get a reading. He may say that everyone can relax, she isn't pregnant. If he says that she is, several decisions have to be made. Should the girl have the child or have an abortion? If adoption is the route she intends to follow, who should carry out the procedure? Should she tell her partner, her parents, her friends? Where should she go for guidance?

Abortion

Many take the abortion route. This is a controversial decision, of course. At least some of the members of almost every religious faith consider it a sin to terminate the life of a fetus. In their view, the woman who has an abortion is killing her own child. There are the embarrassment, the cost, the emotional upset for the girl to contend with. Some girls have had mental breakdowns and have even attempted suicide over the procedure. But there are others who prefer this course of action to bearing an unwanted child.

Abortions aren't nearly as hard to obtain as they once were. And, when legally performed, they're not truly threatening to life or health. The U.S. Supreme Court simplified the problem on January 22, 1973 by ruling on *Roe* v. *Wade* and *Doe* v. *Bolton*. In effect, the decisions rendered most state abortion laws unconstitutional and set the following limitations on state regulations:

1. The woman's physician can decide whether an abortion should be performed during the first trimester of pregnancy.
2. States may regulate abortion procedures for the second trimester. But the regulations have to relate to the woman's health.
3. A state may prohibit abortion during the third trimester, unless it's necessary to preserve the mother's life.[19]

Some women try to induce abortions on themselves, have boyfriends induce them, or pay nonmedical personnel to bring them on. This is foolish! The estimated mortality rate for abortions of this type ranges from 100 to 250 deaths per 100,000. When abortions take place under medical supervision, the risk is almost nonexistent.

Nonmedical abortions usually involve inserting a foreign object into the womb. Soap solutions, pastes, rubber catheters, a variety of chemicals—the kinds of foreign objects are unlimited. These agents usually force the womb to contract and force out part of the embryo. But the womb often doesn't empty entirely, and infection is common. Sometimes particles of soap solution or paste enter the venous circulation and travel to the brain or lung. Death can be instantaneous.

Adoption

But the girl might have a lot of doubts about abortion—social, religious, medical—and decide to carry through with her pregnancy. This, of course, involves a totally different set of problems. Perhaps she would like to get married and keep the baby. This isn't always possible or even desirable. One parent may want to keep the baby, to cope with the infinite number of problems that arise from this situation. But quite often neither parent feels he or she can keep the child and provide the type of environment necessary for wholesome growth. So the decision is to put the child up for adoption. Clergymen of all faiths will provide help in this area. If they don't have the information desired, they'll usually try to obtain it. And there is the state welfare department, a branch of the Jewish Family Service, or a branch of the Catholic Family Services, Inc., in all states. Also, there are the two national agencies—the Florence Crittendon Association and the Child Welfare League—that deal with the care of unwed mothers.

If there are any doubts about the adoption or abortion procedure, others with more information and experience should be consulted. Can parents help? Sometimes. A lot depends on the family relationship. The same applies to the prospective fathers. Some are helpful and considerate. Some will try to avoid responsibility, even smear the girl's reputation. This obviously doesn't help matters. But it's usually best if the problem is discussed with someone. There are consulting services, religious organizations, sympathetic peers. This is a big step in someone's life, usually too big to be handled alone.[20]

A word about the unwed father. He's often the forgotten man in this pregnancy situation. The accepted image is that he's only incidentally involved, someone who has little responsibility, other than financial, for the child, and someone whose responsibilities to his sexual partner, to society, to himself don't have to be examined in depth. This is nonsense. Even in this current era of changing attitudes and values, problems associated with out-of-wedlock births and pregnancies are deep-rooted. They leave scars on both partners that can affect lives for several generations. The vast percentage of unwed fathers aren't irresponsible delinquents who take advantage of innocent girls. The relationship wasn't a hit-and-miss affair, but one that was meaningful to both. A large number of the potential fathers are concerned about their future children's well-being and want to act in a responsible way. But there are problems of guilt, fear, and immaturity. Pregnancy comes as a shock, often causing a complex identity crisis. Girls have little difficulty envisioning themselves as mothers. With males, it's somewhat different. "Me a father? You're kidding!" Young men don't give a lot of thought to this role until the role is suddenly theirs. Sometimes seeing their babies helps them adjust to the reality of the situation, but not always. Who likes to be forced to grow up suddenly? But sometimes a young man, with a little support, will do what he feels he should and become a better person in the process.[21]

Venereal Disease

Intercourse can cause complications other than pregnancy. There are venereal diseases that are almost never contracted in any other way. Toilet seats and towels have been blamed for spreading VD in certain instances, but the instances have been extremely rare. Is the malady widespread? You bet, particularly among the young. Only the cold is a more common communicable infection in the United States than syphilis and gonorrhea, the two most common venereal diseases. There were 3,000 teenage cases of syphilis and 150,000 teenage cases of gonorrhea reported in 1970, causing VD to outrank the incidence of hepatitis, measles, mumps, scarlet fever, strep throat,

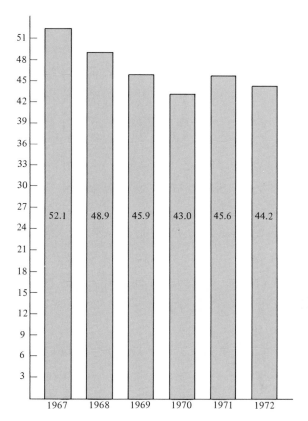

SOURCE: Health Education Services, Wichita-Sedgwick County
Department of Community Health, 1973.

FIGURE 2-7. *Syphilis case rates per 100,000 population
in the United States.*

and tuberculosis combined. And this doesn't really tell the story, since it's estimated that three out of four venereal disease cases aren't reported to public health authorities.[22]

No birth control device, other than the condom, protects against VD. And the condom isn't 100 per cent effective. When a sore appears, usually in the genital area, between 10 days and 3 months after intercourse, the individual should visit a physician immediately. The sore, which is often small, and may not even hurt, could be the first symptom of syphilis. If this symptom is untreated, it will disappear in several weeks. But the disease doesn't disappear. At a later date a rash may come out on all parts of the body. The rash also may disappear. But the disease may then enter a latent stage, with no obvious clues to its presence. Five to 50 years later tragedy can strike. Syphilis germs can attack the heart or the nervous system, causing paralysis, blindness, death. And the disease may be passed on to newborn children. A syphilitic woman will often bear a stillborn or blind child if she's not treated early in pregnancy.

The male with gonorrhea will usually experience severe burning during urination approximately 3 to 9 days after exposure. He also emits a thick,

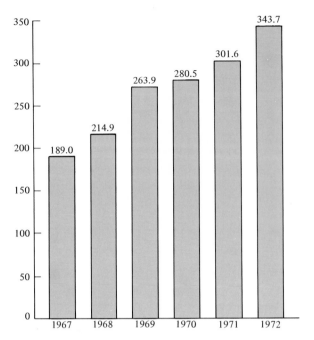

SOURCE: Health Education Services, Wichita-Sedgwick County
Department of Community Health, 1973.

FIGURE 2-8.   *Gonorrhea case rates per 100,000 population in the United States.*

yellow discharge. Females can emit the same discharge, but 80 per cent with gonorrhea have no noticeable symptoms. They should receive treatment, though. If untreated, the disease can cause sterility, eye infections, arthritis or joint irritation, and inflammation of the bladder.

Syphilis can be easily diagnosed by a blood test, and the presence of gonorrhea can be found in a bacterial culture. Doctors in 24 states can test and treat minors with these afflictions without the consent of parents. If these diseases are caught in their early stages, they can usually be cured easily by penicillin or other types of antibiotics. Someone suspecting that he has VD, if he doesn't seek treatment immediately, is not only risking his own health, but also the health of loved ones and offspring.[23]

Changing Sex Roles

There is more to sexuality than biological phenomena. Much more. The sex roles we play and how we come to terms with these roles have as great an effect on our relationships with others as our bodies do. Certainly a girl can physically mate, physically give birth without getting involved in this role thing. But what about learning to be a wife, a mother, an effective sexual partner? The sex roles we're acting out are changing drastically. Not only has the scenery shifted from the girl's front parlor and a pitcher of lemonade to a drive-in movie and a six-pack of beer—the parts we're playing have different characterizations as well. The concept of masculinity is different from the nineteenth-century concept, when it was equated with independence, dominance, and aggressiveness. Is the sissy having his day at last? How about the female—that twittery young lady who becomes faint in the presence of true masculine virility? Has she vanished as well? She most certainly has, assuming that her stereotype ever existed.

Since early times, manhood has been linked with physical strength, physical courage, feats of military bravery, sometimes brutality. But male occupations in today's Western world, including the occupation of student,

FIGURE 2-9. *The female ideal of the 1970s is a little different from grandad's demure, blushing bride.*

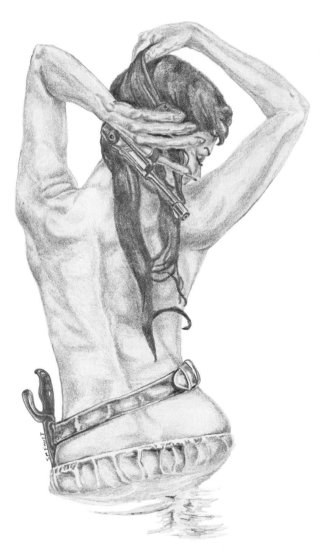

place small premium on physical strength. Most men follow pursuits, blue collar or white collar, that do little to develop the he-man role of yesteryear. Of course, young men can join the Marines or the Army to bolster feelings of virility. But today's warrior is often just another version of the General Motors foreman or the Western Electric management trainee. The odds are much greater that a young man will be killed in an auto crash than lose his life or limbs in combat, despite the Korean and Vietnamese conflicts. A man can live his whole life and never know whether he's a coward or hero. Aggressiveness? This is becoming almost out of place in the American occupational world. Congeniality is the male mood of the times. You've got to get along with your fellow man in order to economically survive.

As to that specific facet of the masculine role called sexuality, older America had some clear-cut traditions. Physical satisfaction for the man was the prime goal of intercourse, and his prowess in seducing a varying number of prim young ladies was a highly sought-after skill. Yesterday's man—probably today's as well—was quite a vain creature. He took pride in gaining women's admiration, regardless of whether seduction entered the relationship. But man now has a new sexual ideal. Masculinity is measured largely by his ability to sexually satisfy his partner. And the female has a new ideal as well. Isn't it her duty to see that a man becomes sexually aroused? She just might be "turning him off." Everyone knows that just shouldn't be.[24]

Part of the problem has been the industrial revolution. There weren't enough men to fill the needs of this new corporate society, so women entered the work force. Then they decided to vote. Then they challenged the concepts of masculinity and femininity. What's wrong with a man pushing a broom or doing the dishes? Just who has the exclusive right to decide how money will be spent and where? Women even started wearing pants—rather decorative pants, called slacks, to be sure. But this represented a freedom that Grandma didn't have. Modern woman has influence over the design of the office where she works, the car she drives, the goods she buys, and definitely the house she lives in. She realizes that she, too, has sexual needs. And she can do something about them without being labeled "lost," "loose," or "easy."[25]

Where does this no longer segregated, no longer inferior, no longer dependent female leave American masculinity? According to New York psychiatrists Ginsberg, Frosch, and Shapiro, she leaves it quite battered. They've reported a noticeable increase in impotence in young males and a growth of complaints from young females that their lovers lack sexual enthusiasm and ability. Ginsberg and colleagues feel that aggressive female attitudes are causing the problem. Young men, instead of being predators, are now expected to measure up to certain standards in the copulation game. This has created feelings of fear, inadequacy, and resentment, making some young tigers pussycats.[26] However, other authorities in this area don't agree. Modern man, according to them, with his longer hair, preoccupation with the arts and social action, lack of interest in business and economic competition, open enjoyment of companionship with the opposite sex, deep antagonism to war and other types of hostility, is every bit as virile as Granddad was—probably more. He doesn't visit a prostitute as often. He has a deeper affection for his sexual partner than Granddad did, and he's not as puritanical or as squeamish about sex as his World War I or World War II predecessors. Sex, to the young man of the 1970s, is something to be appreciated, not joked about; something to share, not get; something to accept as part of life, not fear.[27]

Sexual Variancy

There are homosexuals and nymphomaniacs. There are voyeurs, fetishists, exhibitionists, tranvestites, sadists, sodomists, and masochists. These are the "odd" people, the ones who create shock, disgust, curiosity, pity, fear, and, in a few instances, sincere understanding. A lot of myth and folklore surround this behavior, and even the well educated often have a twisted view of it. Many prefer to ignore it. Sexual variancy scares us, makes us wonder about ourselves. But people with these problems are human. And this status calls for something more than hatred. Also, any sexual act carried on with uncertainty, with doubt, without complete love and understanding of the partner, is somewhat perverse. Who has the right to cast that first stone?

Homosexuality

There's no variant behavior more widespread or misunderstood or more feared than homosexuality. It's been around for quite a while, despite the fear, having existed in every culture since the dawn of history. What is it? It's a sexual compatibility pattern between people of the same sex. Both females and males can become involved with it, and the pattern isn't always exclusive from heterosexual behavior. There are bisexuals who have relationships with members of both sexes. What causes this behavior pattern to develop no one really knows. Some claim it's inheritance. Some claim it's environment. Some claim it's a combination of the two.

No one knows how many homosexuals there are in the United States. And no one knows whether the pattern is growing or receding. But homosexuality has become a more open pattern on some college campuses in recent years. The first college "gay" groups began in the 1960s. Most students hesitated to join them, but today some campuses have turnouts of 50 or 60 people at weekly or biweekly meetings. In May 1970, the Gay Student Union of the University of California at Berkeley sponsored a dance. Over a thousand people turned out, and the dance was ranked as one of the bigger social events of the year. Of course, campus homosexuality existed prior to this Berkeley dance, but it was much less public.

Not all male homosexuals are effeminate, and not all female homosexuals look like linebackers for the Green Bay Packers. Only a small minority exhibit these characteristics. And homosexuality isn't predominant among the better educated. The greatest percentage of homosexuals is found among people who never graduated from grade school. And the variancy rate of high school dropouts is significantly higher than the rate of college graduates.

There is a myth that homosexuals don't do manual work. Not so. There's a high incidence of this type of activity among cattlemen, prospectors, lumbermen, miners, hunters, and farmers. Homosexuals often claim that they're a highly joyous group, sensitive, well adjusted. Nope. Possibly because society shuns them, most are very lonely people who have trouble forming long-term, intimate sexual relationships. Especially with the males, there can be a lot of narcissism in their personalities, creating competition between partners over who is the more attractive. They often try to confirm their sexual appeal with others, destroying any type of a stable affection model. Also, most homosexuals seem to be looking for an ideal that no human could possibly live up to. They deal with others more in terms of fantasy than realism. So they're constantly looking for new partners. They patronize public lavatories, bars, steam baths, street corners, hotel lobbies. There are homosexual meeting places and homosexual communities in almost any city of reasonable size.[28]

Lesbianism, the female form of homosexuality, isn't nearly as widespread as the male variety. And the lesbian seems to adjust to American culture better than her male counterpart. She's often less open with her sexual desires, less aggressive. And much of society doesn't put the stigma on the female it does on the male. After all, there is an affection between women that the social code encourages. Most people aren't shocked when two women embrace, hold hands, or dance. Lesbianism implies something else, of course. But it seems more in line with what most think of as being ethical than love between men.

But be they male or female, homosexuals aren't mentally ill—according to the American Psychiatric Association. They're people who, for an infinite number of reasons, prefer sexual and emotional partners of the same sex. Some argue the term should be "homoemotionality," not homosexuality. Some don't agree. It's a problem and an attitude society won't solve in the 1970s.

Promiscuity

Promiscuity describes people who have indiscriminate sexual relations. In women, an extreme of this sexual pattern is called nymphomania. In men, the extreme is satyriasis. These people usually don't recognize sexual partners as human beings—they're shadowy figures, bit players in an intricate, erotic dream.

Fetishism

Fetishism involves becoming sexually aroused by an object, an act, or something that isn't a complete person. Some men get excited by women's high heels or tight corsets. There are skin diving suits, and boots and spurs, and women's underclothes. Some steal these items and use them when masturbating.

Voyeurism

Voyeurs get their kicks from observing sexual acts or objects. They peek in windows (peeping Toms), hoping to see people scantily clad or carrying on intercourse. Sometimes they frequent stag movies and peep shows.

Exhibitionism

Exhibitionism is the act of exposing one's genitals to someone else in public. People who do this type of thing are usually inept in heterosexual relations and feel they are drawing attention to their masculinity or femininity.

Transvestism

A transvestite gets sexual satisfaction by putting on clothes of the opposite sex. This can be totally independent from homosexuality. The person gets his sexual satisfaction from the clothing, and that's it.

Sadism and Masochism

Sadists get sexual gratification by inflicting pain. Masochists get their pleasure by receiving pain. And, oddly, a person who gets gratification from one of these activities often gets gratification from the other. Whips, chains, and matches often play a big part in the sexual relations of these people.

Sodomy

Sodomy is the act of anal intercourse. It can be carried on by two homosexual men or by a man and a woman. Some states word their sodomy laws so that they also apply to mouth-genital contact and the act of intercourse with animals (bestiality).[29]

Population Explosion

Some forms of sexual variancy have one virtue that heterosexual copulation doesn't. Two males or two females can't produce offspring. Many ecologists consider this a tremendous blessing. There were around 1 billion people in the world in 1830. By 1930 there were 2 billion people. In 1960 the number had become 3 billion. And it's estimated that the fourth billion will be around in 1975 and that there will be 5 billion people in 1985. The United Nations has warned that world population is increasing by approximately 70 million per year or about 8,000 people per hour. Has the United States played a part in this explosion? It most certainly has. We grew our first 50 million people between the years of 1620 and 1880. Just 35 years later we added another 50 million people to our census. Thirty-four years after that another 50 million were added. It took only 18 years to add a fourth 50 million. During this last growth period the population increase was equivalent to the entire population of France. But hasn't immigration had something to do with this growth? Not much. Between 1850 and 1915, a third of the increase was due to immigration. Since then, only an eighth of the rise has been due to something other than an excess of births over deaths. If this trend were to go unchecked, the United States would soon have an 800 million population, as China has.

Of course, we could support 800 million people, maybe a billion or more. But there is a question as to just what level these people could be sup-

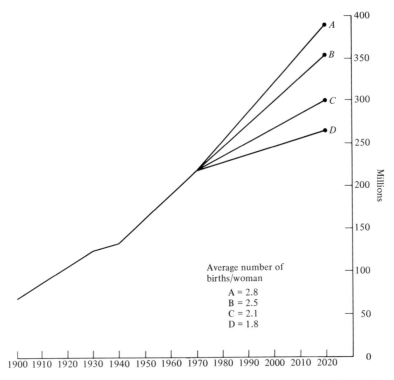

The four population projections are based on four different assumptions concerning family size. *A* assumes that women now entering childbearing years will have an average of 2.8 children; *B* assumes they will have 2.5 children; *C,* 2.1; and *D,* 1.8. Mortality rate is assumed to improve slightly to the year 2020. Net immigration is projected at 400,000 persons per year.

SOURCE: *Social Indicators 1973* (Washington, D.C.: The Social and Economic Statistics Administration, U.S. Department of Commerce), p. 233.

FIGURE 2-10. *Population explosion in the United States, 1900–2020.*

ported at and through what adjustments. Famine would occur if our food production weren't dramatically expanded. There would have to be a drastic curtailment of per capita consumption of all items, life sustaining as well as luxury. Masses of people would have to be relocated. The federal government would surely apply local zoning laws, and there would be a stifling bureauracy. Consider how unmanageable our large cities are today. Can you imagine how 800 million people could be organized, controlled, administered to in a completely democratic way? And think of pollution. Our air, our streams, and our landscapes are waste-ridden now. Certainly more people would produce more waste. Obviously, the United States could provide for a much larger population than it currently has. But ecologists question what the social, moral, and aesthetic costs would be.

The population growth in the United States has slowed down, though. In 1850, the average number of children per family was 6.0. By 1970, the average was 2.45. Our population growth will stop entirely when 2.1 to 2.2 children per family is reached.[30] The sex revolution, if there is such a thing, has its advantages.

Notes

1. Pitirim A. Sorokin, *The American Sex Revolution* (Boston: Porter Sargent, 1956), p. 3.
2. Ira L. Reiss, "Premarital Sexual Standards," in *The Individual, Sex, and Society,* ed. by Carlfred B. Broderick and Jessie Bernard (Baltimore: Johns Hopkins Press, 1969), pp. 109–111.
3. William R. Reevy, "Vestured Genital Apposition and Coitus," in *Advances in Sex Research,* ed. by Hugo G. Beigel (New York: Harper and Row, 1963), pp. 27, 32.
4. Arthur J. Yander, James H. Sherman, and Dorothy S. Luciano, *Human Physiology* (New York: McGraw-Hill, 1970), pp. 452–456.
5. Ibid., pp. 454–458.
6. Ibid., pp. 443–450.
7. William H. Masters and Virginia W. Johnson, *Human Sexual Response* (Boston: Little, Brown, 1970), pp. 3–8.
8. Thomas R. Schill, "Need for Approval, Guilt and Sexual Stimulation and Their Relationship to Sexual Responsivity," *Journal of Consulting and Clinical Psychology,* Vol. 38, No. 1 (February 1972), 31.
9. Ira L. Reiss, *The Family System in America* (New York: Holt, Rinehart and Winston, 1971), pp. 156–160.
10. James Leslie McCary, *Sexual Myths and Fallacies* (New York: Van Nostrand Reinhold, 1971).
11. J. T. Landis and M. G. Landis, *Building a Successful Marriage* (Englewood Cliffs, N.J.: Prentice-Hall, 1963).
12. Alfred W. Melton, Jr., "Human Sexual Response," in *The Individual, Sex, and Society,* ed. by Carlfred B. Broderick and Jessie Bernard (Baltimore: Johns Hopkins Press, 1969), p. 225.
13. Masters and Johnson, *Human Sexual Response.*
14. Melton, *The Individual, Sex, and Society,* p. 226.
15. Ibid., pp. 226–228.
16. "Teen-Age Sex: Letting the Pendulum Swing," *Time Magazine,* August 1972, p. 34.
17. Donald Mosley and Herbert J. Cross, "Sex Guilt and Premarital Sexual Experience of College Students," *Journal of Consulting and Clinical Psychology,* Vol. 36, No. 1 (1971), 27–31.
18. *The Student Guide to Sex on Campus,* Student Committee on Human Sexuality, Yale University (New York: New American Library, 1971), pp. 51–92.
19. *The Official Associated Press Almanac,* 1974, p. 251.
20. Howard Osofsky, "Adolescent Out-of-Wedlock Pregnancy: An Overview," *Clinical Obstetrics and Gynecology,* Vol. 14 (June 1971), 442–445.
21. Rueben Pannor, "The Forgotten Man," *Nursing Outlook,* Vol. 18, No. 11 (November 1970), 36–37.
22. *Time,* "Teen-Age Sex."
23. Helen M. Wallace, "Venereal Disease in Teen-Agers," *Clinical Obstetrics and Gynecology,* Vol. 14 (June 1971), 432–441.
24. Nelson N. Foote, "Changing Concepts of Masculinity and Femininity," in *The Individual, Sex, and Society,* ed. by Carlfred B. Broderick and Jessie Bernard (Baltimore: Johns Hopkins Press, 1969), pp. 141–153.
25. Robert R. Bell, "Some Emerging Sexual Expectations Among Women," in *The Social Dimension of Human Sexuality,* ed. by Robert R. Bell and Michael Gordon (Boston: Little, Brown, 1972), pp. 158–165.
26. George L. Ginsberg, William A. Frosch, and Theodore Shapiro, "The New Impotence," *Archives of General Psychiatry,* Vol. 26 (March 1972), 218–221.

27. Foote, "Changing Concepts of Masculinity and Femininity."

28. Mary McIntosh, "The Homosexual Role," in *The Social Dimension of Human Sexuality,* ed. by Robert R. Bell and Michael Gordon (Boston: Little, Brown, 1972), pp. 176–188.

29. James E. Moore, "Problematic Sexual Behavior," in *The Individual, Sex, and Society,* ed. by Carlfred B. Broderick and Jessie Bernard (Baltimore: Johns Hopkins Press, 1969), pp. 362–372.

30. Walter Pitkin, Jr., "Too Many People: Can Education Find an Answer?" *Phi Delta Kappan,* Vol. 49, No. 9 (May 1968), 473–479.

3 The Family

It was love. There's no other explanation for it. Both of them had known their share of young men and young women before they had met. And even when they did meet there weren't bells or tremors or the earth stopping. But then there was that day at the beach. Suddenly they knew. Each had found the perfect partner to satisfy his dreams, his needs, his passions. There was no one else in the world for either of them. This was really going to be a marriage made in heaven.

The idea of romance has been around a long time. But it didn't hit its stride in the marriage field until a couple of centuries ago. Prior to this, girls had to have dowries, and marriages of nice girls and proper young men had to be arranged by their families. But then came Columbus, George Washington, and the new permissive land of romance called America.[1] Free choice became the name of the game in mate selection. There were a few cynics who claimed that this freedom was just an illusion. But, after all, there will always be cynics. It's true that the boy did seem to end up marrying the girl next door, or the girl who lived on the next farm, or the girl who was a friend of his younger sister. But what did that have to do with limiting freedom? What's wrong with marrying the girl who lives in the same community, eats the same kind of food, goes to bed about the same time, and has the same kind of ideas about church and politics as you do? Heard of a Baptist who married a Presbyterian once—and everybody knows that's not so good.

Mate selection isn't as regimented as it once was. Free choice is a lot freer than it was in great-granddad's day. But total freedom? Of course not. All of us are bound, to a greater or lesser extent, by a conformist system called culture. It's worth looking at this American culture, not that it will keep us from conforming with it. Or maybe we want to conform with it. But knowing the rules of any game we play can make us better players, more independent players, players who get more happiness from the sport.

Mate selection is about as big a decision as we can make. Our homes, our families are usually the centers of our lives, and everything else moves around them. Often this everything takes in some confusing, painful, and erratic experiences. But a good marriage can be a stable core that makes the worst day a great day, a big loss a big win. And there can be the bad marriage, the one that turns the successful executive into an alcoholic, the beautiful bride into a pill-taking neurotic. What are the critical incidents that build success or failure in this intimate jungle? How about premarital sex? Can this make you unhappy once the vows have been taken? How about Catholics? Can they be happily married to Jews? How about the personal characteristics you should look for in a partner? Certainly everyone doesn't

FIGURE 3-1. *The strongest political unit, the most stable social unit, the most binding legal unit that man has devised. The family can turn losses into wins, regrets into pride, misery into fun. The unit will probably exist as long as there are people.*

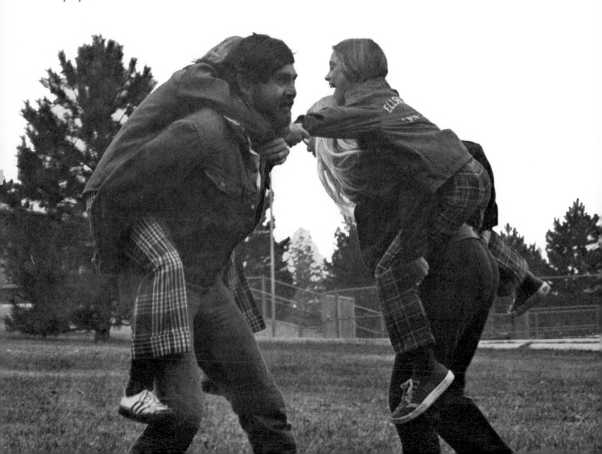

want or need the same kind of intellectual and sexual ideal. Questions like these are about as meaningful as any we can ask. The right answers won't assure a happy marriage, of course, or even a happy engagement. But they get us to thinking about things we should think about and often don't think about enough.

Dating

It came with the industrial revolution. But no one's sure that the revolution caused it. Maybe it was coeducation, women's lib. Or it could have been the rising standard of living, the growth of urbanization, increased leisure time that brought on the dating phenomenon. But, whatever, dating wasn't widely practiced until after World War I, and it didn't become completely established until after World War II. Now, of course, junior high and middle school children have dates. It's even a fairly common practice in some elementary schools.[2] The young are enjoying a growing intimacy with the opposite sex, a certain freedom from parental control, and having a lot of fun.

One of the purposes of dating is to select a mate, of course. That's why most parents approve of the procedure. But young people sometimes have other ideas in mind that the parents don't approve of. Young men often pursue young women in order to "make out." And young women often date the really "exciting" men, the kind who will be an asset to their social status. It's probably a kind of defiance against the older generation. But dating, in any form, usually helps boys and girls learn to relate to each other. There's a game involved—a competitive kind of game—between the two sex groups. Who can date the best-looking girl? Who can date the girl who likes to "play around"? Who can date the boy with the best car, the quarterback, the president of the student senate? Who can "make out" with the most girls on campus?

But a lot of dates aren't too wrapped up in this peer status thing. They're just a couple of young people who genuinely enjoy each other's company. None of this football hero or free love bit. There have been several studies showing that young people have about the same tastes in picking dating partners that their parents do in picking friends and acquaintances. Sincere maturity is one of the most important characteristics young people look for, and they value a good disposition, consideration, pride in personal appearance, and dependability. And, not surprisingly, they've indicated that they're looking for the same traits in marriage partners.[3]

So dating can involve some conflicting emotions. The struggle for status can get in the way of seeking a spouse, and most young people, despite women's lib and the new morality, are husband and wife hunting. We're a bizarre group, we humans, particularly during our fertility rites.

Selecting the Marriage Partner

There are the Bontok people of the Philippines. They're not about to allow the process of falling in love to be subject to the whims of the young, so they place their eligible young girls in special living quarters called the olag.

Lovers may come at will, sex play is free, and it is hoped that marriage will result. There's a tribe called the Ekoi in Nigeria. Ekoi men like their women fat. All eligible young girls are sent to a special location where they concentrate on eating and doing almost no exercise until they're properly fattened for the marriage process.[4] There's a tribe in another part of the world called Americans. This tribe sends young girls to finishing schools and colleges, gives them dancing lessons, and buys them nice clothes. The tribe sends young men to college as well, encourages them to play football, get active in student leadership roles, and get trained for the right kinds of jobs or professions. Young men then attract the types of females whom this American tribe considers desirable. Marriage is too important a factor for any culture to leave to the whims of chance.

Endogamy and exogamy have a lot to do with the American mate selection process. Endogamy means that we should select our mates within certain groups. According to exogamy, we shouldn't select our spouses from certain other groups. These are just cultural norms, of course, and usually aren't formalized into law. But the norms exert overwhelming pressure on the young people concerned. Endogamy standards, although not as strong as they once were, still discourage Christians from marrying non-Christians. Jews also have the same kind of endogamist restriction. Interracial marriage is considered absolutely taboo by many elements of society. As to exogamy, incest usually isn't permitted beyond the first-cousin relationship.[5]

There's a more restrictive cultural pressure yet called homogamy. Homogamy implies that like should marry like. We should select mates from our own social status, who have similar interests, similar intelligence, and similar ethnic backgrounds. Here are some of the more common homogamist characteristics:

Age Homogamy

Teenage girls usually don't marry men in their 90s, usually don't marry those in in their 30s or 40s, either. And this holds regardless of the subgroups the teenagers belong to. It involves Puerto Ricans, Blacks, and Whites, rich and poor, the well educated and people who quit school in the fifth grade.

The age homogamy thing is itself affected by age. It's strongest during the teenage years and the early 20s. But the homogamy doesn't become nearly as rigid as people grow older. When men marry at age 20, their brides, on the average, are about a year younger. There's a 3-year difference, though, when men are 25 years old. At age 30, the difference becomes 5 years, and the difference becomes ten when the man reaches 60.[6]

Social Status Homogamy

People used to select mates with similar family backgrounds, similar occupational and educational levels, and they still do—but not nearly to the extent that they once did. Some students, particularly those living on campus, claim they pay little attention to the social status of the people they want to spend

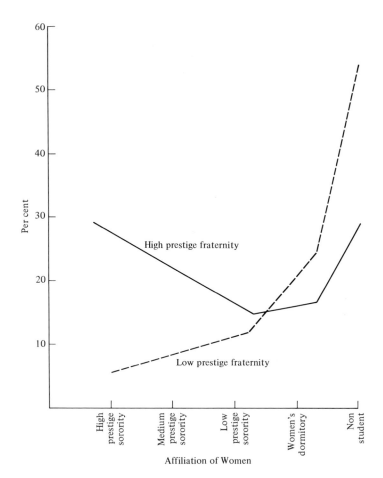

SOURCE: J. Richard Udry, *The Social Context of Marriage* (Philadelphia:
J. B. Lippincott, 1971), p. 106.

FIGURE 3-2. *Fraternity prestige influences who pins whom.*

the rest of their lives with. But it is still a factor in the mate selection process,
sometimes a very meaningful factor.

Also, there's the concept of the "mating gradient." This describes the
tendency in men to marry downward. Despite women's lib, men like to
marry girls younger than themselves, those with slightly less education and
slightly lower IQs, and those from a slightly lower social status.[7] This isn't
always the case, of course. There are wives much smarter and more gifted
than their chauvinist husbands—even though the husbands won't admit it.

Race Homogamy

Is race homogamy still a big issue in American society? It most certainly is.
Interracial marriages, in most cases, are in no way illegal. But a large part of
society mightily frowns on the process, thereby keeping the racial intermar-
riage rate so low that it's almost impossible to measure. Some claim these

marriages don't work out. Others, defending them, point out that marriages, whether between Oriental and White or Black and White, have certain strains and tensions. But all marriages have certain types of adjustment problems. By and large, interracial couples interviewed seem happy and stable, and express few regrets. The relationships with parents and friends seem to be as good as any couple could expect and seem based more on the partners' personal characteristics than the races they identify with.[8]

Religious Homogamy

Religious homogamy isn't as strong as racial homogamy, but it is strong. Jews have a tendency to marry Jews, Catholics to marry Catholics, and Protestants to marry Protestants. One study reported that 97 per cent of Jewish, 94 per cent of Catholic, and 74 per cent of Protestant marriages were religiously homogamous.[9] Young people often ask how this affects marriage survival. Do people who practice religious homogamy have a better chance of staying married than those who don't? By and large, yes they do. This isn't saying that religiously homogamous marriages are more successful, happier, or better-adjusted marriages than interfaith marriages. But the rate of survival is greater when Catholics marry Catholics, Protestants marry Protestants, and Jews marry Jews. Divorce rates are lowest among the Catholic and Jewish homogamous unions, higher among Protestant couples, and higher yet when there is no religious affiliation. And the divorce and separation rates among mixed Catholic-Protestant marriages are more than twice the rates of the homogamous variety.[10]

Personal Characteristics

Do football players marry girls who are interested in skiing and swimming and playing tennis? Do research chemists marry girls who like to play chess, attend concerts, and read poetry? Some say likes marry likes. Others feel we marry people who complement our needs. If we're aggressive, we like to marry someone who's submissive. If we like to give sympathy and care for others, we marry someone who needs to be nursed, loved, and protected. And there are those who claim we marry someone similar to the parent of the opposite sex. "I want a girl just like the girl who married dear old Dad." This is such a broad area, and personal characteristics are so varied, that it's not surprising there isn't much agreement.[11]

Love

You can love your boxer dog, love your country, love a good ice cream sundae. And there's also conjugal love. This is the kind between men and women, and it leads to marriage. It's probably more important in American culture than in any other culture in the world. If you're unloved in the United States, you're unwanted. Who wants to be marked with that kind of stigma? Also, American folklore dictates that in this great, expansive world there is just one person—one only—who is our ideal soul mate. This is nonsense, of course. There are probably thousands of people in this world who would make us happy, and whom we could make happy.[12] But it does seem kind of ego satisfying to say that each one of us is so individual, so special, that only one other human being can meet our needs.

Love is a real emotion, though, an exciting, painful, frightening, euphoric feeling that can make the world a carnival or cabaret. This love may not take place at first sight. It may not have to prove itself by being tested, as American folklore dictates, and love probably won't conquer all. Alcoholic soul mates, drug addicts, or ones who are sexually promiscuous can destroy our lives, no matter how much we love them. But the emotion does exist in one form or another. And though it won't guarantee a happy marriage, lack of it will guarantee boredom, self-pity, and regret.

A lot of people have tried to define this love thing, to explain what makes it up. No one has succeeded, of course, in the complete sense of the term. It's far too complex and individualistic an emotion to be described by checklists and rating scales. But there are a few key components of most love relationships.

The first is "idealization." This deals with the extent to which the loved one impresses the opposite sex with certain attractive qualities. A lot of us have undesirable traits, of course, that don't appeal to our mates. But if the idealized qualities are strong enough, and really prized, the undesirable ones can be ignored.

Another component is "respect." You just can't love someone you don't have a basic admiration for, someone you can't accept on an individual basis. Personal faults our soul mates may have. But it's hard to say that we truly love them when these faults interfere with our feeling of pride in and approval of their behavior.

"Sexual attraction" is a love component that's almost a must for the young. We all need physical satisfaction in one degree or another, and anticipation of this satisfaction has something to do with the warm and tender feelings we experience. This doesn't mean that love is a rationalization of the sex urge. There's much more to the feeling than that. But sex does enter the picture.

"Companionship" is a component that doesn't reach the intensity of sexual attraction, but it's probably more important than sex after the love relationship has existed for a while. A couple should enjoy being together, sharing experiences, thoughts, and plans. This companionship doesn't have to exclude others. Sometimes it exists to a greater degree when others are present.

"Selflessness" is a love component describing one partner's ability to recognize the other's needs and trying to satisfy them at the expense of his own. Personal preferences and desires get put aside. The other person's sense of well-being, sense of personal worth and happiness, takes priority.

And then there's "maturity." No one is quite sure of what this is, but we are sure that our mates are never quite as mature as we are. Maybe one way of looking at the idea is considering it the ability to deal in an adult way with varying contingencies. There are a lot of situations a couple have to accept, a lot of wins, a lot of losses. Does the wife call her mother every time the couple has an argument? Does the husband go to the local bar to drown frustrations and disappointments? Does the couple go for weeks without speaking to each other? This isn't maturity, and it's not a component of what people usually think of as love.[13]

Premarital Sexual Adjustment

"I loved Charlie. Didn't just like him. It was love, fellow, I mean the real thing. Go to bed with him? Absolutely not! Not yours truly. This is one of those girls who comes from one of those towns where sex is something you spell, whisper about, giggle about. You definitely don't do it. Nope. Charlie wasn't about to get in bed with this young lady. But he did, of course. Like I said, it was the real thing—love. That's the way things are these days. We even talked about getting married. Nothing definite, of course, but we thought about it. Like I said, there was this love thing. What better reason? This is 1976, and there's a lot of living to do in 1976. Guilt? Don't be ridiculous. That kind of thing interferes with living. I know Charlie feels the same way. We've had fun. What more can you ask?"

Is this the typical American coed talking? Who knows? There's no such thing as a campus attitude toward sex. Young people look on this relationship in a lot of different ways. And there are thousands of years of history shaping the attitudes we feel.

The Western world for a long time has said that sex and marriage go together. Neither of them belong alone. The ancient Hebrews had stern punishment for betrothed couples who had intercourse. To them, this was adultery, a violation of the Ten Commandments. And the Romans, free-swinging as they were, punished premarital intercourse almost as stringently as the Hebrews did. Then Rome fell, and sex took on more of an evil connotation yet. Even married sex had its sinful side. And sex outside of marriage was a blasphemous orgy brought on by the devil. This attitude was widely accepted during the Dark Ages, the Middle Ages, the days when chivalry reigned.

Then came Jamestown, Dolly Madison, and Americans. The medieval attitudes toward sex persisted. Fornicators were punished. There were fines, branding, imprisonment, sometimes forced marriages. But our great-grandmothers and great-grandfathers began to take a new interest in the relationship. They did a lot of clucking of tongues and shaking of heads, but they began whispering and chuckling and winking, too.[14]

And now it's America in the 1970s. The jokes aren't quite as free as they once were. The chuckles aren't quite as loud. You have to feel a little guilty about something to laugh at it. And a lot of the guilt, the shame, and the fear of sexual relations is gone.

Premarital Sexual Standards

Petting seems to be the norm in today's America. Practically all young men and young women get involved in the act before they're married. A large percentage carry it through to the point of sexual climax. Then there are some who look on it as a prelude to premarital intercourse.

Some claim there's a lot of this premarital intercourse going on. It's a sex revolution, a national orgy, a mass fornication brought on by the pill, permissive parents, and women's lib. But researchers haven't found this to be so. Apparently, men participate in no more premarital coitus today than they did for years and centuries prior to this date. There has been a change in whom young men are having intercourse with. Prostitutes played a major role in the lives of young rakes of prior centuries. But many young men today find they can satisfy their sexual desires with girls from their own social level.

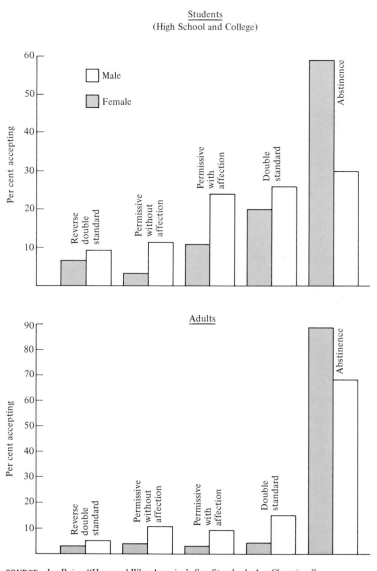

SOURCE: Ira Reiss, "How and Why America's Sex Standards Are Changing," *Transaction,* 5 (1968): 26–32.

FIGURE 3-3. *Most women still believe in premarital sexual abstinence.*

The premarital intercourse revolution, if there is such a thing, has largely involved women. Less than half the number of girls born prior to the turn of the century carried on premarital coitus as did their daughters and granddaughters of the following decade. And there's been no social, no educational level that has been unaffected. Girls who spend their summers at Cape Cod, girls whose families are on welfare, girls who earn scholarships to Vassar and Smith are more likely to engage in premarital heterosexual relations than their great-grandmothers were. Over half of the young women of the 1970s have sexual intercourse prior to marriage. But a lot of this intercourse takes place just a year or so prior to marriage, and a lot of it takes place with the fiance only. There are girls who have intercourse with other men as well as with their future husbands. And there are those who have relations with other men but refuse to have intercourse with their finaces until after receiving the blessings of the church. But these aren't common behavioral patterns. Promiscuity isn't the norm on most campuses or anywhere else.[15]

Religion plays quite a role in this situation. Campuses abound with tales of young Sunday school teachers who carry on wild antics during the rest of the week. There may be a case or two like this, but they're definitely the exception. Girls who take the church seriously, the truly devout ones, are far less likely to become sexually involved than those who take their religion casually. Inactive Protestant, Catholic, and Jewish women all have a high incidence of affairs with the opposite sex. And it's relatively unimportant which religion the women follow. Differences within faiths between the devout and the inactive are far greater than differences in sexual practices between members of the different faiths. The devout, in all categories, appear to have a high degree of chastity.[16]

Effect on Later Marital Relations

How does all of this relate to marital adjustment? Do "bad" girls make "bad" wives? Do males who are virgins at marriage become cold, domineering, rather childish husbands? And how about sexual adjustment after marriage? Couldn't premarital promiscuity make men or women more passionate in the marriage bed? There are no answers to questions like these that aren't partisan views. Although there are research findings, it's almost impossible to analyze findings in this area in an unbiased way. One study, in the 1930s, showed that premarital intercourse definitely interfered with marital happiness.[17] Another one, a little later, showed that premarital intercourse correlated with a high divorce rate.[18] And another yet indicated that couples who were chaste at the wedding had happier and more fulfilling marriages.[19] Then there were studies indicating that girls who had relationships with their husbands prior to marriage had much more satisfying sexual relations after marriage.[20] And another study indicated that the most happily married couples were those who had found meaningful sexual relationships prior to saying "I do."[21] Probably marital happiness, mature companionship, and satisfying sexual adjustment are areas too complex to be analyzed by statistics, dissected by researchers, or moralized about by people other than the participants involved.

Marital Adjustment

Is your life all happiness, all sunshine, all fun? You're lucky if it is, because you're probably the only person in the world who doesn't have feelings of inadequacy, disappointment, pain, humiliation. If you're not this lucky, if you're like everybody else, the odds are that you've adjusted to the situation pretty well. Mature people don't expect life to be perfect. And even the immature ones have a pretty good grasp on this idea. But then there's this idealistic dream world called marriage. Even the wisest, the most sensible people, people with a complete understanding of reality, people with common sense and intelligent judgment, look on marriage as some type of euphoric escape from a bitter and disappointing world. Adjustment between the partners is completely effortless, according to these delusions. There's romance in which sexual excitement never dies; mutual interests that are forever interesting, challenging, fascinating; companionship that is always warm and understanding. Soap and drug commercials have had a lot to do with this dream. Fiction writers probably contributed to it. And probably man himself is an incurable romantic who doesn't need too much help to live in this imaginary Camelot.

The Engagement

There are cynics, of course, even among youth. These dour and rather cold people tell the world that they're entering marriage with eyes wide open. Will there be problems? You bet! They know that there will be heart-breaking quarrels, extreme disappointments with themselves as well as with each other, feelings of frustration and total inadequacy. But then comes the engagement. Even Ebenezer Scrooge would be softened by this state of affairs. Love is the predominant force, and no matter how realistic we might be we just can't resist seeing ourselves in the eyes of our betrothed. We're the glamorous kings of the campus, the most gorgeous, seductive balls of femininity this side of *Vogue* magazine or one of the national TV networks. We're football stars even though we've never gone to a football game. Do we ever say anything inane, foolish, self-conscious? Of course not. Our words are clever, creative, imaginative. Every act we perform is graceful, virile, distinctive. What days, what a time! Can it last? Even the most naive realize that this can't go on—nor can the first few weeks of marriage. There's high sexual tension, followed by new heights of sexual excitement and thrills. There are giddiness, irresponsibility, happiness sometimes too great to understand or even bear.

Disillusionment

But then comes sobriety. Sometimes it creeps into the marriage almost unnoticed, then grows like a cancer. Sometimes it becomes immediately apparent, like financial disaster or a blown piston rod. What goal, once we've attained it, is nearly as significant, as exciting as the anticipation of it? We start slowing down. Each partner sees life in more realistic terms, and eventually

FIGURE 3-4. *The engagement turns us all into gladiators and queens.*

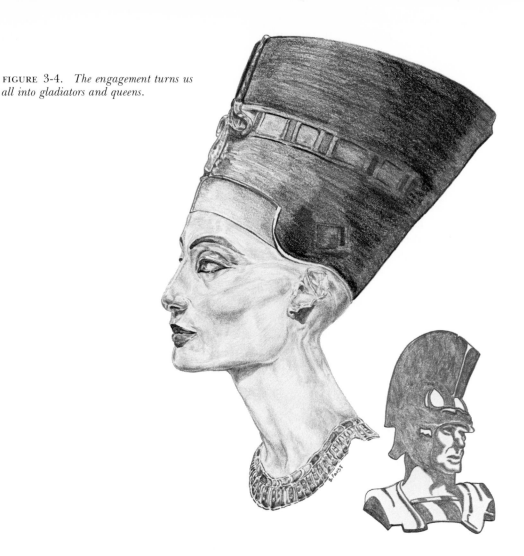

the realism grows into disillusionment. Does it come from realizing that the person we married is human like everyone else, that he has the same short-comings, the same weaknesses our brothers, sisters, friends, and parents have? Maybe it comes from a bigger shock—marriage hasn't really trans-formed us into someone else. We're still us, the same old face in the same old mirror, the same old body in the same old suit or dress, the same old mind that really isn't much like Albert Einstein's, the same old personality that doesn't please the world. Our new-found glamour, our virile prowess, and tigerlike images are gone.

All couples face this disillusionment. Some have a bigger problem than others. There's the stable young couple who have economic security, a wide range of interests and friends, and good relationships with parents and other relatives. And there are couples who look on marriage as a trap, an es-cape from home, or something to try to see if it just might work out. The disillusionment never takes quite the same form for different people. And the problems they have are always solved in individual ways. But some type of early marital adjustment does take place—assuming that the marriage survives. The highest divorce rates in the United States occur during the second and third years of marriage.[22]

Overt Conflict

Most of early marital conflict or adjustment is overt. Young people don't throw beer bottles at each other or use rolling pins or canes. At least, most couples don't. There can be violent word battles. "Why can't I go bowling with the boys?" "You don't want to make love—how come?" "You're not interested in what I have to say. You haven't paid attention to me in weeks." Words can get loud, and they can bite, and they can hurt. People often try to destroy the small fictions that underlie their partners' self-concepts. The husband thinks he's a real charmer with the ladies. The wife says other women are laughing at his childish antics. The woman thinks of herself as a completely gorgeous female. The mate talks about her bowed legs and big hips. Is this destructive? Extremely. Marriage is never quite the same after attacks of this type. But these battles do have their good sides. A couple gets a chance to dissipate some of the pent-up energy caused by disillusionment and frustration. And sometimes these battles bring on a certain amount of understanding and insight. But there's a danger that the couple won't learn to adjust to each other before the destructive effects of the quarreling destroy the meaning of the marriage itself. A conflict that isn't resolved creates hard feelings that carry on to the next quarrel. This makes it more bitter than the one that preceded it, and eventually there's a neverending spiral that leads to permanent alienation.[23]

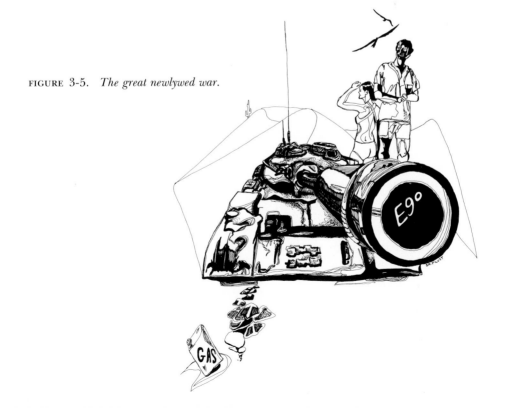

FIGURE 3-5. *The great newlywed war.*

But how about the good marriages, the ones where the partners are still deeply in love after 30 or 40 years? Has there been some conflict there? Probably. But probably the really hateful struggles have been held to a minimum. Then there are marriages that have survived for half a century in which the partners have almost no interaction at all except for an occasional bitter struggle. But most marital adjustment patterns fall somewhere in between. The nuptial state may not be one of perfect bliss, but a lot of the world seems to accept it as a happier state of affairs than going it alone.

Covert Conflict

Even more damaging than open quarreling is covert conflict. Here the couple has reached the stage where they can't or won't discuss their frustrations. They punish each other with "emotional withholdings." There is the frigid wife, the impotent husband. Sometimes there is the surreptitious affair with the girl down the street. When couples fight, at least they're aware that they have a problem, and this awareness can create some kind of solution. But this covert struggle creates punishment that isn't completely understood. There are some marriages that become stabilized around this kind of situation. After all, the relationship is painful, sickening, degrading. But isn't that better than an abrupt divorce, a cruel readjustment? Then there are monetary sacrifice, confusion on the part of the children, and the feelings of the parents and in-laws to consider. There are some "happily married couples" with ulcers and migraine headaches.[24]

Adjustment to In-laws

One of the most common problems young couples face is getting along with the families they've married into. They don't have to face this problem, of course. There are some who get along perfectly with in-laws. They enjoy their company, look forward to evenings together, try to arrange social events so the two families can be included. The anticipation of in-law problems can be a self-fulfilling prophecy. But if you have a few problems of this type, it's best to know that you're not alone. Others have faced them, are facing them, and will face them as long as the marriage idea survives.

Look at it from the parents' standpoint. The offspring isn't a newlywed only. This is the little girl who used to bounce on Daddy's knee, the teenage boy who wouldn't pick up his clothes or take a bath or get a haircut. Parents rear their children, make major decisions for them, and then these "children" get married. Mom's and Dad's words don't carry the weight they once did. And it's hard for them to adjust. Who's at fault? Obviously, the new spouse. Things were just fine before the new girl or new boy entered the picture. Then came an undermining of confidence, of love, even of moral standards.

And how about the worth of offspring? Mom and Dad look on sons as combinations of Kennedy, Einstein, and Johnny Bench. Their girls are Madame Curie, Eleanor Roosevelt, and Zsa Zsa Gabor. Couldn't their children have selected mates who were their equals? Whoever this new mate is must be criticized, chided, told how fortunate he or she is to have done so well in life.[25]

What about adjustment on the part of the poor newlywed? He's had quite a dependent role relationship with parents for years. Dad's and Mom's advice was important. But now this advice can be a threat to a young bride's or groom's perception of his family role. Shouldn't a girl's husband be seeking advice from her and not his mother? She hopes she hasn't married a momma's boy. And does the young man's wife have to call her mother every day? What in the world do they talk about?

And there's a tendency to compare our mates with parents of the opposite sex. Seems kind of unfair. After all, how can the bride cook as well as the groom's mother? Mom has been fulfilling this role for the last 30 years. But newlyweds don't always think or act in a fair way. So marriage can become a breeding ground for in-law disagreements. There are some well-adjusted people who rise above this quagmire of conflict and never face an unpleasant in-law situation. These people are rare, though. Cynics claim that they're nonexistent.

Wives are more likely to have in-law problems than husbands are. The roles of mother-in-law and daughter-in-law are pretty similar. Each has her own way of doing things. The wife has trained under her own mother, and this training often conflicts with advice a meddlesome mother-in-law gives.

FIGURE 3-6. *Appearances might change, but the little girl who bounced on daddy's knee goes on forever.*

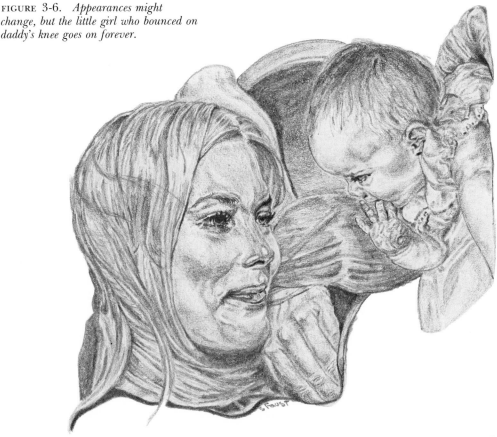

The mother-in-law is hurt when the advice isn't freely accepted. And if it is accepted then the wife's mother feels a sense of rejection. The poor girl is caught in a battle between two experienced hands—a game that she's just learning to play. And all the while there can be an even fiercer battle going on—the wife and the mother-in-law are competing for the husband's affection. Daughters-in-law replace mothers-in-law in the most sensitive areas of husbands' love as the marriage grows. But mothers-in-law won't give up their stake in this love without a struggle.

Despite all the jokes, the strife between mothers-in-law and sons-in-law isn't nearly as great as it is between mothers-in-law and daughters-in-law. There are different sexes involved, and there are two totally different roles in life. This makes it hard for role rivalry to develop. Problems can come up when the husband doesn't treat his wife the way the mother-in-law thinks he should. And sometimes the husband feels threatened when his mother-in-law has too much influence on his new bride. Problems in this area can become severe if the wife has a deep emotional dependency on her mother. And they can be downright unbearable if there's an economic dependency between the two families, such as sharing the same household. But in most cases husbands get along with their mothers-in-law acceptably, if not happily.

Fathers-in-law fare quite well in this in-law game. By and large, there isn't too much friction between fathers-in-law and sons-in-law, fathers-in-law and daughters-in-law. Problems can develop in these areas, of course, just as they can between sisters-in-law and brothers-in-law. But they're usually short-lived problems, ones that aren't too violent.[26]

Marital Sexual Adjustment

Despite the sexual revolution—if there is such a thing—it's about twice as likely that young men have had intercourse before marriage than their brides have. And about seven times more young men than young women have had orgasm prior to marriage. But then come the wedding vows, and the couple has to seek some type of sexual adjustment.[27]

This can be difficult, even though intercourse is a frequent act with young married couples. The average, if there is such a thing, seems to be about three times a week for married teenagers. By the time the couple reaches age 30, the average becomes two times a week. By age 60, the average becomes once every 12 days. But numbers of this type really don't mean too much. The key question involves how enjoyable the experience is. For some young wives, and a few young husbands, the experience isn't quite as enjoyable as it should be. Many brides have difficulty attaining orgasm; although this isn't a must for a satisfying relationship, the attainment of it occasionally can be desirable. About 25 per cent of all brides never attain orgasm during the first year of marriage, but the vast majority have no problem in this area after the marriage has lasted a few years.[28]

Family Size and Marital Adjustment

About half of all couples have a child during their first year of marriage. And 90 per cent produce offspring before the end of their reproductive years. Some couples want to have large families; some don't want to have any children at all. There's nothing wrong with either goal, just so the goal is genuine, not someone else's ideal.[29] This can easily be controlled, of course, with contraceptive techniques.

Today's wives don't want to have the number of children that wives once did. In 1957, the average number of children per family that women wanted was 3.77. In 1972, this average fell to 2.05. This is slightly below the 2.1 children per family demographers say is necessary to maintain zero population growth in the United States. But modern family planning, by both husbands and wives, makes sense. Most research indicates that parents of small families are happier than parents of large ones. This is particularly true during the early years of marriage. Even childless couples who want children have excellent marital adjustment. It's couples who have more children than they want who seem to have problems.[30]

Religion plays a role in this picture. Roman Catholics usually have larger families than Protestants. And Protestants have larger families than Jewish couples. Income and education influence the picture, too. Low-income and low-education groups don't use contraceptives as effectively as their more affluent brethren. So larger families, and often the more poorly adjusted ones, are found among the lower socioeconomic levels.[31]

The Unmarried

There's an unwritten, but changing, statute in American law stating that marriage is a major goal—perhaps the major goal—for both men and women. It's the normal way for adults to live. But there are people who don't obey this statute, so society punishes them by speaking of them in derogatory terms. There's Sam, the old bachelor. Everybody knows that he's "frustrated," "eccentric," "odd." The same goes for Mabel, the librarian. Ever notice how flustered she gets when she talks to a man? Probably both are a little "queer." These people usually have friends who try to save them from their horrible fate. They're constantly searching for suitable partners for their unfortunate brethren. And sometimes the search is successful, so new members are initiated into the fraternity of nuptial culture.

But there are some people who don't want to get married, just can't get married, shouldn't get married. Maybe they don't meet the right members of the opposite sex, or maybe they don't interest the right members of the opposite sex. Sometimes they're looking for the perfect mate, but they look so long that marital opportunities pass them by. There are careers and education that can delay, and sometimes prevent, marriage. There are health-related problems. There are problems involving the willingness to accept family obligations. There are some who don't marry because they don't want to—nothing more, nothing less. Can someone who doesn't tie the knot lead a happy, creative, and fulfilling life? Sure, no matter what the unwritten statute says. Some single people get more out of and give more to life than their married sisters and brothers could ever hope to. Some have troubles and regrets, of course. But whatever marital path someone decides to follow, he shouldn't feel guilty about it, feel different, unusual, or inadequate. No one should try to make him feel that way, either.[32]

The Family Role

There's nothing new about the American family. The model we follow was popular in the Middle Ages, could be found in Jamestown, in Atlanta after Sherman's march to the sea, in Chicago during the Roaring Twenties. True, the American family of today has a heavier sprinkling of Archie Bunkers, Gloria Steinems, and Ringo Starrs than some of the earlier models. But the family ideal, vague as it is, seems to change at a very slow pace.

Some claim that today's American family has come a long way from the patriarchal kingdom of the 1800s. This was the day when men were men, when wives trembled at the sight of their husbands' frowning, bushy eyebrows. Companionship is now the marriage style, and so are intimacy, intellectual and emotional closeness, sexual compatibility, and equality of the work that holds the marriage together. But even the proudest family revolutionary admits that this is somewhat of a theoretical change. A lot of wives vote, but a good number of them—probably most—think that their husbands know more about politics than they do. A lot of husbands and wives have similar educational backgrounds, but they still feel that the man is innately better equipped to drive the car, handle the finances, replace fuses, and fill out tax returns. Careers? It's his that primarily counts, not hers. If the company he works for wants to move him to a new location, the wife is the one who must quit her job and look for employment near the new homestead. Sometimes there's a sharing of household chores before the children come. But then the children do come, and it's decided that the wife should stay home on a full-time basis to take care of them—and take care of those chores that had been previously shared, too. Waxing floors, washing windows and dishes now become female responsibilities. Male responsibilities suddenly become telling the wife that the husband has to go out of town on business or work late at the office; giving suggestions or approval involving parental discipline, vacations, and entertainment. The man begins to act more and more like his father, and the wife begins to cajole, wheedle, and tease a lot the way her mother used to. The American family model, imperfect and unfair as it is, is a prototype that changes only slightly from generation to generation.[33]

A lot of women, of course, are looking for a change. There are some pantyhose radicals who preach that women's only salvation lies in government-operated nurseries and dissolution of all legal ties with men. Marriage, like slavery and the death penalty, must be abolished. But most women would like to see change take place within the matrimonial framework. What they really want is to be treated as equals. They want respect, not indulgence; help, not criticism; love, not fornication; appreciation, not syrupy words. They would like the right to pursue a career, if a career happens to be what they really want. They would like to be full partners, not junior partners. And this ideal is making inroads. But cultural change is slower than many would like.[34]

Divorce

A lot of couples feel that the pain of marriage, the struggles, the frustrations and disappointments just aren't worth it. When something isn't worth it, you get rid of it. Ergo, there's a divorce. The going rate for this phenomenon is about 3.7 divorces per thousand population. This isn't as bad as it was right after World War II, when the rate ran at 4.3 per thousand. But it's higher than it was in the 1960s, when the rate reached 3.2. The divorce rate in the United States is high, and it seems to be growing higher. There's no other country in the world that keeps records on this kind of thing that reports such a high marriage failure rate.[35] Or are we talking about failure? Divorce doesn't have to mean that the couple was much unhappier than couples who stayed married. This is the day when love and companionship are considered musts for living together. You shouldn't cohabitate with someone you don't respect, don't feel affection for, do want to scream at. Possibly, and only possibly, the failure is greater when the couple stays married rather than having each go his separate way. Also, public opinion has changed. No longer is the divorced woman looked on as the scandalous vamp of the neighborhood. Divorced men aren't considered unstable risks for entanglements, and women don't have to rely on their husbands' paychecks the way they once did. They can support themselves.

But divorce, no matter what the reason, is an emotionally draining experience. It's also financially draining and socially embarrassing. There

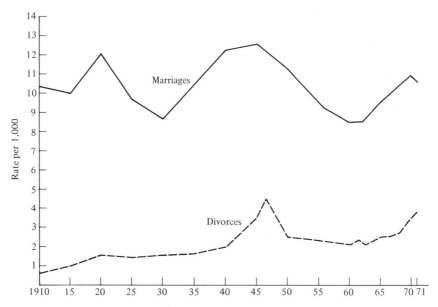

Notice the rise in the divorce rate shortly after World War II. This figure hasn't been reached since, but we're getting close.

SOURCE: U.S. Public Health Service, 1972.

FIGURE 3-7. *Marriage and divorce rates in the United States.*

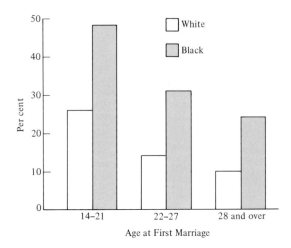

SOURCE: Adapted from Paul C. Glick, "Health, Wealth, and Marriage." Presented at the annual meeting of the American Sociological Association, San Francisco, California, 1967.

FIGURE 3-8. *Men married before age 21 have high divorce rates.*

are usually guilt, usually resentment, and usually fear—if not downright panic. If there are children involved, they can be pulled in two directions, feel responsible for the divorce themselves, become insecure, confused, resentful.

Divorce is more common among city dwellers than it is among those who live in rural areas. It's more common among lower-income families than those with tax problems. And it happens more often with couples who have been married 5 years or less than with those married longer. Also, when one or both parties is under 20 years old when the marriage takes place, the odds of divorce are greater than if the partners are older.[36] There are some who look on divorce as a casual, almost inevitable occurrence in the marriage cycle. But to most a successful marriage is essential to self-fulfillment and a sense of well-being.

Violators of the Code

Marriage usually implies that there will be sexual exclusiveness between one man and one woman. But there are people who claim that this is a reactionary idea. Why can't you have a little variety after you're married as well as before? Most infidelity takes place on a surreptitious basis. There's the secretary whom the wife doesn't know about, the milkman who drops by after the husband has left for work. Affairs of this type can take place on a one-time basis, or they can repeat themselves over and over. People who do this kind of thing often feel quite a bit of guilt and invent elaborate justifications for their actions. "Sally never wants to make love anymore. I'm human, fellow. What am I supposed to do?" "Harry loves me—really loves me. Phil doesn't know I'm around the house most of the time." Behavior of this type can destroy a marriage if the partner finds out. And sometimes the sense of guilt destroys the marriage without the innocent party's being a bit the wiser. Then there are marriages in which the spouse overlooks affairs, or even encourages his mate to have them. These are "swingers," couples who carry on extramarital relations openly, with complete approval of each partner. People who do this kind of thing often have neurotic needs, have sexual problems, or have such extremely weak egos that they're completely subject to the whims of their mates. They often claim that they have good marriages, love their spouses, that their comarital relations make their marriages stronger, not weaker. Most authorities don't agree.[37]

There are also the nonlegal and the group marriages. The nonlegal variety, the kind in which a couple decides to live together without benefit of clergy, became accepted on the college campus a few years ago. This type of relationship isn't common, even among the poor, where its incidence is highest. But it is a relationship that isn't as shocking as it once was and that often leads to a formal marriage contract.[38]

Group marriage is the kind of thing that goes on in communes. A lot of boys live with a lot of girls, and there's a lot of switching of partners. A few communes include married couples or couples who are conventionally faithful, but most go in for sexual collectivism. This isn't as widespread a movement as the amount written about it, both fiction and nonfiction, would lead you to believe. Less than $\frac{1}{10}$ of 1 per cent of the U.S. population is engaged in this group marriage relationship. And though it does eliminate boredom, loneliness, and the success-status-position syndrome of the "straight world," it creates a few problems you don't find in the conventionally married set. How can you find four people, six people, or more who can live together harmoniously? This sometimes seems like an insurmountable problem for just one man and one woman. Then there are problems of leadership, jealousy, and love conflicts. And there are all kinds of problems over sharing the work. It's not just a husband arguing over who should help with the dishes. There are lazy people in communes, energetic people in communes, dirty people and clean people, foolish people and smart people. It's hard to get them to pull together. But the biggest problem of this kind of relationship is the shallowness of the interpersonal involvements. Sexual freedom and universal love are great ideals, but they don't lead to stability, deep personal sharing, empathy. Apparently, the human animal wants these feelings or needs them.[39]

Notes

1. Arlene S. Skolnick and Jerome H. Skolnick, eds., *Family in Transition* (Boston: Little, Brown, 1971).
2. Harold T. Christensen and Christina F. Gregg, "Changing Sex Norms in America and Scandinavia," in *The Social Dimension of Human Sexuality*, ed. by Robert R. Bell and Michael Gordon (Boston: Little, Brown, 1972).
3. Hallowell Pope and Dean D. Knudsen, "Premarital Sexual Norms, the Family, and Social Change," in *The Family and Change*, ed. by John N. Edwards (New York: Knopf, 1969).

4. Gerald R. Leslie, *The Family in Social Context* (New York: Oxford University Press, 1967).
5. Claude Levi-Strauss, "The Family," in *Family in Transition,* ed. by Arlene S. Skolnick and Jerome H. Skolnick (Boston: Little, Brown, 1971).
6. Richard N. Adams, "An Inquiry into the Nature of the Family," in *Family in Transition,* ed. by Arlene S. Skolnick and Jerome H. Skolnick (Boston: Little, Brown, 1971).
7. Milton Yinger, "The Changing Family in a Changing Society," in *The Family and Change,* ed. by John N. Edwards (New York: Knopf, 1969).
8. Anselm, L. Strauss, "Strain and Harmony in American-Japanese War-Bride Marriages," *Marriage and Family Living,* Vol. 16 (May 1954), 99–106.
9. Robert R. Bell, *Marriage and Family Interaction* (Homewood, Ill.: Dorsey Press, 1971).
10. Jerold S. Heiss, "Interfaith Marriage and Marital Outcome," *Marriage and Family Living,* Vol. 23 (August 1961), 228–223.
11. Ellen S. Karp, Julie H. Jackson, and David Lester, "Ideal-Self Fulfillment in Mate Selection: A Corollary to the Complementary Need Theory of Mate Selection," *Journal of Marriage and the Family* (May 1970), p. 269.
12. Bell, *Marriage and Family Interaction,* pp. 109–111.
13. Ibid.
14. Leslie, *The Family in Social Context.*
15. Christensen and Gregg, The Social Dimension of Human Sexuality.
16. Harold T. Christensen, "Value-Behavior Discrepancies Regarding Premarital Coitus in Three Western Cultures," *American Sociological Review,* Vol. 27 (February 1966), 66–74.
17. Lewis M. Terman, *Psychological Factors in Marital Happiness* (New York: McGraw-Hill, 1938).
18. Harvey J. Locke, *Predicting Adjustment in Marriage: A Comparison of a Divorced and a Happily Married Group* (New York: Holt, 1951).
19. Ernest W. Burgess and Paul Wallin, *Engagement and Marriage* (Philadelphia: Lippincott, 1953).
20. Eugene J. Kanin and David H. Howard, "Postmarital Consequences of Premarital Sex Adjustments," *American Sociological Review,* Vol. 23 (October 1958), 560.
21. Alfred C. Kinsey et al., *Sexual Behavior in the Human Female* (Philadelphia: Saunders, 1953).
22. Paul H. Jacobson, *American Marriage and Divorce* (New York: Rinehart, 1959).
23. Talcott Parsons, "The Normal American Family," in *Family in Transition,* ed. by Arlene S. Skolnick and Jerome H. Skolnick (Boston: Little, Brown, 1971).
24. Leslie, *The Family in Social Context.*
25. Bell, *Marriage and Family Interaction,* pp. 315–320.
26. Ibid.
27. Kinsey et al., *Sexual Behavior in the Human Female.*
28. Robert R. Bell, "Some Emerging Sexual Expectations Among Women," in *The Social Dimension of Human Sexuality,* ed. by Robert R. Bell and Michael Gordon (Boston: Little, Brown, 1972).
29. Ibid.
30. Ernest W. Burgess and Leonard S. Cottrell, Jr., *Predicting Success or Failure in Marriage* (New York: Prentice-Hall, 1939).
31. Ronald Freedman, Pascal K. Whelpton, and Arthur A. Campbell, *Family Planning, Sterility and Population Growth* (New York: McGraw-Hill, 1959).
32. Ralph H. Turner, *Family Interaction* (New York: Wiley, 1970), pp. 50–53.
33. Bert N. Adams, *The American Family* (Chicago: Markham, 1971).

34. Bell, "Some Emerging Sexual Expectations Among Women."
35. Richard H. Klemer, *Marriage and Family Relationships* (New York: Harper and Row, 1970).
36. Seymour M. Farber and Roger H. L. Wilson, *Teen-age Marriage and Divorce* (Berkeley, Calif.: Diablo Press, 1967).
37. H. A. Otto, "Has Monogamy Failed?" *Saturday Review,* Vol. 53 (November 21, 1970), 23–25, 62.
38. Ibid.
39. R. M. Kanter, "Communes," *Psychology Today,* Vol. 4 (July 1970), 53–57, 78.

4 Mental Health and Illness

Mental Health

She was pregnant; she was an only child, she couldn't bear facing the recriminations, the shock, the histrionics. The police found her, though. She had known they would. And then came the tearful reunion, the abortion, two more pregnancies, and three more hitchhiking escapes before she left home for good and set up housekeeping with a hospital orderly. There was pot, but no heroin, cocaine, or "speed." There was sex, but only with her boyfriend. There was isolation from her parents. She never visited, seldom telephoned, and wrote on birthdays and holidays only. She respected her parents, liked them in a sense, certainly didn't resent them. There were thoughts of suicide occasionally—just fleeting thoughts. There was self-satisfaction, sometimes exaltation in being a healthy human animal in an interesting and free world. Was she sick, mentally healthy, maladjusted, a pioneer in a new social experiment, one of the few happy escapees from a conformist society that secretly envied her?

A Healthy Mind

What really is mental health? To the banker, responsibility in money matters has a lot to do with it. To the preacher, Christian morals play a key role in the definition. And education has something to do with it if you ask the schoolteacher. And the football coach, the political activist, the bartender, the salesman have views on the matter, too. Mental health is pretty much of a value judgment. Certainly the Buddhist monk who douses himself with gasoline and lights a match wouldn't be looked on as emotionally stable in Wichita, Kansas. In Vietnam, this kind of behavior is idealistic heroism. The same analogy applies to South Sea natives who dress in loincloths. In New York City they'd be arrested for streaking. And there are members of religious sects who mutilate their bodies, sometimes cripple themselves to atone for sins. These groups definitely consider themselves mentally stable, look on the rest of the world as deviant, irrational, emotionally ill.

The mentally healthy person, in the broadest sense, is someone who copes effectively with himself and his environment. If he adjusts well to the people, events, and things in the world around him, if he gains approval from this world and seems to be reasonably happy, then his mind is considered sound. This is kind of a fluid state, though, because both the individual and his surroundings constantly change. Good mental health isn't a condition that's permanent. The world can be ours in the morning. Afternoon can bring rain and darkness and cold.

And there's a learning factor to mental health. The human mind is adaptable, strong, pragmatic. It will overcome pain, if possible. If not possible, it will avoid it. And emotional illness, even in its most mild form, is painful. So we try to be mentally healthy. We modify our attitudes, our values, our self-concepts, our ideals, our behavior an infinite number of times, bringing them into line with the ideals of society and the goals, limitations, and experiences of who and what we are.[1] Mental health is a lifelong pursuit. And, like the Holy Grail, we never quite find it. But the quest makes us stronger, better, and happier people.

Human Motivation

Why do we campaign for a certain candidate, sign up for a certain class, play football, or take a shower? Because we want to get something for our efforts. Maybe it's money we're looking for, maybe prestige, maybe just relaxation. Our motives are limitless, and any list of them is totally inadequate. But motives can be grouped in order to discuss them. Granted, this type of grouping is arbitrary, but it brings a little organization to the behavioral jungle.

One way of breaking motives down is putting them under two major categories: affiliation oriented and prestige oriented. Our affiliation-oriented drives deal with the gregarious sides of our natures. We prefer friendship to loneliness, living with someone or some people to being by ourselves, working with others instead of doing it alone. Affiliation-oriented motives explain why man forms corporations, raises families, joins the Elks. It explains why we interact, or sometimes prefer to interact, with people of mutual backgrounds and mutual interests. Teenagers like to relate with teenagers, businessmen with businessmen, and housewives with housewives. And the relationship is more satisfying when there's a common language so we learn the native tongues of those we're associated with, pick up their slang and colloquial expressions. These motives can range in degree from casual acquaint-anceship to close friendship and love.[2]

AFFILIATION-ORIENTED MOTIVES

We probably inherit these affiliation-oriented motives, but learning refines them. After all, without people none of us would have survived infancy. People gave food and warmth, removed irritants. So people at an early age learn to like people. This matures into a type of dependence, a feeling of depression when we're deprived of human contact over an extended period. One of the most severe punishments anyone can receive is solitary confinement. Prisoners dread it, report delusions, nightmares, depression, feelings of shame and inadequacy when they go through it.

There are people who like to be alone, of course. But most of them have affiliation-oriented motives to some degree. They have a few friends, a member or two of their families they're intimate with. Sometimes they read a lot or watch TV, getting human contact in an indirect way.

We work hard to win the approval of our fellow man. Disapproval can bring rejection, and rejection can be terrifying. So we conform to activities our cultures approve of. We hold responsible jobs, dress conservatively, marry—if our culture encourages this kind of behavior. If the culture we belong to, or want to belong to, encourages smoking pot, living with someone without benefit of clergy, condemning the establishment, living on welfare, then this might be how we live. Man really does need other people, and he works hard at satisfying this need.[3]

PRESTIGE-ORIENTED MOTIVES

We don't just want to associate with our fellow man; we want to outdo him. It's not just the social climber who wants the house with the swimming pool, the Cadillac, the membership in the country club. Everyone is looking for a Cadillac of sorts. Maybe they want their names in print, an election to an all-America team, membership in the student council, a reputation as being popular. But whatever form this dream machine takes, it's got to be the biggest and shiniest one on the block. Did you ever hear just one joke at a party? Never! One fellow gets a laugh, then someone else tries to get a bigger laugh, then someone outdoes the second person, and so on. Each builds his storytelling prestige by outdoing the storyteller who went before. The same goes for gossip, fishing yarns, and tales of athletic and girl-chasing prowess. We're status seekers, we Americans, and the same applies to Germans, French, Englishmen, Israelis, Cubans, and natives of Pago Pago.

But different cultures respect different kinds of achievement. The successful entrepreneur is a big success in American culture. In Russia or China he has almost no status whatsoever, assuming such a person exists. The matador in Spain is a national idol. In America, it's the pro football quarterback, the winner of the Indianapolis 500, the big-league pitcher with 30 wins for the season. And even in a given country or culture, there are subcultural patterns with their own prestige values. The hippie at Haight-Ashbury certainly didn't see much prestige in having the best sales record or biggest Chevrolet agency in Oakland. The insurance salesman doesn't find status in beating bongo drums or reciting idealistic poetry. Each of us, though, wants to comply with some cultural ideal, comply better than anyone else who has the same kind of ideal. Maybe being content and adjusted to your lot in life is the only ideal you have. But chances are you want to be less dissatisfied, less neurotically ambitious, less covetous of your boss's country home than any other "perfectly stable" garage mechanic, housewife, or schoolteacher.[4]

STATUS SYMBOLS

We become aware of status symbols at an early age. "Quitters never win and winners never quit," Dad counsels. "Winning isn't the most important thing; it's everything!" says the coach. "You can do anything you really set your mind to," says Mom. And then there are the teacher, Aunt Agnes, and Uncle Joe who tell us that we ought to "hitch our wagons to stars," "there's plenty of room at the top," "whatever you do, you should do with all your might." Little girls are supposed to be cuter than most other little girls, prettier, more ladylike. Little boys are supposed to be the toughest little boys in their neighborhoods—aggressive, manly, daring. For adolescents, status comes on the football field, at proms, at the beach. It comes from the classroom and the church, too, of course. But these are more sober status symbols, ones that are part of the teenage culture, but not the glamorous part.

There's a subtle part of adolescent status that involves establishing independence from Mom and Dad. The young fellow who has to be home by midnight, has to get a haircut occasionally, and depends on Dad for his allowance may not have much respect in the eyes of his peers. The girl who dates only the boys Mom and Dad approve of may have a respect problem, too. So the teenager most independent from his family, who sets his own rules, answers to himself and no one else, is often the peer group idol.

Different people, regardless of age, sex, race, or religion, place different values on athletic, social, and intellectual achievement. If he's 6 feet 10 inches, weighs 250 pounds, and can run 40 yards in $4\frac{1}{2}$ seconds, probably his heroes are in the sports world. The girl who is homecoming queen, a cheerleader, and president of her sorority probably looks on achievement in the social arena as the ultimate in status. We tend to value proficiencies we think we have or think we can develop. After all, this builds our self-concepts, makes college professors feel superior to bankers, bankers feel superior to politicians, and politicians feel superior to everybody. You don't have to excel at everything to be proud of yourself. Success in just one or two areas, or striving for success, can satisfy prestige-oriented drives.[5]

MOTIVE MODIFICATION

Of course, be they affiliation oriented or prestige oriented, we have to adjust our motives to the world as we find it. People don't always give us what we're looking for. Maybe the girl you like can't stand you; maybe your friends have gone away for the summer; maybe you've moved to a new neighborhood and haven't been able to make new friends. And prestige can be harder to find than friends. To get it you have to excel, which means you have to do better than the competition. Because the competition is trying to do better than you, you'll run into your share of losses. But if you're healthy, you adjust. Like the rest of the human race, you modify your motives through experience, learn to cope with an infinitely complex environment.

Human Needs

Another way of explaining human behavior is by listing what seem to be human needs. We want to fulfill these needs, so our actions, our thoughts, our personalitites get shaped accordingly. Of course, we need many and varied things, so no human need list could be complete. But Abraham Maslow compiled the following, which many regard as classic:

PHYSIOLOGICAL NEEDS

We get hungry from time to time and thirsty. We need sleep, and we need sexual expression in one way or another. Thwart these needs, and all others seem relatively unimportant. When you're starving, you don't have much interest in that new car you might think you need when you're well fed. When you're sleepy, you don't get much emotional satisfaction out of the concert you're attending. When you have a strong sex drive, which most young people do, there is a tendency to think about little else.

SECURITY

Security or safety is important to children. They frighten easily, become upset when parents quarrel, often become withdrawn and depressed when the family moves. Older people are concerned with security, too. But they try to hide these feelings from others. Flunk a final? No problem. You can always take the course over. Lose your job? Who cares? There'll be better ones. The same applies to family quarrels and social disasters. We don't feel secure about the consequences even though we don't cry and fret in front of friends. But we want that security; we need it, whether we're 6 or 60.

LOVE AND BELONGING

Some people find it hard to form close, personal relationships. Maybe society is at fault. Maybe the people are. Parts of our culture imply that deep feelings of affection are signs of weakness. This is nonsense, of course. And other parts of our culture imply that love and sex are the same thing. This is nonsense, too. Love is extremely complex, possibly relates to sex in one way or another, but it certainly doesn't have to encompass the act. Children can love their parents deeply, priests their congregations, soldiers their country. Sex, in the true sense of the term, doesn't enter the picture. Prostitutes usually don't feel much love for their partners, and sex is what that relationship is all about. Love isn't an easily definable emotion, but it does exist. And even the most backward sense it, recognize it, need it.

ESTEEM

All of us have to believe in ourselves. Some believe more than others do. Some emanate self-confidence, genuine pride, personal strength. And there are "losers," who are afraid to ask for a date because they might get turned down, know they're no good at basketball and dancing, and know they don't have the personality to be a salesman or manager, or to enter politics. But everyone believes in himself to some degree. He can lace his shoes, eat his breakfast, perform an adequate role in certain types of routine jobs. People without a basic degree of self-esteem can't function in society, often can't function at all. We need this belief in ourselves almost as much as we need food and water. And we need the esteem of those around us as well. The truly self-confident person may not need the number of compliments and approving smiles that the insecure fellow does. But there's no one who can get by on constant frowns, badgering, and complaints. Probably we build self-esteem by winning the approval of others; probably the self-esteem we have has a lot to do with winning others' approval. It's a never-ending cycle, which contributes to the rich getting richer, students who got A's in high school joining Phi Beta Kappa, teenagers picked up for auto theft eventually doing life terms for bank robbery. Someone who finds himself in the wrong direction of this cycle can change things. Losers really can become winners. But it takes some self-discipline, determination to succeed in some constructive area, determination to change the way you think about yourself.

SELF-ACTUALIZATION

Writers have to write, dancers have to dance, football players have to push pigskins. But self-actualization implies that participation in these activities and all the others human beings get involved in isn't enough. Whatever your potential is, you have to realize it or come close to realizing it. Joining the football team isn't enough if you have the speed, size, and desire to be a great defensive lineman or quarterback. You have to work at it until you're exhausted, think about it when you're tired of thinking about plays and formations, sacrifice when you're sure you've already sacrificed too much, and keep trying during setbacks and discouragement. The same is true for musicians, professors, managers, and housewives. You don't have to be the best in any given field, but you have to be the best that you can be—adding your own individuality and approach to the endeavor.

This is the ultimate of all human needs. Many certainly don't satisfy it. Many rationalize that no such need exists, settle into a comfortable rut, and laugh at "climbers," "drivers," people who can't settle for what they've got. But these people who don't really try are often preoccupied with more basic needs like hunger, love, and security. Or maybe they're foolish enough to deny themselves, to accept frustration and feelings of inadequacy as part of living.[6]

Characteristics of the Emotionally Healthy Person

There is no such thing as perfect emotional health, of course. All of us have our moments of feeling insecure and depressed, moments of being irrational, unstable, irresponsible. And some personalities are a little less healthy than they should be all the time. There is the constant worrier, the timid housewife who escapes into soap operas, and the arrogant manager who gets his fun out of belittling and threatening subordinates. But when or where mental illness begins isn't quite clear. What mental health is isn't quite clear, either. There's no precise line dividing the two conditions. There are some characteristics, though, that emotionally healthy people exhibit more readily than do people society labels as ill.

THE ABILITY TO WORK PRODUCTIVELY

There are people who can't hold jobs; housewives who can't keep up with the washing, vacuuming, and wild children; students who flunk their courses or drop courses they know they'll flunk. All of these people aren't ill; many have good reasons for failing, for setbacks, for lack of accomplishment. But when failing becomes failure, setbacks become a way of life, emotions can be causing the problem. Many feel the key indicator of mental health is the ability to work efficiently and productively. There are the chronically unemployed who are mentally healthy, of course. The same applies to dropouts. But many need help—the emotional kind.

THE ABILITY TO FACE REALITY AND DEAL WITH IT

It's an unfair world, sometimes a selfish and cruel one, often a painful one. There's a temptation to fantasize your way out of it, drink your way out of it, escape with a needle or a pill. Mentally healthy people face reality, though—at least most of the time. They overcome problems they can overcome, bear those they can't.

THE ABILITY TO CONTROL EMOTIONS

There are women who fly into jealous rages, men who threaten and shout when they don't get their way, men who cry and women who pout. Sometimes a little loss of control can be good. But, by and large, runaway emotionalism signifies serious mental and nervous problems. The emotionally healthy face disappointment with mild dejection, not depression; react to good news with elation, not euphoria; occasionally get angry, never hate; are occasionally suspicious, never paranoid.

ABILITY TO BALANCE INDEPENDENCE AND DEPENDENCE UPON OTHERS

Some people know that they're always right. Or maybe they're afraid to admit they're wrong—to others or to themselves. This might show weakness, and they know that's bad. There are others who can't make up their minds about even the simplest matters. What clothes should they wear? What movie should they see? Should they watch a variety show or Monday night football? If criticized, they feel guilty. There's no chance the other fellow was wrong. Neither of these extremes represents good mental health, of course. The well-adjusted person isn't afraid to think for himself, be it on a short-term or long-term basis. But he's willing to listen to advice, even criticism, from people with the experience and background he respects. He has enough personal security not to become paralyzed by fear of mistakes or to close his mind to an idea.

ABILITY TO BUILD TOWARD LONG-RANGE GOALS

No one likes to save money when there's a dress, car, or television set he'd like to buy. No one likes to study instead of go to a dance, mow the lawn instead of go to the beach, practice the piano instead of watch television. But even though they don't like to, mentally healthy people, in varying degrees, sacrifice immediate pleasure for long-range goals. The mentally disturbed often grab their fun where they find it, are incapable of planning for next month, next week, tomorrow.

ABILITY TO ADAPT TO CHANGE

Who wants change? No one, if the change converts his win to a loss. Change to the man who's made a fortune may mean that he gives up part of his fortune, his power, prestige. Change to the young can mean they grow old. And no strong person wants to think of himself as becoming weak. But changes do take place, whether we want them to or not. There are new roles we have to assume, new challenges to meet, new disappointments to adjust to. The mentally healthy accept change as inevitable and adapt accordingly. Maybe they wish change wouldn't come, but they don't waste a lot of energy in futile resistance and regret.

THE ABILITY TO LOVE

Most of us have loved ones we cherish—our families, close friends. A few love no one at all, not even themselves. Obviously, this latter group isn't too well adjusted. And neither is another group of people who superficially love their own kind but distrust and hate everyone else. There are "superpatriots" who know the communists, fascists, Japanese, or Germans will attack any day. There are Whites who hate Blacks, Blacks who hate Whites, Reds and Orientals who know that Whites are shifty. Some women look on men as degenerate beasts ("They're only looking for one thing"). Some men are afraid of women, don't understand them, don't want to have anything to do with them. Then there are young who hate the old, old who judge the young, and middle-aged who are convinced that all other generations have lost their senses. The emotionally well adjusted love all people, regardless of creed, race, or nationality. Of course, they love some more than others. But they spread their love around. They don't reserve it for a chosen few, for a select elite.[7]

A Healthy Philosophy

But characteristics only describe what a mentally healthy person is like or does. Can't mental health be cultivated? To some extent, yes it can. There's no formula or rigid procedure you can follow, of course. It's way too vague an area. But here are a few suggestions which some people find helpful:

1. If you've got a sense of humor, use it. If you don't, develop one. Life can be funny, and probably there's no one funnier than you. Have a laugh on yourself.
2. Get some real friends. They're rare and extremely precious. With them, we can share troubles and fortunes. Without them, we share a lot of loneliness.
3. Face your troubles, your worries. But don't face them for too long. After you've thought and done what you could, turn your attention to more pleasant things.
4. Don't be an extremist. Enjoy sports, politics, poetry, business—in moderation. A balanced personality can have a lot of fun and bring a lot of fun to others.
5. Have several major goals in your life. One usually isn't enough. But make sure that they're your goals, not just some nice ideals.
6. You're going to have impulses and emotions. Although you can't give them free rein, don't try to suppress them, either. Guide them into desirable, creative channels.
7. Get in the habit of appreciating the beauty, the nobility, the excitement of the world around you. Work at enjoying the present. Yesterday, good or bad, can't be relived or changed.
8. Time heals a lot of wounds and wounds a lot of heels, too. Don't exaggerate today's setbacks. That great day in the morning will probably come.
9. Believe in yourself, or no one else will. And help the other guy believe in himself. The two of you, or three of you, or four of you can make quite a team.
10. Believe in something greater than yourself. Then you can grow greater than you are.
11. Be genuine, the unique you. Imitations never work. If people don't like the real article, that's their problem.[8]

Coping with Stress

The world's a threatening place, even for the most self-confident and strong. There's a boss who threatens to fire us, a teacher who threatens to flunk us, health that threatens to fade, youth that threatens to age. If we let ourselves dwell on our problems, anxiety would dominate our personalities, fear would be our life style. So we humans practice what are called "defense

TABLE 4-1
Summary Chart of Ego Defense Mechanisms

Denial of reality	Protecting self from unpleasant reality by refusal to perceive or face it, often by escapist activities like getting "sick" or being preoccupied with other things
Fantasy	Gratifying frustrated desires in imaginary achievements
Rationalization	Attempting to prove that one's behavior is "rational" and justifiable and thus worthy of self and social approval
Projection	Placing blame for difficulties upon others or attributing one's own unethical desires to others
Repression	Preventing painful or dangerous thoughts from entering consciousness
Reaction formation	Preventing dangerous desires from being expressed by exaggerating opposed attitudes and types of behavior and using them as "barriers"
Undoing	Atoning for and thus counteracting immoral desires or acts
Regression	Retreating to earlier developmental level involving less mature responses and usually a lower level of aspiration
Identification	Increasing feelings of worth by identifying self with person or institution of illustrious standing
Introjection	Incorporating external values and standards into ego structure so that individual is not at their mercy as external threats
Compensation	Covering up weakness by emphasizing desirable trait or making up for frustration in one area by overgratification in another
Displacement	Discharging pent-up feelings, usually of hostility, on objects less dangerous than those that initially aroused the emotions
Emotional insulation	Reducing ego involvement and withdrawing into passivity to protect self from hurt
Intellectualization	Cutting off affective charge from hurtful situations or separating incompatible attitudes by logic-tight compartments
Sublimation	Gratifying or working off frustrated sexual desires in nonsexual activities
Sympathism	Striving to gain sympathy from others, thus bolstering feelings of self-worth despite failures
Acting out	Reducing the anxiety aroused by forbidden desires by permitting their expression

Source: James C. Coleman, *Abnormal Psychology and Modern Life,* 3rd ed. (Chicago: Scott, Foresman, 1964), p. 107.

mechanisms." These mechanisms calm us down, help us face life in as productive and easygoing a way as we can. They keep us from seeing life as it truly is, which can be good. Complete honesty is painful and destructive. But avoidance of reality can bring on punishment of its own. Defense mechanisms, if practiced to too great a degree, can make us irresponsible, childish, self-centered. Practice them not at all, and it's time for tranquilizers and counseling. Like food, too little can make you weak, unproductive, and ill; too much can make you lazy, dull, self-indulgent, and flabby. Here are a few of the most important of these mechanisms. There are hundreds more, possibly thousands. The human mind will never lack for ways of telling it like it isn't, concentrating on something other than facts.

RATIONALIZATION

No one likes to accept total blame for his own failure. If he flunked an exam, possibly he didn't study the way he should, but the teacher really didn't cover the material too well, either. If he got fired, maybe he could have worked harder, but the boss really had it in for him and didn't give him much of a chance. Some people carry rationalization to an extreme. Nothing is ever their fault; someone else has caused their woes. This lack of personal honesty can interfere with development and maturity.

DAYDREAMING

Daydreaming is fun. We become quarterbacks in the Super Bowl, get crowned Miss America, make a fortune the envy of Howard Hughes and Rockefeller. It's also creative. Without a dream, you can't really have a goal or growth. Even practical achievements probably start with an escapist fantasy. But daydreaming can be destructive. It's one thing to take a few minutes out from a tough study routine, a hard job, a personal disappointment and go to that castle in escape land. It's another to make too many trips or get locked in the castle and not be able to return. Some people can't distinguish between reality and fantasy. They think they have won the Nobel Prize, run the 3-minute mile, mastered thought travel to Mars. This calls for professional help.

FIGURE 4-1. *Daydream.*

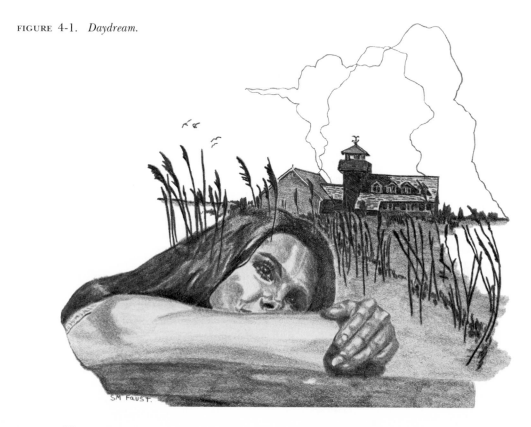

SM Faust.

REPRESSION

Where did all the good times go? Right into the forefront of our memories. We never forget our wins, successes, and compliments. Then what about the bad times? We tend to screen those out. After all, if you waste your energy on regrets, self-pity, and resentment, you'll never concentrate on opportunities for fun and achievement. But repression of unpleasant experiences can get out of hand. If you don't let yourself think of a truly painful time, even for an instant, you can have feelings of anxiety and guilt and not know why. You won't let yourself think about the real problem. This is too painful. This pain usually won't fade until the sufferer makes up his mind to face the truth.

PROJECTION

Do you know the fat girl who speaks of a friend who can't stick to a diet, the dropout who talks about "dumb" athletes, the "loner" who talks about the "in-group" on campus? All of us see our own faults in other people. The shy person is often convinced that everyone else is shy; the drunk knows he's not the only person in the world with a drinking problem; the selfish fellow knows he'd better get his before the rest of the world cuts him out. Projection has its good side, too. Self-confident people usually think of others as self-confident; friendly people think of others as friendly; sincere people believe what they hear. Apparently, our thoughts about ourselves get passed on to others.

IDENTIFICATION

There's no one without a hero. For a young child, this hero might be Mom or Dad. For Mom or Dad, this hero might be a political figure, a boss, or possibly some nebulous ideal, like the code of the Optimist Club, like the goals of women's lib. Without this identification with who or what we would like to be, there would be no pattern to organize us or direct us. But sometimes this identification gets carried to an extreme. We look on our families, our schools, certain clubs, our codes as all that matter in life. Others and others' needs and ideals are ignored or held in contempt. This can make us shallow, self-centered, boring.

REGRESSION

He yells; he throws things; he hits at the air. She becomes sullenly silent, carps, cries, and hints at divorce or suicide. Teenagers or grownups sometimes act like children because this seems to solve an emotional need. Sometimes it helps them get something they want, this regression to childhood. Someone pacifies them, cajoles them, or babies them. But too much of this kind of behavior can cost a lot of respect, a lot of self-respect.

DENIAL

Denial is something like whistling in the dark. We tell ourselves we're not afraid, in hope that the fear will disappear. This is good if we're building needed courage, bad if we're eliminating needed fear. All of us should be afraid of cancer and get annual physicals, be afraid of leaving our families destitute and take out insurance. Denial to too great a degree can turn courage into foolhardiness and irresponsibility.

SUBSTITUTION

None of us gets everything he wants in life. If you're not big enough to make the football team, tall enough to be good at basketball, maybe distance running or wrestling can substitute. Or maybe you're not athletic, so you substitute playing in the band, working on the school newspaper, working in student government. Substitution is fine as long as we substitute healthy alternatives. Substitution of martinis, "speed," or promiscuity for a disappointing life isn't usually healthy.

AVOIDANCE

If you're afraid of flying, you might avoid airplanes. If you're afraid of swimming, you can stay away from the water; afraid of dogs, don't own one. Everyone has fears, and there's nothing wrong with giving into the harmless ones. Some people are so afraid of germs, though, they won't kiss, or even touch, another person. Some are so afraid of accidents they won't leave their homes, so afraid of being fired they won't get a job. Avoidance, like any defense mechanism, is a sensible and healthy way of dealing with life; or it's crippling, destructive, irrational. Sickness or health depends on how much, how often.[9]

Psychological Development

How do we get to be the way we are? Obviously, each of us is unique, has a personality that's a little more outgoing, a little more studious, a little more insecure, a little more creative, a little more friendly than that of anyone else who is, who has been, who ever will be. And, obviously, certain personalities adapt to the world around them better than other personalities do. If we understood what made people glib politicians, lion tamers, research chemists, possibly we could make more of the same; possibly we could keep people from becoming heroin addicts or larcenists or prostitutes. Possibly we could make everyone happier, make the world less chaotic, eliminate wars, famine, and greed. It's knowledge worth having. And, considering the state of planet Earth, it's knowledge we don't have to any major degree as yet. Possibly we will have it in the 1980s or 2080s or the 2180s. Possibly, upon acquiring it, we'll find that it's knowledge we really don't want. Perfect human beings and idealistic societies can create demons and nightmares the laissez-faire emotional world can't envision. But, whether for better or for worse, man will continue to philosophize and research about what makes individuals the peculiar types of individuals they are. Here are some of the thoughts and findings in this area to date:

INSTINCT

We're willing to accept the inevitability of having brown eyes, being 5 feet 10 inches tall, having red hair, having an average IQ, an average ability to play the piano. But it's hard to accept the inevitability of being shy, being cranky, or being a bore. Americans, particularly, feel this way. "You can be the man you want to be," we tell our sons. "Learn to be a lady" or "Develop style," we tell our daughters. The American dream says we're in control not only of what we become but also of who we are. There are other dreamers, though, mostly Europeans, who disagree. They cite studies of identical twins, who have the same genetic makeup, and fraternal twins, whose genetic patterns are no more similar than those of other siblings. The characterisics of identical twins are much closer than those of the fraternal variety in the following areas: self-confidence, stubbornness, brain wave patterns, response to music and color, smoking habits, susceptibility to mental illness. These doubters of the "self-made man" philosophy founded the science of ethology. In the Darwinian tradition, they study animals in their natural habitats.

Ethology. Animal behavior, of course, is largely instinctive. There's little, if any, introspection involved. And ethologists feel the same is largely true of man. Our environment shapes us, of course, but not in the complex way many philosophers imagine. Konrad Lorenz, one of the leaders in ethology, argues that environment "imprints" various behavioral patterns on man during critical periods of his development. Like goslings that attach themselves to any person or object that satisfies their needs of the moment, men do the same. And, like those of geese, our behavioral patterns grow from these attachments and last for a lifetime. There are children who were isolated from adults during critical stages of development, such as 6 months to 2 years. When they got older, these children had problems in relating to other people, sometimes had difficulty speaking, often had trouble controlling emotional reactions. The same often is true of children institutionalized for extended periods shortly after birth. Could the trouble be that little or no imprinting took place between these children and other human figures?[10]

INSTINCT PERSONALITY THEORIES

Ethologists realize that humans are extremely complex, that observations made in the animal kingdom can't be automatically applied to people. Critical stages in the development of geese, rats, guinea pigs aren't hard to isolate. Critical stages in the development of humans are. But in spite of this, or because of it, several personality theories have grown around the critical-stage concept. A good example is the psychoanalytic theory of Sigmund Freud.

Sigmund Freud. Freud believed that children pass through five distinct phases in which they relieve their sexual tensions by stimulating erogenous zones such as the mouth, the anus, and the genitals. Gratification has to take place during each stage or the individual becomes so seriously frustrated that his personality is warped. For instance, a person who smokes a lot, chews a lot, or talks a lot might have been frustrated during his oral stage. If the anal stage wasn't gratified, the grownup might be stingy and stubborn. And then there's the "Oedipus complex," in which the child wants to join the parent of the opposite sex in the marriage bed. If this isn't properly resolved, the grownup might be incapable of carrying out heterosexual relations.

Freud uses instinct as a basis of development and emphasizes critical periods, just as ethologists do. Actually, he divides all instincts into two categories—the life instinct, exemplified by sexual drive, and the death instinct, which we show largely through aggression.[11]

Erik Erikson. Erikson studied under Freud's daughter, Anna, and agreed with most of the basic elements of psychoanalytic theory. Sex instincts, or life instincts, he agreed, supply the basic energy for human emotions; these emotions are never in harmony with society's code. Erikson feels there are more than just five critical stages of development, though. Personalities form and change as people get older, just as they do during youth. So Erikson essentially accepts the five periods outlined by Freud and adds three of his own. Freud's theoretical human goes through his last critical stage during adolescence. Erikson's model goes through personality modifications during early adulthood, middle adulthood, and late adulthood.

Erikson labels his theory "psychosocial" rather than "psychoanalytical" in order to emphasize society's role in shaping what we become. The world we live in presents problems of infinite complexity. How we solve or adjust to the problems determines how we live, who we are.[12]

Robert White. White has no quarrel with Freud or Erikson over the number of critical stages we go through, but he questions the motivating force behind them. The sex urge, he feels, is important, but it's not an all-encompassing drive. We have a need to master our world, White feels. We must become competent in fields such as language and self-locomotion, in interaction with other people and things. We humans are curious; we're explorers, we're achievers. We want to make an impact on ourselves and the world, even if we have to increase our sexual tension a little in the process.

White weaves his "competence theory" through most of Freud's and Erikson's development models. For instance, there's Freud's "oral stage." A child less than 1 year old identifies pleasure in his mouth. There are sucking, eating, biting, chewing, and spitting. White doesn't quarrel with this but feels there are other activities, such as playing and trying to feed himself, that bring on pleasure as well. The child is instinctively trying to gain competence. Weaning, of course, would be an overwhelming tragedy if the child didn't get some type of gratification from drinking from a cup. The same is true of toilet training and the mastery of sexual roles. Achievement in these areas motivates us as strongly as the urge to reproduce, the urge to love.[13]

ENVIRONMENT AND LEARNING

Albert Einstein wouldn't have been much of a physicist if he had been raised in a jungle. There's never been a track star who didn't have to train, a quarterback who didn't have to learn how to pass and read defenses. Those who believe environment is the key ingredient in making us doctors, lawyers, merchants, what-have-you don't ignore heredity. They admit that there's no guarantee of turning out heavyweight champions in a gym, Charles Darwins in a university. But they focus on ways we learn to become strong, weak, kind, selfish, genuine, insincere. A human's potential isn't their prime interest. Neither are his instinctual drives. How he becomes what he can become and how society can help him are.

Learning Theory. Learning theorists feel we become what we become because of the way the world rewards us and punishes us. According to the theory of "operant conditioning," we increase behavior that brings reward and decrease that which brings pain. And to make it more complex, there's the concept of "classical conditioning." This states that we associate pleasant and unpleasant experiences with what's going on at the same time. For instance, a child might find making a bed a pleasurable experience if he got a piece of candy every time he did it. And he might consider cuddling up to his mother unpleasant if she rapped him on the head when he came close. So habit patterns might be formed that turn him into an obsessively neat hermit.

This theory is very precise and logical, with one major exception. What in the world is a reward, and what in the world is a punishment? For lower forms of life, these terms can be pretty clear. For man, even when he's extremely young, no one can be sure whether a piece of candy, a token, or a compliment is a big reward, a small reward, no reward at all. Value systems in people are as variable as their heights, their weights, their incomes. Reinforcement really doesn't explain behavior. It accounts for it, though, bringing a little order to the confusing actions of *Homo sapiens.*[14]

Social Learning Theory. Social learning theory stresses the concept of "modeling." We don't just look like our parents; we generally speak the same language they do, gesture like them, have the same religion they have, the same politics, the same types of friends. This also applies to brothers and sisters and peers. We imitate those we admire, those with status, those who seem to be getting rewards. Possibly we imitate those we don't admire, too. Have you ever noticed how someone with a new job, who has just been elected to student government, who has just made a certain team has taken on a new personality? Sometimes a girl seems totally different after she's gotten married. We're imitators, and who we're imitating determines who we become.

Albert Bandura and Richard Walters have done some interesting research in this field. They arranged for some children to watch an adult kick a large, plastic doll. Sure enough, the children began doing the same. They found that motorists were much more likely to stop and help someone fix a

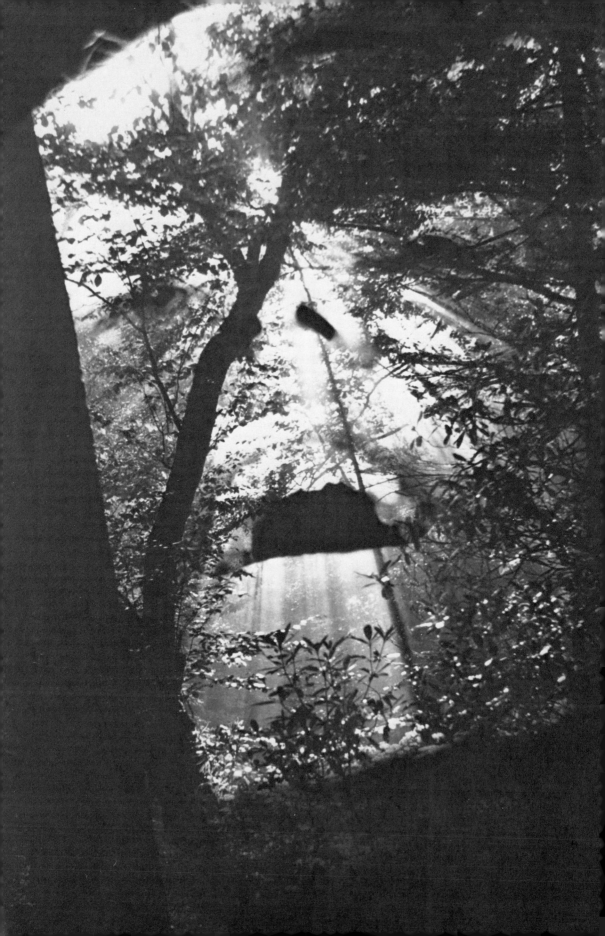

flat if they saw another motorist helping someone else. And the likelihood of someone's contributing to the Salvation Army depended on whether he saw someone else contribute. Apparently, if you want to be like someone, associate with him. Some of it does rub off.[15]

Cognitive Development. Jean Piaget, a Swiss psychologist, agrees that people learn from modeling and from reward and punishment. He feels that an important something has been left out of the human equation, though—the mind. Thoughts, or cognition, shape us as much as, maybe more than, heroes and compliments. You certainly can't learn to solve math problems by imitation, by being told that you're doing fine. You have to think about them, think about various approaches to solutions, reject the unworkable, accept the workable. The same applies to solving problems of life. You select what seem to be workable solutions, adjust or shape yourself the way you think you should, make infinite variations in the way you act, who you are. According to cognitive development theory, the main motivating force in our lives is the need to know. Like Robert White, Piaget feels that man has an insatiable hunger to understand his world and control it. So he develops cognitive structures that improve his comprehension and supply receptacles for new information.

There is emotion, of course. In no way is the cool, calculating individual the prototype of mankind. We often act before we think. We often base our actions on feelings instead of reason, often rationalize our mistakes instead of learn from them. If man were a perfectly logical creature, wars, poverty, prisons would have disappeared centuries ago. Piaget and his followers recognize this. But they feel the important part of emotion is how we interpret it. A mother's scolding can be rejection, discipline, love, eccentricity, funny. It depends on the makeup of the person; his makeup depends on how he thinks; how he thinks determines who he is. The same applies to most experiences in life. We emote about them; but, in one way or another, we do interpret them. A low grade can make someone a better student or a dropout. An election to the student council can produce a responsible leader, a self-conscious snob. A traffic ticket can make you drive more cautiously or see what you can get away with. We reflect, we think, we change, we become.[16]

Mental Illness

He screamed at the sky. There was the chattering of an owl before the scream, and crickets chirping. Some leaves were rustled by a passing deer. But the scream stopped all other noise. The forest, where the man was lying, was used to screams of death, shrieks of pain, cries of fear and anguish. But this was a different sound—something hollow, something mystical, something that belonged in a dimension that nature didn't encompass. He had had a dream, this screamer, only he hadn't really been asleep. There had

FIGURE 4-2. *The scream.*

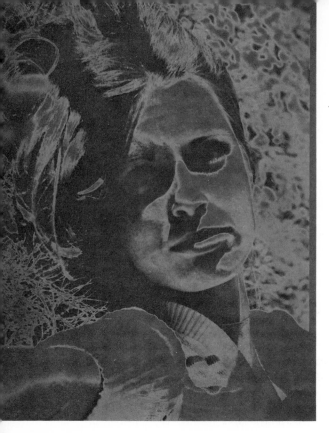

FIGURE 4-3. *Feeling low? All of us do from time to time.*

been shadowy, diabolical shapes reaching for him. There had been sounds that really weren't words, but he understood them. They penetrated his being, distorted it, defiled it. He beat at the ground, clawed at it, bit into the dirt—or was it his hand on a rock? Teeth snapped, but the pain seemed almost welcome. It was a contact with reality, a reminder that there was environment with which he could interact. There was order, consciousness. After all, he could control himself. Hadn't he mastered his surroundings? Tools, fire, shelter he had made in this new age of enlightenment. This was 10,000 B.C.

Mental illness is as old as man. If there weren't such a thing, certainly we'd imagine it. It's a bizarre concept, something haunting, deeply frightening, yet a fascinating idea, exciting to think about. College students consume limitless amounts of fiction and nonfiction on the psychologically twisted. So does the rest of America. Yet despite the interest in the topic, few understand it. There are lots of conflicting viewpoints in this field, and a lot of what passes for information is distortion or just plain error.[17]

There was the movie *Psycho*. Here the image of insanity was linked with murder. The "mad killer" is an exciting and dramatic idea, but it doesn't describe the majority of the insane, who are really confused, deeply depressed, deeply fearful. The movie *Freud* repeats the trite tale of the patient who is magically cured when he remembers a painful childhood experience. This is great for celluloid and sound tracks but has nothing to do with the everyday treatment and help for the mentally disturbed. What to believe? Certainly not most fiction. Novelists and short story writers aren't obliged to give lessons in abnormal psychology. Popular nonfiction? There are some interesting articles and books that tell us how to solve marital and emotional disorders through autoanalysis, psychoanalysis, yoga, self-hypnosis, psychotherapy, Zen Buddhism, and the right kind of diet. A lot of commercial writing has the goal of entertaining rather than educating, providing hope rather than facts. Here are some of the facts, or at least what authorities think are facts.

Mental Illness Categories

Who is sick? You are, of course, and all of your friends. There's no such thing as a person who is completely physically healthy. We have our sore toes, our toothaches, our bad eyesight. The same applies to mental health. We're not happy all of the time. We're not as self-confident as we should be. And most of us are anything but truly efficient. We waste a lot of our lives in dreams, regrets, self-pity, and just plain laziness. This is a mild form of illness that all of us have to some degree. If it's a mild enough case, the person is looked on as an "individual" or, at worst, an eccentric.

Prior to this century only "madmen" or "maniacs" were considered mentally ill. But now the boundary between illness and health has shifted. What used to be looked on as character weakness or just unwise behavior is now labeled psychological maladjustment. Take the boy who is flunking his courses because he would rather party than study, the girl who feels the need to discuss her most intimate relations with anyone she meets, the man or the woman who can't get through lunch with less than three martinis. Mental illness today encompasses the 800,000 people divorced yearly, the 700,000 children brought to court as delinquents, the 200,000 women who bear illegitimate children. It includes 9 million or more alcoholics, uncountable millions with migraine headaches or colitis, the friendless, the deeply bored. By this criterion, one out of every ten Americans is emotionally sick.[18]

NONCRITICAL EMOTIONAL ILLNESS

Most of these fall into the category of noncritical emotional illness. This takes in people who are constantly dissatisfied with their work, no matter what they do in life; people who seldom make friends, yet complain about and bicker with the few friends they have; people who are afraid to make the most routine decisions; people totally irresponsible with money; people who make their families miserable with unreasonable demands and criticism. These are irritating and unhappy people, but they do get along. Many of them hold fine jobs, are respected members of their communities. Some even envy them. They don't get lost in a world of fantasy. They don't think people are going to poison them. They don't think they're Napoleon or Jesus Christ.

CHARACTER DISORDER

A more serious type of mental illness is called character disorder. People in this category don't have the same standards of conduct or achievement as the rest of society. They cheat, steal, lie, perform acts of sexual deviancy, take drugs, commit assault—and don't feel a bit guilty about it. They're like impulsive and selfish children who haven't developed an adequate conscience. These people are sometimes called psychopaths. But some prefer the term "sociopath," arguing that character disorder really isn't emotional illness at all. It's just antisocial.

PSYCHOSOMATIC DISEASES

There are people who get diarrhea before an important business conference, people who get headaches after fighting with their friends or loved ones, people who break out in a rash during an important examination. These are passing versions of psychosomatic diseases. But there are longer-lasting versions of the same ailment. Peptic ulcers, urticaria, and asthma are typical of this type of problem. They don't have to be caused by emotional stress only; they can have organic causes. Or maybe the mind and the body interact to cause the sickness. But, regardless of the cause, the sickness does exist. A person suffering from a psychosomatic disorder isn't a "hypochondriac," someone who doesn't have a thing wrong with him but who is sure he's ill. Psychosomatic disease creates a need for medical as well as psychological treatment.

These illnesses can symbolize underlying emotional problems. There is the woman whose husband threatens to leave her, so she develops crippling arthritis. There's the insecure professor who develops mouth ulcers. These keep him from having to teach his classes. There's the child whose mother

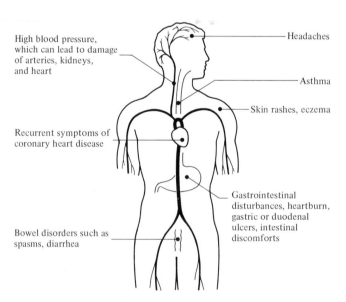

High blood pressure, which can lead to damage of arteries, kidneys, and heart

Headaches

Asthma

Skin rashes, eczema

Recurrent symptoms of coronary heart disease

Gastrointestinal disturbances, heartburn, gastric or duodenal ulcers, intestinal discomforts

Bowel disorders such as spasms, diarrhea

FIGURE 4-4. *Some disturbances that may be psychosomatic (or emotional) in nature.*

neglects him. When he becomes a man, he develops stomach trouble, has a constant need to be pampered with special foods.

NEUROSIS

But there are lots of people who feel pretty bad who don't have tangible physical symptoms. They worry a lot. They're sure that the worst is about to befall them. They eat constantly or almost never, walk in their sleep, or are insomniacs (people who have trouble falling asleep). There are the "neurotics," people constantly cursed by a sinking feeling that uses up their energy and sometimes fills them with dread. They're not happy people, not nearly as happy as they should be. And their efforts to love, to work, to play are usually feeble.

They're similar, these neurotics, to people with noncritical emotional illnesses. But their anxieties are much greater and interfere more with the way they live. Some neurotics have to be hospitalized. But most earn a living, usually quite painfully, have a home life of sorts, and carry on most activities in an acceptable way.[19]

PSYCHOSIS

While neurosis can be extremely painful, people who suffer from it have a grasp on reality. They don't get a friend confused with an enemy, a room confused with a castle, the 1970s confused with the Middle Ages. There are people called "psychotics" who lose this type of orientation. These are the most ill of the mentally ill. They can't get along in the world, even in the suffering and limping way of the neurotic. The majority of hospitalized mental patients are diagnosed as having this illness.

The most common type of psychosis is schizophrenia. Sadly, people afflicted with it are usually in their most productive years, between the ages of 15 and 45. The term means "split personality," and it applies to a great variety of conditions. There is no set of symptoms that describes all schizophrenic patients. But some of the more common symptoms are:

1. Major fluctuations in behavior. The person may sit motionless for a while, then rush around.
2. Complete disregard of personal appearance.
3. A broad range of talk. The person may be mute, then burst into meaningless chatter, then suddenly stop.
4. Delusions and hallucinations. The person may think he's a victim of a plot. He may hear voices, see visions, smell peculiar odors.

A lot of schizophrenic patients have spent lifetimes vegetating in back wards of mental hospitals. It's a long-duration psychosis, but recent use of psychoactive drugs has allowed many schizophrenics to function productively in society rather than be institutionalized.

Another psychosis is labeled depression. This is characterized by disturbances in mood. It is sometimes labeled "manic-depressive," as people suffering from this problem have periods of mania (elation) and periods of depression ("down" feelings, pessimism, and so on). Most have extreme mood changes, but some have permanent mania. They're constantly in a state of euphoria. They talk incessantly and never sit still. And there are those who suffer constant depression.

This illness usually develops slowly, with neither the victim nor his family being aware of what's taking place. As psychotic signs become more severe, the victim has trouble doing his usual jobs. He looks at life in a more and more pessimistic way. Feelings of guilt begin to grow. Physiological difficulties develop as well. The victim loses his appetite, has severe constipation, and suffers from insomnia. One of the major dangers of this psychosis, of course, is suicide. Many of the 22,000 Americans who kill themselves each year suffer from this condition.

TABLE 4-2
The Truth About Suicide

Fable	Fact
People who talk about suicide don't commit suicide.	Of any ten persons who commit suicide, eight have given definite warnings of their suicidal intentions.
Suicide happens without warning.	Studies reveal that the suicidal person gives many clues and warnings. Almost no one commits suicide without letting others know how he is feeling.
Suicidal people are fully intent on dying.	Most suicidal people are undecided about living or dying, and they "gamble with death," leaving it to others to save them.
Once a person is suicidal, he is suicidal forever.	Individuals who wish to kill themselves are "suicidal" for only a limited period of time.
Improvement following a suicidal crisis means that the suicidal risk is over.	Most suicides occur within about 3 months after the beginning of "improvement," when the individual has the energy to put his morbid thoughts and feelings into effect.
Suicide strikes much more often among the rich—or, conversely, almost exclusively among the poor.	Suicide is neither the rich man's disease nor the poor man's curse. Suicide is very democratic and represented in all levels of society.
Suicide is inherited or "runs in the family."	Suicide does not run in the family. It is an individual pattern.
All suicidal individuals are mentally ill, and suicide always is the act of a psychotic person.	Studies of hundreds of genuine suicide notes indicate that, although the suicidal person is extremely unhappy, he is not necessarily mentally ill.

Source: E. S. Schneidman and N. L. Farberow, *Some Facts about Suicide*, PHS Publication No. 852 (Washington, D.C.: U.S. Department of Health, Education, and Welfare).

There's not much agreement about what causes psychosis. Some believe that society's external pressure brings it on. Others think that an individual's internal psychological weaknesses are at fault. But most think that both inheritance and environment play their parts. Also, there are a large group of psychotics whose behavior is almost entirely caused by organic problems. They've damaged their brains with alcohol or drugs; they have brain tumors; or maybe there's hardening of the arteries that carry blood to the brain. But, even though the causes are tangible, the behavior of such people is almost indistinguishable from the behavior of those with psychologically caused psychosis. These people can fly into wild rages or laugh hysterically. Sometimes they huddle silently in a ball. They can't or won't hear, can't or won't comprehend. Sometimes they lose bladder or bowel control as though they were still infants. They're confused, suspicious, angry, depressed. Some medical treatments help organic psychosis. Some only calm the patients, make them comfortable or comatose.[20]

Treatment of Mental Illness

There are a thousand therapies designed to make the mentally sick mentally well. Maybe ten times ten thousand is a better number. But all treatments for mental and emotional illness can be grouped. One of the more popular groupings is into psychological, physical, and social.

PSYCHOLOGICAL TREATMENT

The term describing psychological treatment in any form is "psychotherapy." This describes treatment by words. The patient and the practitioner talk; and there are words of advice, evaluative words, and words that probe. Psychotherapy has nothing to do with shock treatment, drugs, brain surgery, or physical restraint. These can be used in connection with psychotherapy, of course. But because they don't involve words, they're not in the psychotherapeutic domain.

Psychotherapy can be used to relieve a momentary spell of depression or to remake an entire personality. The span of treatment may range from one 30-minute session to hundreds of hours over a period of 6 or 7 years. The simplest type of treatment is often performed by a minister or a doctor or a teacher, using a form of mental first aid called "ventilation." This lets the person blast at the world, tell about his troubles, complain about his no-good girlfriend or father-in-law. The listener won't sympathize or show disapproval. He'll just give the patient a chance to get rid of his rage, panic, or gloom and get himself under control. If the patient is relatively healthy, this is probably what will happen.

Ventilation and reassurance have nothing to do with looking into the dark and twisted caverns of our minds. They're used to help us get a better look at the problems we're already aware of. But there's reparative therapy, which has a deeper goal. It seeks to remold our personalities by focusing on problems we're not aware of. Sometimes external stress, such as the death of a parent, flunking out of school, or losing a job, can cause emotional problems. These probably don't call for probing types of treatment. But people who get upset by everyday arguments, are constantly worried about acceptance by peers, resent their classes and their families might benefit from treatment of this type.

How does it work? The patient talks, and the therapist tries to get an angle on the unconscious motives behind the patient's behavior. The patient may never know what the therapist comes up with. But the therapist guides the discussions and asks leading questions that can help the patient gain insight into his real problems. Also, a therapist often tries to change the patient's external situation. There's the bossy wife, for instance, whose husband dreams of Tahiti for himself or crocodile pits for her. The therapist might help her get the type of job that can gratify her domineering needs.

Social workers do a lot of counseling of this type. It's used a lot with marital problems, problems of child rearing, and problems involving employment. But there are deep-seated neuroses, psychosomatic conditions, and severe cases of mental illness that call for still deeper psychotherapy. This is where the clinical psychologist or the psychiatrist becomes involved.[21]

"Reconstructive psychotherapy" or "psychoanalysis" is the most ambitious of the psychotherapeutic methods. There is Freudian psychoanalysis, with the couch, the notebook, and the expressionless doctor. This is the archetype. But there are other types, including "analytically oriented psychotherapy," "existential analysis," and "ego analysis." And there are particular facets of psychoanalysis that followers of Harry Stack Sullivan, Carl Jung, Otto Rank, Karen Horney, and Alfred Adler subscribe to. There's some disagreement among the various schools as to what causes emotional problems and how they should be treated. But all of them try to get the patient to examine his thought and behavior patterns, to get some idea of how his concealed wounds have distorted his personality. And all psychoanalytic schools agree that insight and conscious thought by themselves won't cure emotional illness. People have to mentally relive certain formative life periods in order to reshape their psychological makeup. Take the timid young lady who tries to avoid her classmates. She doesn't want to feel like a fool when she talks to them. Take the young man with the uncontrollable temper. He's constantly in a rage over trivia. Don't these people realize how irrational their behavior is? They often do, but it takes more than awareness of our fears and frustrations to change how we act.

Most psychoanalysts encourage their patients to "free-associate," to speak naturally without concealing, modifying, or connecting thoughts as we do in normal conversation. If the thoughts seem irrelevant or shameful, fine! They can give the therapist information about the patient's psychological patterns and help explain causes of the emotional problem. The next step is to help the patient become aware of why he's acting as he does, help him reshape his personality along more mature and stable lines.[22]

PHYSICAL THERAPY

People were analyzing, reasoning with, and reassuring the mentally ill long before the days of Sigmund Freud. But the words didn't always produce desired results, so madmen were flailed with whips, thrown into snake pits, and dashed with cold water. Medicine men in the days of Cleopatra came up with brews and herbs that seemed to calm the insane. Greek and Roman physicians had their own brands of sedative drugs. And in the Middle Ages trepanning (cutting out a section of the skull) got to be quite the technique. Today we treat the minds through the bodies as well, and we think we get better results than our ancestors did. We sometimes put people in warm tubs of water for prolonged periods. There are "wet packs," which involve putting a person under restraint in a laced-up sheet and then spraying the sheet alternately with hot and cold water. There's electroconvulsive therapy, sometimes called "electric shock." Here a patient gets a series of treatments of about 80 to 100 volts each. This brings on uncontrollable convulsions and renders the patient unconscious. Insulin-coma shock treatment produces similar effects. Both are used to relieve depression or help people suffering from schizophrenia. Then there's prefrontal lobot-

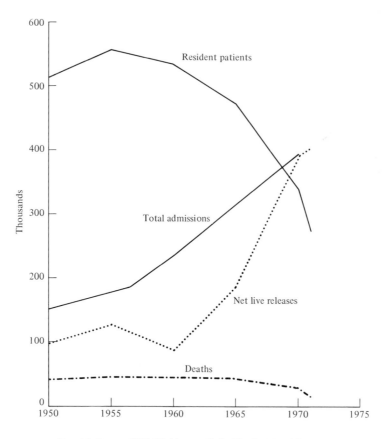

SOURCE: *Social Indicators 1973* (Washington, D.C.: The Social and Economic Statistics Administration, U.S. Department of Commerce), p. 12.

FIGURE 4-5. *Patients in state and county mental hospitals: 1950–1972.*

103

omy. Here certain brain fibers are cut so that highly excited patients can calm down. But, even though abnormal behavior and emotions disappear, the patient often becomes reduced to a vegetable-like state.

In 1955, the era of psychoactive drugs was born. Chlorpromazine and reserpine, the first of the tranquilizers, were introduced to American mental hospitals. Wild, abusive, and confused patients improved dramatically. They began associating with other patients and hospital personnel and even assumed some of the responsibility for running their institutions. Some of the "hopeless" psychotics were able to leave the hospital in just a few weeks. Apparently, the drugs achieved results sought by drastic physical shock therapy in a much simpler, surer, and safer way. Physical treatments, other than drug therapy, are still used. But drugs, by far, seem to be the preferred approach.

Drug therapy, by itself, can cure psychosis. But it usually doesn't. The drugs can put a damper on the patient's fear, though, help to hold down his hallucinations and wild ideas. This gives his mind a chance to repair itself, and probably works something like a doctor's dressing on a wound. The dressing doesn't heal the wound, but it tips the balance in favor of natural healing processes.[23]

SOCIAL TREATMENT

Social treatment involves changing the patient's environment. Of course, it can be a nice term for putting him in a mental institution. But mental hospitals of today aren't the nightmare torture chambers of an earlier era. They're designed to help patients grow, bit by bit, into a world of reality. They can be friendly and understanding worlds, better than the alarming ones patients flee from. They can provide a chance for someone to rebuild himself, rebuild his thoughts, rebuild his relationships with others.

But social treatment encompasses more than mental institutions. It takes in the entire concept of modern humanitarianism, which looks on mental illness as a community problem rather than something brought on by evil spirits or mean mothers. There are three social therapies that have become popular among mental health workers in recent years.

There's "group therapy." Here a half dozen or so patients get together with one therapist and discuss each other's problems and feelings. The group method is better than the individual method for some patients. It resembles the social interaction they face in the real world, and some people need this badly.

There is "family therapy." Here the family becomes the patient; the members of the family meet with the therapist as a unit, and interact with each other as well as with the therapist. The concept is that something in the family relationship caused the illness. Therefore, the family, not just the individual, has to be treated.

One of the more dramatic developments in mental health since the 1950s has been the rapid rise of "community therapy." Efforts here are aimed at high-need members of the community, such as disturbed children.

Techniques used include social planning, cooperative consultation between health care professionals, and public health education.[24]

The Therapists

There are all kinds of people available who claim to be able to treat mental and emotional illnesses. But there's a wide variation in the services they offer and the kind of training they've had. People working with the mentally ill run the gamut from the recently hired hospital attendant, with no training and almost no experience, to the psychoanalyst, who has usually spent about a dozen years preparing for his work. There are several specialists in between, some medical, some nonmedical.

PSYCHIATRISTS

Psychiatrists are the most broadly trained of the mental health practitioners. They're physicians who have completed medical school and have taken additional training involving the study of illnesses of the mind. They're trained to treat severe disturbance, as well as mild neuroses and character disorders. They can prescribe drugs and use a wide variety of physical as well as psychological therapies. Most psychiatrists devote the majority of their time to private practice. But around 25 per cent work exclusively for clinics, social agencies, and hospitals.

PSYCHOANALYSTS

Although most psychiatrists use psychotherapy with their patients, they're not equipped to practice psychoanalysis without further training. The American Psychoanalytic Association requires that members be physicians, have successfully completed courses and seminars for around 6 years in one of the recognized training institutes, analyze at least two patients under the supervision of an experienced psychoanalyst, and submit to analysis themselves. Also, there are some nonmedical practitioners called lay analysts. These have had psychoanalytic training in institutes that require a Ph.D. in clinical psychology or a related discipline for admission rather than an M.D. Partly because of these stringent requirements, there are only a few thousand recognized psychoanalysts in the country.

CLINICAL PSYCHOLOGISTS

Only about a third of the psychologists in the country are clinical psychologists. These are the ones who have received extensive training in psychotherapy. They hold master's degrees, often Ph.D.'s, and have specialized in diagnostic testing and all forms of psychological treatment. They can't prescribe medicines, though, or other types of physical treatment. And they often work under the supervision of psychiatrists. They work in mental hospitals, family service organizations, and mental health clinics, as well as in private practice.

SOCIAL WORKERS

Around a fifth of the nation's social workers are trained to do psychotherapy. These have master's degrees from accredited schools of social work and have taken special courses in counseling. Few have the background and experience neccesary for more than brief supportive therapy, but all are trained to recognize serious emotional problems and to make referrals.

PASTORAL COUNSELORS

A large percentage of people who seek help for emotional problems consult their clergymen. Most clergymen are qualified to deal with surface problems, but only about one out of 25 has had special training in pastoral counseling. They often arrange for people to receive proper help, though, when their problems are more than a clergyman can handle.[25]

Notes

1. Lealon E. Martin, *Mental Health/Mental Illness: Revolution in Progress* (New York: McGraw-Hill, 1970), pp. 55–58.
2. Ledford J. Bischof, *Adult Psychology* (New York: Harper and Row, 1969).
3. Ibid.
4. Ibid.
5. O. Spurgeon English and Gerald H. J. Pearson, *Emotional Problems of Living,* 3rd ed. (New York: Norton, 1963).
6. Abraham H. Maslow, *Motivation and Personality,* 2nd ed. (New York: Harper and Row, 1970).
7. Richard S. Lazarus, *Psychological Stress and the Coping Process* (New York: McGraw-Hill, 1966).
8. Frederick C. Thorne, *Tutorial Counseling* (Brandon, Vt.: Clinical Psychology Publishing Company, 1965).
9. Lazarus, *Psychological Stress.*
10. N. Sanford, *Issues in Personality Theory* (San Francisco: Jossey-Bass, 1970).
11. Sigmund Freud, *Psychopathology of Everyday Life* (New York: Macmillian, 1917).
12. Erik H. Erikson, *Childhood and Society,* 2nd ed. (New York: Norton, 1963).
13. Robert W. White, *Lives in Progress* (New York: Holt, Rinehart and Winston, 1966).
14. Clifford T. Morgan and Richard A. King, *Introduction to Psychology,* 3rd ed. (New York: McGraw-Hill, 1966).
15. L. J. Soul, *Emotional Maturity* (Philadelphia: Lippincott, 1960).
16. Ibid.
17. Thomas S. Szasz, *The Manufacture of Madness* (New York: Harper and Row, 1970), pp. 3–27.
18. U.S. Department of Health, Education, and Welfare, Public Health Service, *Major and Minor Emotional Problems* (Washington, D.C.: Government Printing Office, 1971), p. 36.
19. Martin, *Mental Health/Mental Illness,* pp. 17–28.
20. Ibid.
21. E. Berne, *A Layman's Guide to Psychiatry and Psychoanalysis* (New York: Simon and Schuster, 1968).

22. Ibid.
23. S. Cohen, *The Drug Dilemma* (New York: McGraw-Hill, 1969).
24. Martin, *Mental Health/Mental Illness,* pp. 47–52.
25. F. N. Arnhoff, E. Rubinstein, and J. C. Speisman, *Manpower for Mental Health* (Chicago: Aldine, 1969).

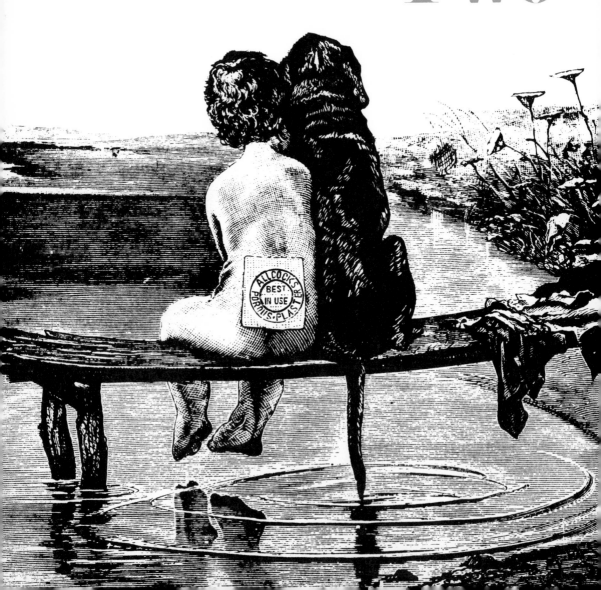

Part
Two

Health
Escapes

5 Drugs

"They ought to kill those kids. They're mad dogs, that's what they are. What do you do with mad dogs? You kill them, that's what you do." "Poor babies! They don't know what they're doing. My heart just bleeds for them." "That's the king, man. See him up there shining on his throne, all nice and bright and wet and shimmery? He's beautiful, man, just beautiful, beautiful, beautiful, beautiful."

The drug cult has arrived on the American scene. The reaction to the bearded, beaded, unwashed longhairs has been as mixed as feelings on the Vietnamese War. Some have claimed that the flower of American youth has been perverted, that American culture has become a Haight-Ashbury version of Sodom and Gomorrah. There are others who want to help the poor innocents retreating from a status-conscious, success-conscious, materialistic world. And there are those who have found a new religion, a new dimension to existence, a guru demanding a faith far deeper than Job's or Daniel's.

Not all have long hair, of course. And many are scrupulously clean. But the drug culture has been assigned a stereotype, just as the Army officer has, the college professor has, and the accountant has. The stereotypical drug freak shops at "psychedelicatessens" and "head shops." His dress is extremely bizarre, with trinkets, beads, headbands, and earrings—something like the tribal adornments of a primitive culture. His music comes from a multitude of levels at a volume that forces all other sound from the con-

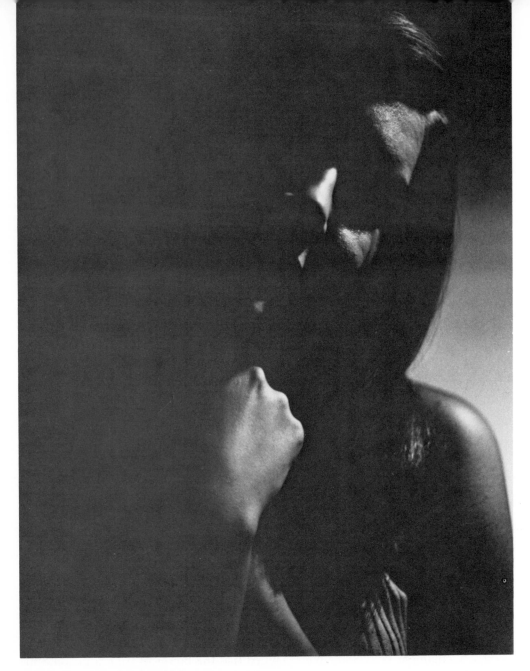

FIGURE 5-1. *Beautiful, beautiful, beautiful . . .*

sciousness. And he uses stroboscopes, light machines, multiple projection cameras, and ornate wall posters to brightly illustrate his new sensory frontier.

The stereotype isn't what all members of the drug culture conform to, of course. There are crewcut quarterbacks who smoke "pot," management trainees who pop an occasional "benny." But the stereotype represents a kind of symbol that most members of the cult accept and that many members of the straight world detest.[1]

The "turned-on" generation has established headquarters on many a college campus. There are "freakouts," there are "love-ins," there are "psychedelic light shows." There are "golden leaf," and "hash," and "meth," and "Panama red," and "sugar cubes," and "splash"—all available for a price. And sometimes they're available without a price. Like most fanatical sects, they're looking for converts, people who can be shown the real truth, the bliss of nirvana. New members shouldn't have to pay a price for this.

Then there are students who sample the wares, those who want to get a look at the show just to see what it's all about. Saying that you got "stoned," that you're "tuned in" or "turned on" can be the "in" thing to say. It doesn't mean that you have to participate in the rites on a daily or weekly basis. And there are young people looking for a buffer against society. Human relationships can be painful, humiliating, defeating. Here's a way to ease the pain a little. But this doesn't mean you're giving the cult an all-out commitment.

Drug escapists often claim that the unhooked society tries to escape, too. They have their cigarettes, their beer and Scotch, their tranquilizers, aspirin

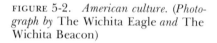

FIGURE 5-2. *American culture.* (Photograph by The Wichita Eagle *and* The Wichita Beacon)

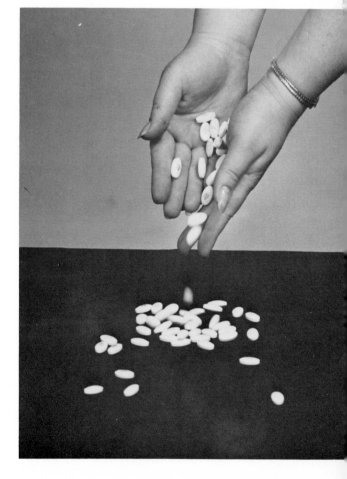

tablets, and hay fever pills. And this argument is hard to fault. The person who smokes three packs a day, has a couple of martinis for lunch, a highball before dinner, two or three after, takes a seconal to be sure that he has a good night's sleep, takes a "diet pill" with a couple of cups of coffee to get himself going during the day is probably every bit as much turned on as the pot smoker and the occasional "speed freak." But this reactionary Timothy Leary is turning on legally. He's using drugs that can be purchased openly in any community with a physician's prescription, and some that are legal without a prescription. The "acid heads," the "mainliners," the "trip takers" are getting high on things purchased in violation of the law.[2]

There are some members of this world who don't bend their minds at all. And there are some who twist them to a modest degree only. Are they members of the drug cult? Words like "addict," "dependence," and "abuse" have gotten to be fairly common. But a lot of people who use them aren't quite sure of what they mean. Here are some definitions which can clarify things:

1. *Drug dependence.* This can involve psychic dependence or physical dependence or both. Sometimes it happens when someone uses a drug occasionally, sometimes when he swallows, sniffs, or injects himself daily. It's a concept that can mean different things, depending on the type of drug the person takes. The World Health Organization breaks dependence into the following types: morphine, barbiturate, alcohol, cocaine, cannabis (marijuana), amphetamine, Khat, and hallucinogen (LSD).

2. *Drug addiction.* This is a type of drug dependence with the following characteristics:

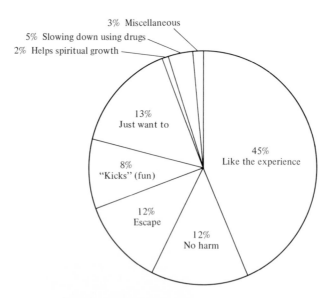

SOURCE: Edward M. Scott, *The Adolescent Gap* (Springfield, Ill.:
Charles C. Thomas, 1972), p. 40.

FIGURE 5-3. *Why drug users use drugs (research from group of drug users).*

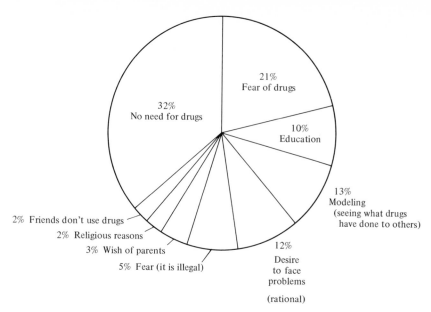

32%
No need for drugs

21%
Fear of drugs

10%
Education

13%
Modeling
(seeing what drugs
have done to others)

2% Friends don't use drugs

2% Religious reasons

3% Wish of parents

5% Fear (it is illegal)

12%
Desire
to face
problems

(rational)

SOURCE: Edward M. Scott, *The Adolescent Gap* (Springfield, Ill.: Charles C. Thomas, 1972), p. 23.

FIGURE 5-4. *Research with non-drug-using teenagers: the principal reason for not having started drug use.*

    a. An overpowering need for the drug. The addict will do anything possible to get it.
    b. Physical as well as psychic dependence.
    c. Detrimental effects on society as well as on the individual.
    d. A tendency to increase the drug dosage.

    3. *Drug habituation.* This is another type of drug dependence, but it isn't as physically destructive as addiction. It's characterized by

    a. A strong desire to keep taking the drug. But the user doesn't have an overwhelming compulsion he can't control.
    b. No physical dependence on the drug, but a strong psychic dependence.
    c. Detrimental effects on the user only. Society doesn't pay a major penalty.

    4. *Tolerance.* Someone who has developed a tolerance for a drug feels compelled to take increasing quantities. If he's looking for the same effect he got last week, he'll need a bigger dose of heroin, alcohol, or what have you. Sometimes people build tolerance for doses that would kill occasional users or nonusers of the drug. Also, there's cross-tolerance. In this case, tolerance for one drug carries over into tolerance for another. Heroin produces a cross-tolerance for morphine. LSD does the same with mescaline.
    5. *Abstinence syndrome.* Here a person who has developed tolerance for a drug stops taking it. Because the drug has altered his metabolism, he needs

it to function normally. Take alcohol or barbiturates. Eight to twelve hours after the beginning of abstinence the person with the tolerance often has delirium tremens. There are hallucinations, violent shaking, sometimes convulsions. People on skid row call these the "rum fits," the "horrors," or the "shakes."

6. *Anesthetics.* This class of drugs brings on relaxation, sometimes coma. Physicians use them to relieve pain and condition patients for operations. Some of the traditional drugs in this category are alcohol, laughing gas, and ether.

7. *Narcotics.* These are pain killers, many of which come from opium. There are heroin, Dilaudid, codeine, and morphine. Cocaine is sometimes categorized as a narcotic, sometimes as a hallucinogen. And there are synthetic narcotics, those made in a laboratory, such as Demerol, Percodan, and methadone. Narcotics can bring on euphoria, hallucinations, complete relaxation, total unconsciousness, or death.

8. *Sedatives.* These quiet people down, relax them, bring on sleep. Barbiturates are a type of sedative; so are tranquilizers such as Miltown.

9. *Stimulants.* These speed us up, elevate our spirits, make the rest of the world look lazy. They're at the other end of the scale from sedatives. Amphetamines are typical stimulant drugs.

10. *Hallucinogens.* Some call these "psychedelics." They bring on hallucinations, loss of self-identity, and mystical perceptions. There can be reverie; there can be hysteria. LSD is the most popular drug in this category.

11. *Drug abuse.* It's the continued use of any drug, legally purchased or not, that brings on physical or psychological dependence or both. Abuse can make people deviate from accepted behavior patterns.[3]

Types of Drugs

There's an almost unlimited number of drugs the cult uses. Some, of course, are more popular than others. Here are a few of the favorites:

Marijuana

There are 300 million people on this planet who puff on marijuana or swallow it. Sometimes they call it "pot," "maryjane," "hemp," or "grass." There are about 20 million people in the United States who have tried it. It comes from a plant called *Cannabis sativa,* which produces a resin that in pure form is called "hashish." Hashish, known as "hash" by users, is about ten times as powerful as marijuana and is very popular in some parts of the world. But it hasn't caught on in this country. Marijuana, of course, has. About $100 million worth of it crosses the Mexican border into this country each year. Users roll it into cigarettes called "joints," or they eat it. Also, there are "roach" pipes. A lot of marijuana users use these so that they can get their last few ecstatic puffs from butts that have become too small to hold in the fingers.[4]

Users of marijuana report euphoric sensations, and there are users who

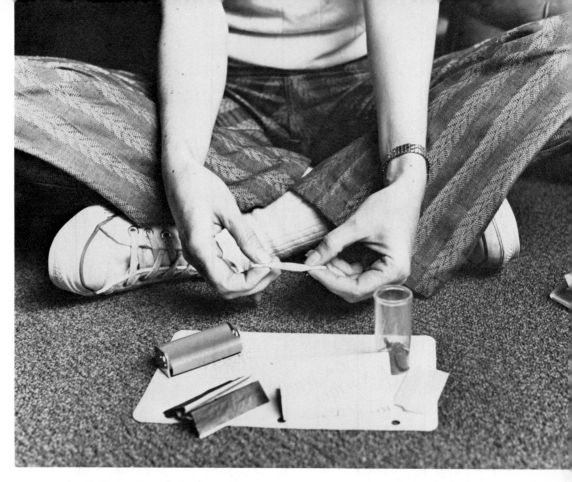

FIGURE 5-5. *Rolling a funny-looking cigarette.*

say it makes them sleepy or dull. And there are users who say they get no sensation at all. A lot depends on how long the person has been smoking marijuana, his psychological and physiological makeup.

People trying marijuana for the first time often fall into the "no sensation" category. They get a bigger lift from a normal cigarette or a bottle of beer. This is probably because of an ineffective smoking technique. You can't puff on grass the way you do on a Salem. But once the new technique has been mastered the participant often experiences a sudden sense of relaxation, something like floating. The senses seem sharper; time seems to slow; the world seems like a brightly colored fishbowl with water that barely ripples. There's a sense of well-being, the appetite increases, fears and feelings of inadequacy slip away.

So what's wrong with that? Why all the fuss by parents and police and politicians? The world is less than perfect, kind of dehumanized really, with its industrial, governmental, and academic regimentation. Is a chemical escape so bad, particularly if it's on a temporary basis? Probably not, if we're sure about the temporary state of affairs. But the case over what kind of harm marijuana does to the system is still before the jury. Some researchers claim that it causes permanent brain damage, others that it causes emotional

TABLE 5-1
Marijuana Psychoses Among U.S. Soldiers in Vietnam, 1967–1968: Twelve Cases

Case No.	Age	First Exposure to Marijuana	Physical Symptoms	Impaired Cognitive Functioning	Mental Symptoms	Delusions	Premorbid Personality	Duration of Symptoms
1	26	+*	+	+	Paranoid, anxious	+	–	36 hr
2	19	+	+	+	Paranoid	+	–	3 days
3	24	+	+	+	Paranoid, anxious	+	Aggressive	7 days
4	21	+	+	+	Paranoid	+	Psychopathic	2 days
5	20	+	+	+	Paranoid	+	–	2–3 days
6	22	+	+	+	Anxious	–	–	1 day
7	21	+	+	+	Anxious	–	–	2 days
8	21	+	+	+	Paranoid	+	–	3 days
9	22	+	+	+	Suicidal, paranoid	+	–	11 days
10	22	+	+	+	Anxious, paranoid	+	–	2 days
11	19	+	+	+	Anxious, paranoid	+	–	3 days
12	19	+	+	+	Paranoid	+	–	2 days

*+, Indicated positive; –, negative.

Source: Adapted from John A. Talbott and James W. Teague, "Marijuana Psychosis," *Journal of the American Medical Association,* Vol. 210, No. 2 (October 13, 1969), 300.

instability, others that it does no harm to the human body whatsoever. As to psychological effects, the drug can lead to dependency. It's not addictive, as some of the harsher drugs are. But a user can become afraid to face difficult situations without having a joint or two, feel that he can't relax or really enjoy himself without the help of maryjane. And then there's the problem of how somebody acts when he's high. Some become very gentle, loving, and permissive. Some become highly aggressive, want to fight or hurt. Marijuana, like alcohol, cuts down on inhibitions, creates exaggerated versions of the personalities we have. While under the influence, people can do things they later regret.

Many used to believe, and some still believe, that using marijuana automatically leads to the use of hard drugs, such as cocaine and heroin. This isn't true. But someone under the influence has lower resistance than someone who isn't. He can be tempted to experiment with things he later finds he can't give up.[5]

Amphetamines

She had red hair, a perky chin, and well-shaped legs. And her eyes sparkled, and she giggled a lot. Her cheeks were much too orange, though. And every so often her hands would tremble. She would shriek, too. It would start as one of her giggles, but then the pitch would rise, and she would be shrieking. Heidi hated the establishment, even though she talked about it through her giggles. She would make little "O's" with her mouth and big, dancing "O's" with her eyes. She was animated like a child. It was a silly, mean world. It wanted to own you, like Mommy and Daddy. Daddy used to take her to the park and the movies and for long walks. Mommy used to make her puddings and fix her hair. They wanted to own her, though, possess her. You can't be owned. There was a time when Heidi got her kicks from a lick from a chocolate cone. There were cotton candy and roller coaster rides and a slurp from her dog. Now the kicks come from methamphetamine. Heidi is a "speed freak."

"Speed" has become a highly popular way to turn on. Many LSD users have turned to it because of the genetic and mental harm they think LSD can do. Some people swallow speed, some people "skin pop" it, some shoot it straight into the vein. This brings on a quick euphoric "flash." Someone who's taking a "journey" instead of a "trip" mainlines for days without sleep. Then he gets "strung out" and "crashes" and goes into a long, comalike slumber. When he wakes up, the journey starts again. This isn't the best way to improve your health, of course. Lack of sleep, rest, and food can make fine-looking people look like vampires, act like they're in an air raid.[6]

Benzedrine and dexedrine are amphetamines that are usually taken orally. Doctors sometimes prescribe them in mild forms as diet pills. And truck drivers and pilots often use them to stay awake during long, tedious nights. The pills replace fatigue with energy and can produce a sense of self-confidence, too. Some feel they can handle mental and physical tasks more efficiently with help from these pills. But depression can set in after they've been taken for an extended period. And so can fatigue, headaches, delirium, dizziness, and agitation. Sometimes a person escaping from a mood finds

TABLE 5-2
Drugs, Medical Uses, Symptoms Produced, and Their Dependence Potentials

Name	Slang Name	Chemical or Trade Name	Pharmacological Classification	Medical Use	How Taken
Heroin	H, horse, scat, junk, hard stuff, joy powder	Diacetylmorphine	Depressant	Pain relief	Injected or sniffed
Morphine	White stuff, Miss Emma, M, dreamer	Morphine sulfate	Depressant	Pain relief	Swallowed or injected
Codeine	Schoolboy	Methylmorphine	Depressant	To ease pain and cough	Swallowed
Methadone	Dolly	Dolophine, amidone	Depressant	Pain relief	Swallowed or injected
Cocaine	Speedballs, gold dust, coke, bernice, corine, flake, star dust, snow	Methyl ester of benzoylecgo-nine	Stimulant	Local anesthesia	Sniffed, injected, or swallowed
Marijuana	Pot, grass, Mary-jane, hashish, tea, gage, reefers	Tetrahydrocan-nabinol	Stimulant or depressant, or hallucinogen	None in U.S.	Smoked, swallowed, or sniffed
Barbiturates	Barbs, blue devils, candy, yellow jackets, phennies, peanuts, blue heavens	Phenobarbital, nembutal, seconal, amytal	Depressant	Sedation, to relieve high blood pressure, epilepsy, hyperthy-roidism	Swallowed or injected
Amphet-amines	Bennies, dexies, copilots, wakeups, lid proppers, hearts, pep pills	Benzedrine, preludin, dexedrine, dexoxyn, meth-edrine	Stimulant	To relieve mild de-pression, control appetite and nar-colepsy	Swallowed or injected
LSD	Acid, sugar, Big D, cubes, trips	*d*-Lysergic acid diethylamide	Hallucinogen	Experimen-tal study of mental function, alcoholism	Swallowed
DMT	Businessman's high	Dimethyltrypta-mine	Hallucinogen	None	Injected
Mescaline	Cactus, peyote	3,4,5-Trimethoxy-phenethylamine	Hallucinogen	None	Swallowed
Psilocybin	Mushrooms	3-(2-Dimethyl amino)ethyl-indol-4-ol dihydrogen phosphate	Hallucinogen	None	Swallowed

120

Usual Dose	Duration of effect	Initial Symptoms	Long-term Symptoms	Physical Dependence Potential	Mental Dependence Potential
Varies	4 hr	Euphoria, drowsiness	Addiction, constipation, loss of appetite, convulsions in overdose	Yes	Yes
15 mg	6 hr	Euphoria, drowsiness	Addiction, impairment of breathing	Yes	Yes
30 mg	4 hr	Drowsiness	Addiction	Yes	Yes
10 mg	4-6 hr	Less acute than for opiates	Addiction	Yes	Yes
Varies	Varies	Excitation, talkativeness, tremors	Depression, convulsions	No	Yes
1 or 2 cigarettes	4 hr	Relaxation, euphoria, alteration of perception and judgment	Usually none	No	?
50–100 mg	4 hr	Drowsiness, muscle relaxation	Addiction with severe withdrawal symptoms, possible convulsions	Yes	Yes
2.5-5 mg	4 hr	Alertness, activeness	Delusions, hallucinations	No	Yes
100 mcg	10 hr	Exhilaration, excitation, rambling speech	May intensify existing psychosis, panic reactions	No	?
1 mg	4-6 hr	Exhilaration, excitation	?	No	?
350 mcg	12 hr	Exhilaration, anxiety, gastric distress	?	No	?
25 mg	6-8 hr	Nausea, vomiting, headaches	?	No	?

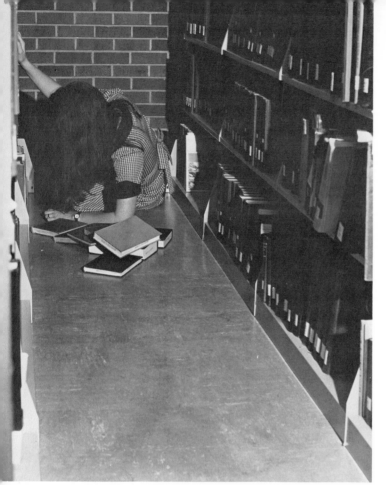

FIGURE 5-6. *The trip is over.*

himself in a deeper form of the same old mood again. The escape was only temporary.

There are some fine people who use benzedrine and dexedrine. There are some successful executives who want that extra drive, some professional athletes who want that extra effort, and some people in show business who want extra spark. Some people use the pills to supplement their liquor supply at parties. They're having a high time. There's no reason why their guests shouldn't. Occasionally someone has a crying fit or starts to shake and can't control it, but he's the exception.

Because of widespread use, there hasn't been a lot of public disapproval of amphetamines other than speed. A lot of speed takers have problems with paranoid psychosis and have various organic disabilities. Some suddenly die.[7] Then comes public disapproval. Enjoying a party or putting a little extra effort into a job is one thing, kind of a desirable thing in a way. But death and insanity aren't desirable.

Barbiturates

Another class of drugs widely used and abused by everyday people are barbiturates. These were first made in the nineteenth century from barbituric

122

acids. Over a quarter of all mind prescriptions that physicians write come under this category. There are phenobarbital, mephobarbital, methabarbital, amobarbital, and others.

Medically, these drugs are used to relax nerves and muscles, lower blood pressure, and slow down the heart. Side effects are euphoria, drowsiness, and interference with concentration and the ability to think. Users claim they like these side effects. They help them escape worry and attain a feeling of well-being. Also, some users claim barbiturates improve their sexual competence.

Amphetamines, dangerous and harmful as they might be, don't cause physical dependence. Barbiturates do. A person addicted to any of the drugs in this category normally withdraws only under professional supervision. And the withdrawal can last for many painful weeks, bring on epileptic seizures, or bring death.

Barbiturates are an extremely popular way of committing suicide. Many, though, who die from an overdose do it accidentally. Barbiturates are unpredictable drugs, and a lethal dose can be pretty small for some people. Also, there are absent-minded souls who can't keep track of which pills they've taken and when. So they take a double dose or triple dose just to be sure they're getting their proper medication. Sometimes people wake up half-drugged in the night and don't realize what they're doing. They grab for the pill bottle and have a good last swallow. And there are people (quite a few young people) who mix barbiturates with alcohol. This is a way of getting a real high, the kind that makes you float and dream. The only problem with highs of this kind is that you sometimes don't come down. Alcohol and barbiturates interact synergistically. Their total depressant effect is a lot greater than the sum of the two effects individually.[8]

Hallucinogens

Hallucinogens aren't as widely used as marijuana and amphetamines, but there's a group who feel that "acid trips" are the only way to add a little zest to a boring and superficial world. They see music; they hear pictures; they touch sunshine and taste love. They see walls wave, see colors sharpen, sense ecstasy so intense that it transcends reality. They can sense a hell that's intense as well. And sometimes they feel both emotions at the same time. They can walk on water, they sometimes think. They can fly without wings or run faster than a car. They're greater than the world, totally in control of environment. Some trip takers have stepped out of ten-story windows, jumped in front of speeding trains to prove their invincibility.

Psychiatrists became interested in these drugs in the late 1930s and early 1940s in order to produce mild psychoses for study. They also used them to treat alcoholism, impotence, and general personality disorders. But the results haven't lived up to expectations.

People usually take these drugs in small groups. They like the cult kind of companionship, and this makes someone available to help if they have a "bad trip," also known as a "bummer" or "downer." Here the user becomes delirious and can't pull out of it.

The most popular hallucinogenic drug is *d*-lysergic acid diethylamide-

25, or LSD. It's extremely potent. As little as 1/40,000 of a gram of it can produce a schizophrenic-like reaction. This is about one-fourth the dose usually taken by an "acid head."

LSD raises blood pressure, dilates pupils, can make you vomit, can bring on all kinds of aches and pains. Some claim LSD damages chromosomes. Since these are the things that determine inheritance, problems in this area can cause malformed children or even grandchildren. True, no one has proven that these biological dangers exist, but a lot of authorities think they do exist. Research continues.[9]

There are several other hallucinogens that produce effects similar to those of acid, and many users prefer them. One of these is peyote, which is sometimes called "moon," "P," or "the bad seed." It comes from a cactus plant. Users brew it with tea or chew on peyote buttons while they're drinking wine or some other strong-tasting drink. Peyote tastes terrible.[10]

Another hallucinogen that comes from cactus is mescaline. "Mesc," or "big chief," produces effects that can last for more than 10 hours. But mescaline users get their hallucinations the hard way. There is 1 to 3 hours of cramps, muscle twitching, sweating, diarrhea, and vomiting before the world becomes vividly colored, blindingly lighted, and weirdly shaped. During this kaleidoscopic illusion, the person often loses his sense of identity. There's no longer a him or her. There's a spirit only—not anybody's in particular—which can sense and float and dream, never think or reason.[11]

Psilocybin is a hallucinogen coming from mushrooms in Central Mexico. Indians there have used it for centuries to help them communicate with the gods and the devils. Americans use it to communicate with the "new reality" or the "fifth-dimension world."[12]

DMT, the "businessman's trip," produces illusions similar to those of LSD, but the effects don't last nearly as long. Instead of seeing pretty colors and shapes for hours and days, the DMT user can fly during the lunch hour, even a long coffee break. It can be made in the laboratory, like LSD, or be extracted from seeds of the morning glory plant.[13]

Other hallucinogens, which aren't widely used but produce effects similar to those of LSD, are MMDA, DET, psilocin, STP, and 68 or "sex juice." There are also morning glory seeds, which are about one-tenth as powerful as LSD but can cause suicide or psychotic reactions. South American tribes were using these seeds before the days of Montezuma. They chew them like you would peanuts or rock candy.[14]

Narcotics

The most dramatic of all the drugs, and probably the most harmful, are in the category of narcotics. There are two varieties: synthetic narcotics, such as Dolophine, Demerol, and Percodan, which get manufactured in a laboratory, and a brand Mother Nature produces called "opiates." Here you find opium, heroin, morphine, codeine, and cocaine. Narcotics can relieve pain, free minds from anxiety and depression. And they can be used in large doses to create a sense of euphoria. It's this euphoria, this sense of supreme ecstasy, that most narcotic users are looking for. And usually they find it. But the thrill and elation don't last for long. The user quickly gets dull, withdrawn, and finally he goes to sleep.

Some narcotics can be sniffed or swallowed. But most addicts prefer slipping them into the skin or veins with hypodermic needles. This doesn't give them an inflamed nose, and it does give them that thrilling "kick." A "skin popper" doesn't get the thrill that a "mainliner" does. But the fellow who's satisfied with sticking a muscle instead of a vein is usually a novice. You have to use narcotics a while before you get into the swing of things.

Addicts aren't much at sterilizing needles. This takes time, and they're anxious to get their thrills. So no matter how they make the injection, there's the threat of hepatitis, syphilis, or another disease that someone who used the needle earlier might have had.[15]

OPIUM

Opium comes from a Turkish plant or one grown in India, Mexico, Egypt, Southeast Asia, and some parts of Russia and China. The plant flourishes in hot, dry climates and places with seasonal rainfalls. A lot of people eat the plant's products. Some smoke them in a pipe. This is a popular practice in Oriental countries, but Americans have never taken to that type of thing. They prefer the opium derivatives.

MORPHINE

Morphine is an opium derivative physicians use to kill pain. Addicts accept it, but they really don't like it. They prefer the stronger opiate, heroin, which produces a euphoric high that morphine can't. Peddlers handling morphine have usually stolen it from a pharmacy or a doctor, or have bought it with a false prescription. Because there isn't a lot of demand for the drug, there isn't a regular line of supply.

HEROIN

Heroin is sometimes called "H," "Harry," "joy," "joy powder," "white stuff," or "scott." It's refined morphine, ten times more powerful than the mother drug. But peddlers never sell it in its pure form. They dilute it so that the package the user purchases is about 1 to 5 per cent of full strength. But this is strong enough to build an overwhelming craving. Tolerance develops quickly, and increasing amounts become needed for that short burst of ecstasy or the momentary relief from hell.

Sometimes the heroin addict escapes all further pain and suffering. He drops dead from an overdose. This can happen easily, as heroin isn't packaged under laboratory conditions. A dealer crudely cuts it with milk sugar, or something else, and the procedure is checked by no one other than the user. If he lives, he probably got the amount of heroin he bargained for, or less. If not, the mistake gets buried.

The dealer isn't always at fault when an overdose happens. Sometimes the user's ignorance is to blame. He's not sure how much he should take in order to get his thrill, and he estimates a little too far on the high side.

There are "joy poppers" who use heroin just occasionally. These people get a high from about 5 to 10 milligrams. But people who use the drug regularly build a tolerance and can require around 450 milligrams to get a similar kind of effect. Such a high dose would quickly kill people who hadn't gradually become used to it. Sometimes "junkies" who have been jailed and had their heroin supply cut off for a time lose some of their tolerance. If they don't make allowance for this when they get their next fix, they add to the overdose statistic.

Sometimes heroin users can't get hypodermic needles, so they open themselves up with pins, razor blades, or nails. Then they apply the drug to the lesion with a medicine dropper. Of course, blood vessels won't take a lot of this kind of abuse without breaking down, and veins get covered with scar tissue. So addicts are always looking for new places to stick themselves. When they've used up all the areas in their arms, they inject their legs. When these scar up, they go to the skin between their fingers, on their necks, on their scalps, inside their mouths.[16]

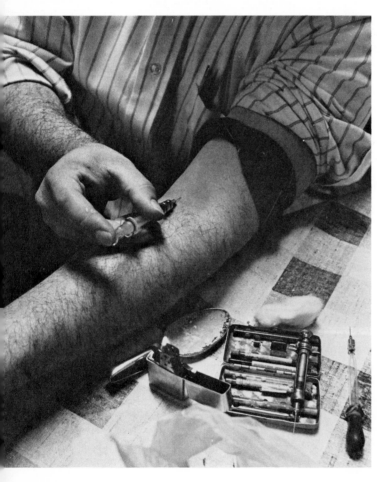

FIGURE 5-7. *The joy popper.* (*Photograph by* The Wichita Eagle *and* The Wichita Beacon)

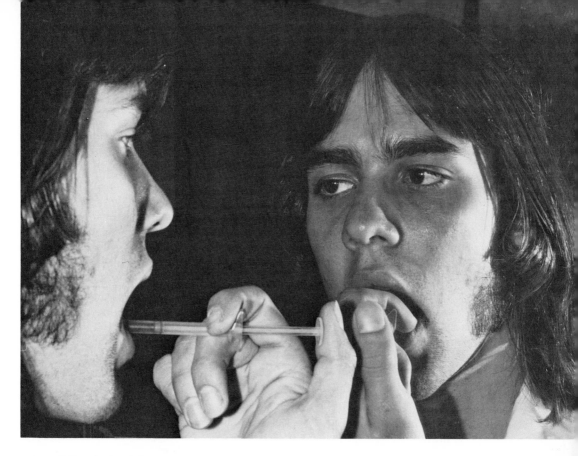

FIGURE 5-8. *A trip of the tongue.*

CODEINE

Codeine doesn't produce much of a euphoric effect, even though it is an opium derivative. But, like other opiates, it is addictive. Heroin users will take it when they can't get their favorite powder. Codeine has been used as a cough suppressant for years, and you can buy a diluted form of it in many states without a prescription.

SYNTHETIC NARCOTICS

Laboratories make synthetic narcotics from coal tars and petroleum products. They are addictive; they can produce euphoria; but they're so hard to get hold of that pushers seldom handle them. Some of the better known ones are methadone, Mepergan, Percodan, Nalline, and Demerol. Doctors use these to control pain and sometimes to treat opiate addiction.

COCAINE

Cocaine is a white, fluffy powder that looks a little like snow. So "snow" is what it's called by the cult. People don't need a needle to take cocaine. The preferred way of getting it into the system is sniffing it. This tempers the effect of cocaine a little, but also prolongs it. To heighten the effect, some mix a little heroin with the cocaine, then take it as an injection. This is called a "speedball."

There's an argument as to whether cocaine is a narcotic or a hallucinogen. According to federal narcotic drug laws, it's in the former category. Like other narcotics, it affects the central nervous system, even though it stimulates rather than depresses.

Someone who comes under cocaine's spell can be one happy fellow. He talks a lot, is filled with energy, and feels such a euphoric love for the world that he sometimes trembles and cries. But there are also the pretty colors and the parade of distorted configurations. Because cocaine brings on these hallucinations, some put it in the hallucinogen category.

The drug originates in Peru and Bolivia, coming from leaves of the coca shrub. Natives have chewed the leaves for over 400 years. They get a relatively mild effect, but Americans get a refined product produced from these leaves that is mild in no way. It can cause dependence, convulsions, extreme anxiety, extreme depression, or no sensation whatever on a permanent basis.[17]

Volatile Solvents

Volatile solvents are chemicals that produce fumes causing euphoria. A person who inhales one of these deeply gets light-headed and drowsy, and has an intense sense of well-being.

Gasoline is one of these solvents. And though it's almost impossible to live in the twentieth century without inhaling your fair share of petroleum-polluted air, you won't get the intoxicated effect unless you inhale the vapors in a concentrated form over an extended period. Fumes from cleaning fluid, lighter fluid, and paint thinner can make you high under similar conditions.

But the favorite for people looking for this kind of treat is model airplane glue or cement. This contains isoamyl acetate, ethyl acetate, benzene, toluene, and carbon tetrachloride. Any of these can kill you if you inhale them for an extended period.

A beginner can usually get a "jag" from inhaling just a few whiffs of glue vapor. But then tolerance sets in, and it takes several tubes of cement to give the "sniffer" that sense of well-being he's looking for. His euphoria usually lasts around half an hour. Then comes drowziness, then sleep. Glue addicts almost always have noticeably bad breath, and they salivate continuously, which makes them spit a lot. Also, they have problems with weight loss, sour stomach, insomnia.

All solvents have a toxic quality that affects the lungs, the skin, the sinuses. And they can harm the heart, liver, bone marrow, and kidneys. In some cases they've caused brain damage, giving users that permanent escape from human society.[18]

Tranquilizers

There are minor tranquilizers, the kind people use to control anxiety, tension headaches, insomnia, and irritability. And there are major tranquilizers used to control psychotic patients in mental institutions. The major type make normal people somewhat depressed and very sleepy. They don't bring on euphoria, so they've never been popular with drug abusers. But they can cause addiction when someone takes them for an extended period. In a lesser sense, this is true of the minor tranquilizers. Sudden withdrawal for someone who's been using them daily can bring on convulsions, twitching, and neurotic anxiety.[19]

Drug Treatment

There are people who use drugs occasionally who'd like to give them up; there are addicts who would like to "kick the habit"; there are families, friends, and counselors of members of the drug cult who would like to see them return to "straight society." What to do? A key step for anyone involved in a treatment program is to realize that he's dealing with individuals, not "junkies," human beings, not sick animals. The key step for the addict is to realize that total freedom from drugs is possible, and that although his enemy is awesome it can be licked. However, there are no sure cures for drug addiction. And maybe it's unrealistic to assume that all who get treatment eventually obtain some kind of ideal goal. What percentage of people can quit smoking, stick to a diet, do a few pushups, and run a mile or two before breakfast? This may be the organization-man society, the conformist culture, the dress and talk like your neighbor in-group, but man is an individual and resents compliance. Be he young or old, athlete or spectator, intellectual or dropout, he resents regulations, even if they're written by Mother Nature. The game is to be beaten, not played. Rules are to be broken, not complied with. In most elements of society, this is good. It preserves human dignity, creativity, a certain amount of sincerity. It creates the feeling (possibly an illusion) that we're not machines. Believers in the Protestant ethic become shocked when treatment programs don't produce massive numbers of total cures. Surely there must be some technique that changes a user's attitude. Can't he realize that what he's doing is destroying

TABLE 5-3
Narcotics Addiction

Item	New Addicts Reported			Total Known Active Addicts Dec. 31, 1971	Total Known Active Addicts Dec. 31, 1972
	1968	*1969*	*1970*		
Addicts (total)	7,219	14,606	12,201	82,294	95,392
Percent using heroin	94.5	96.6	95.8	96.1	94.9
Male	6,136	12,429	10,343	70,260	81,179
Female	1,083	2,177	1,858	12,034	14,213
White	3,785	7,553	6,813	40,299	44,364
Black	3,425	7,008	5,345	41,772	50,779
Under 21 years	1,458	3,380	2,923	9,571	10,328
21-30 years	4,411	8,476	6,874	45,026	56,465
31-40 years	1,069	2,095	1,720	19,249	20,387
41 years or older	281	655	684	8,448	8,212

Source: Drug Enforcement Administration, 94th annual edition, Statistical Abstractment of the United States. 1973 (Washington, D.C.: U.S. Department of Commerce, Social and Economic Statistics Administration), p. 83.

himself, his loved ones, society? Of course, there is no chance this noble stone-caster will change his own views on the world. Why should he? He's right. Anybody knows that.

Statistics involving drug treatment are less than encouraging, less than precise, sometimes less than honest. What percentage of users who try can become drug free? Some statisticians report less than 10 per cent, others more than 40 or 50 per cent. There are questions as to how the statistics are gathered, what the status "drug free" really means, and for how long, whether the researcher is really capable of making a mature judgment about the highly complex discipline of statistics. All who study the field agree, though, that there's no sure cure for addiction or dependence. A lot of fine innovation and treatment has taken place, but a lot more is needed. The following are some of the more common treatments used in the United States in the 1970s. They're certainly not perfect, often not effective. But they do offer hope to the addict looking for a new way of life, offer society a chance to help rather than condemn or punish.

Abrupt Withdrawal

"Cold turkey" may be painful, sometimes lethal, particularly if the person is withdrawing from barbiturates. There can be seizures, which look like epileptic convulsions. There can be diarrhea, fever, vomiting, and delusions. Addicts put in jails sometimes go through cold turkey. Those who desperately want to break the habit sometimes put themselves through it. Usually they seek the help of friends who keep them locked up until the main withdrawal symptoms have passed. Few, if any, could face this ordeal without help.[20]

Gradual Withdrawal

Gradual withdrawal usually takes place in a hospital, often one operated by the United States Public Health Service. USPS hospitals were formed to help merchant seamen suffering from drug addiction, and since their inception over 80,000 "patients" have passed through their wards and counseling programs. There are job training, group therapy, psychiatric evaluation, and, of course, gradual drug withdrawal. The hospitals recommend that the addicts stay for 5 months. Most leave within 30 days. Their physical craving for drugs is broken, so they feel they can handle the psychological dependence without help from aftercare or treatment programs. Many are mistaken.[21]

Therapeutic Communities

Therapeutic communities are complete social systems run largely by ex-addicts. Synanon, established in California in 1958, was one of the first of these and has been one of the more successful. It lists about 1,500 people who once participated in its program who are now completely drug free. Synanon doesn't publish data on its failure rate, though, and it doesn't state what percentage of applicants were turned down for admission. Not just any addict, alcoholic, or drug-dependent can become a member of the Synanon family. A screening committee eliminates people who seem to have little chance of adjusting to around-the-clock supervision and of holding up under the "game." The latter is a kind of intense group pressure designed to break the person's drug desire. Some don't respond, and they're expelled. Those who do respond can move to a higher level of Synanon society.

Other well-known therapeutic communities are Daytop Village, Odyssey House in New York, Phoenix Houses and Gateway Houses in Illinois, and the Tacoma Narcotic Center in Washington sponsored by the federal government. Participants don't have to stay at these centers; they can leave whenever they like. But if they stay they have to comply with community rules.

Of course, it's not uncommon for people to stay away from drugs when they're in these communities. But staying away from them after they've "graduated" is another matter. There are social problems the user has to face when he gets back in his old neighborhood, with his old friends. And there can be legal problems, economic problems, and medical problems that are tough to face, too. So most rehabilitation programs provide facilities for a return to society in stages. There can be short visits home; there can be a half-way house, parish house, work camp, or day-night hospital. These facilities provide counseling on a routine or as-needed basis, vocational services, and therapeutic services. And above all they give people trying to break the habit a sensation that they're not by themselves. Society can be troublesome, even for people adjusted to it. For those trying for a new start, it can be terrifying.[22]

Maintenance Treatment

Doctors Vincent Dole and Marie Nyswander found that an addict's craving for heroin decreased when he received a maintenance dose of methadone. This was in 1964, and since then there have been several treatment programs designed around this form of therapy. They haven't been completely idealistic programs, as methadone itself is a drug, one that brings on deep relaxation and a sense of well-being, creating its own form of dependence. But methadone doesn't have the euphoric effect that heroin does; it doesn't bring on wild craving that distorts morals and ethics. People undergoing maintenance treatment remain addicts. But, theoretically, they can live their lives as productive, responsible citizens instead of slaves to an overwhelming hunger.

There are methadone maintenance programs conducted in hospitals throughout the country, with the largest and most ambitious ones in New York City and Washington, D.C. The addict reports to his treatment center daily to receive 60 to 120 milligrams of methadone, usually served in a cup of orange juice. Within weeks, his craving for heroin subsides, and he can give up the life of crime often necessary to maintain the heroin habit. But there's more to the treatment program than methadone administration. The centers conduct vocational therapy, emotional therapy, recreational therapy, or any type of therapy that seems appropriate to the addicts' needs. There are routine checks of urine to determine whether the person undergoing maintenance has returned to using heroin, other narcotics, barbiturates, or amphetamines. If he has, additional counseling is called for, sometimes expulsion from the treatment program.

There's a cost to this type of program, of course. It can be as little as $500 per year per person treated, or it can run as high as $2,000 per person per year. Although this may seem high, remember that the price of keeping someone in prison for a year is about $10,000, and prison is where a lot of untreated addicts end up. Also, someone on methadone maintenance can hold a job, go to school, pay taxes, make an active contribution to the society that pays for his treatment.

Methadone isn't an easy, complete, or even satisfactory answer to addiction, though. As stated before, it is a drug, and people can become seriously dependent on it. And, as happens with other drugs, some die from an overdose. There are those who enroll in methadone maintenance programs because heroin isn't immediately available. As soon as peddlers put the heroin back on the market, the user withdraws from the treatment program and reverts to his old habits. Also, there's a black market in methadone in spite of, or possibly because of, the treatment centers. The drug has become quite popular, and pushers handle it along with other narcotics, barbiturates, and the like. And there are those who feel that maintenance programs are nothing more than society's way of taking "ghetto rebels" and making them nice, compliant subjects of the organization-man world. After all, does this really deal with the underlying reasons for addiction? Or does anyone really care about lifelong dependence as long as these people don't get in respectable people's way? Even the strongest proponents of maintenance treatment admit that it has its shortcomings. But no treatment at all, or treatment that addicts reject, has its shortcomings, too.

Some maintenance programs use acetylmethadol instead of methadone. It eliminates the craving for heroin as methadone does, it doesn't create a euphoric effect, and it is easily administered. Also, acetylmethadol is effective when taken two or three times a week. Methadone has to be taken daily.[23]

Narcotic Antagonists

An antagonist doesn't prevent withdrawal symptoms. It brings them on, if the person taking the antagonist is addicted to narcotics. Antagonists are structured so similarly to narcotics that they replace them in the nervous system, yet antagonists have no narcotic effect. Nalline is one of the more common of these drugs. It has been used in testing-control programs for several years. Two of the newer members of this family are Cyclazocine and Naloxine. There's been a lot of experimental work done with these newcomers, but the results are inconclusive. One approach has been to build the addict up to a daily dose of 4 to 6 milligrams of Cyclazocine, which theoretically totally blocks the effects of any heroin he might take. But there has to be more to a therapy program than just the administration of a new drug. Social and psychological rehabilitation is essential. After all, the person is going through a learning or "unlearning" process, and there's no pill or injection in the world that by itself can change someone's philosophy of life.[24]

Drug Laws

Drug laws are a fairly recent development in American jurisprudence. Around the turn of the century, you could buy all the narcotics you wanted at pharmacies and general stores. Patent medicines of the day were laced with it, usually in combination with alcohol. There were patent medicine shows, snake oil salesmen, carnival hucksters who sold cures for everything from baldness to impotence and old age.

Then Congress started legislating. There was the Food and Drug Act of 1906, the Harrison Narcotic Act of 1914, the Marijuana Act of 1937, the Boggs Act of 1951, the Narcotic Drug Control Act of 1956, and the Drug Abuse Control Amendment in 1965. Then came December 28, 1970, when President Nixon signed the Comprehensive Drug Abuse Prevention and Control Act—the most far-reaching legislation in this area so far. Here are some of its key points:

1. Anyone caught possessing narcotics illegally may be imprisoned for 1 year and pay a fine of $5,000. Get caught a second time, and the prison term can be 3 years and a fine of $10,000.
2. Narcotic distributors and sellers can get 15 years in prison and a $25,000 fine for the first offense. Penalties are doubled for second and third offenses.
3. A person can get 30 years in prison if he's over 18 years old and gives narcotics to someone who's under 21. This is for a first offense. The second offense can bring 45 years.
4. There are people in the narcotics business on a continuing basis. If they're caught on a first offense, punishment is 10 years' imprisonment to life and a $100,000 fine. If there's a second offense, the prison term and fine are doubled.
5. Penalties for pushers of hallucinogens, barbiturates, and stimulants are similar to those for trafficking in narcotics. Also, the legitimate manufacturer and marketer of barbiturates and stimulants must keep accurate records of all drugs dispensed and received.
6. The law isn't quite as hard on first offenders who possess LSD and other hallucinogens as it is on those possessing narcotics. Someone under 21 caught with LSD or speed or the like can be placed on probation. He can have his conviction erased from criminal records if he stays in good standing during his probationary period. Offenses after the first one, though, can bring a 3-year prison term and a $10,000 fine.
7. Possession of marijuana, even for sale, is a misdemeanor only. The maximum penalty for a first offense is 1 year's imprisonment. It's 3 years' imprisonment for any following offenses. Fines can range anywhere from $5,000 to $10,000.

The Argument

What's wrong with a chemical escape? People wouldn't do it if it weren't fun. Has this free-enterprise, southern fried chicken, love your parents, Coca

Cola world gotten so nauseatingly sanctimonious that fun is now bad? And aren't our bodies ours? Can't we do what we like with them? Or has big brother taken over completely?

Bliss for free, or instantaneous fun is tempting. Sometimes it seems that you can't feel warmth, have understanding, sense excitement or pleasure without a little help. But you can develop a tolerance for pleasure as well as for drugs. Today's ecstasy is tomorrow's routine, next week's boredom. There can always be louder music and stronger wine, of course. There can be a little speed in the acid, some DMT in the pot, heavier doses of heroin to bring on that pulsating rapture. But the search for total euphoria never comes to an end.

So what? So there's been a roller coaster holiday, a cotton candy banquet, a freak show parade. The world's a carnival.

But carnivals do cost. And prices go up when the payment is put off. Eventually they're staggering.

Notes

1. Allen Geller and Maxwell Boas, *The Drug Beat* (New York: McGraw-Hill, 1971), pp. ix–xiv.
2. Leslie H. Farber, "Ours Is the Addicted Society," *New York Times Magazine*, December 11, 1966, p. 43.
3. Sidney Cohen, *The Drug Dilemma* (New York: McGraw-Hill, 1969), pp. 7–10.
4. National Association of Blue Shield Plans, *Drug Abuse: The Chemical Cop-Out* (National Association of Blue Shield Plans, 1971).
5. Edward R. Bloomquist, "Marijuana: Social Benefit or Social Detriment?" *California Medicine*, Vol. 106, No. 5 (May, 1967), 346–353.
6. V. S. Fischmann, "Stimulant Users in the California Rehabilitation Center," *International Journal of Addictions*, Vol. 3, No. 1 (Spring 1968), 113–130.
7. Don A. Rockwell and Peter Ostwald, "Amphetamine Use and Abuse," *Archives of General Psychiatry*, Vol. 18, No. 5 (May 1968), 612–616.
8. Cohen, *The Drug Dilemma*, pp. 83–89.
9. J. Nielson et al., "Lysergide and Chromosome Abnormalities," *British Medical Journal*, Vol. 2, No. 5608 (June 29, 1968), 801–803.
10. Joseph H. Brenner, Robert Coles, and Dermot Meagher, *Drugs and Youth* (New York: Liveright, 1970), pp. 67–68.
11. Ibid., pp. 68–70.
12. Ibid., pp. 70–71.
13. Ibid., pp. 71–73.
14. National Association of Blue Shield Plans, *Drug Abuse: The Chemical Cop-Out.*
15. Jordan Scher, "Patterns and Profiles of Addiction and Drug Abuse," in *Youth and Drugs*, ed. by John H. McGrath and Frank R. Scarpitti (Glenview, Ill.: Scott, Foresman, 1970), pp. 27–32.
16. Franz Bergel and D. R. A. Davies, *All About Drugs* (New York: Barnes and Noble, 1971), pp. 67–77.
17. Cohen, *The Drug Dilemma*, pp. 95–97.
18. Andrew Malcolm et al., "Glue Sniffing May Alter Chromosomes," *Journal of the American Medical Association (Medical News)*, Vol. 207, No. 8 (February 24, 1969), 1441ff.
19. Oliver E. Byrd, *Medical Reading on Drug Abuse* (Reading, Mass.: Addison-Wesley, 1970), pp. 128–129.

20. Julius Merry, "Outpatient Treatment of Heroin Addiction," *Lancet,* Vol. 1, No. 7483 (January 28, 1967), 205–206.
21. H. R. Williams, "Treatment of the Narcotic Addict," *British Columbia Medical Journal,* Vol. 11, No. 1 (January 1969), 11–13.
22. National Association of Blue Shield Plans, *Drug Abuse: The Chemical Cop-Out.*
23. Ibid.
24. Ibid.

6 Alcohol and Tobacco

He's worked hard at preventing childbed fever, smallpox, and rickets. He's developed cures for syphilis, tuberculosis, and duodenal ulcers. And he can perform all kinds of miraculous operations. Heart murmurs can be corrected, crossed eyes can be straightened, broken bones can be mended. He's a genius, man is, at lengthening life and making it more fulfilling, vigorous, and pain free.

But, like many a genius, he has a sardonic twist. Such as manufacturing cigarettes to be purchased by people with lung cancer or emphysema. Young people who have perfectly healthy lungs are taught to smoke. After all, there's plenty of time for the operations and therapy. And death will have its day—just wait.

The waiting may not be too long. There are scotch and bourbon and vodka and gin to speed up the illness and death process. Over 50 per cent of fatal car accidents involve drunken drivers. And there are cirrhosis of the liver, kidney malfunction, and chronic brain damage to get in the way of the good life or any life at all. The tobacco/alcohol situation is totally man made. And, like most of man's creations, it's brilliantly conceived, highly attractive, cleverly touted, and dangerously potent.

Alcohol

The "beer bust" is a big part of the college scene. So is the fifth under the driver's seat of the Chevy, the hip pocket flask at the football game. "Here's to the honor of Colonel Puff," or "Cardinal Puff," or whatever his name happens to be, is a standard game in any tavern near a campus. Marijuana isn't the most abused drug of the young set. It's "booze," ethyl alcohol, the legal mind-bender that has become an integral part of America's life style.[1]

There are numerous innovations to justify the swallowing of liquor. There are the cocktail party, the champagne supper, and the Bloody Mary brunch. There's even a language built around drinks. There are the very feminine, sophisticated sounding ones, such as Pink Ladies, Orange Blossoms, and Brandy Alexanders. There are manly, virile kinds of drinks, too. Take the Rusty Nail, the Stinger, the Screw Driver, the Rob Roy. How do you refill a drink? You have it "spiked" or "freshened up." Or maybe you like "topped up" better. You might want "one for the road," if the party's ending, or maybe you'd rather "put another one under your belt." And just before bed you can have a "nightcap." In the morning, there's the "hair of the dog that bit you" to kill the hangover. Does anyone ever get drunk?

FIGURE 6-1.

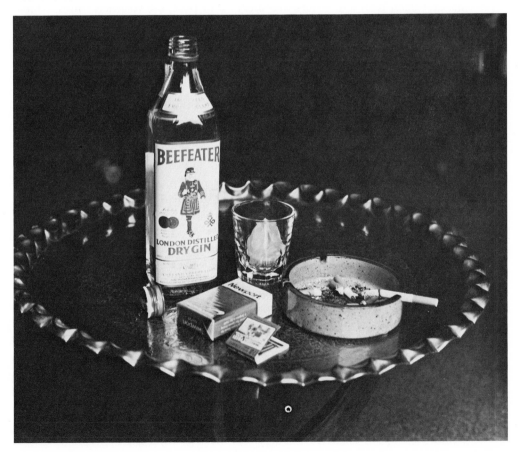

Never! He might get "bombed," "clobbered," "smashed," "tight," "lit," "plastered," "soused," "high." But drunk? That went out with the days of Carrie Nation.

A lot of people don't think of alcohol as a drug. But that's what it is. You can become addicted to it both physiologically and psychologically. It helps loosen us up, helps get rid of the shies, makes us sparkle. It can help us sleep when we're worried, help us to make tough decisions we've been putting off. The drug is quite a depressant that removes some of our more painful inhibitions. But sometimes these inhibitions have a place. Liquor can create a miserable world as well as a happy one.[2]

Scotch, bourbon, rye, vodka, and gin are the things some parties and executive lunches are made of. There are also beer and wine. Beer is the drink for mowing lawns and fishing. Wine is the kind of thing mothers have with dinner, or you get during communion. Beer and wine are mild beverages, some people think. They're like iced tea or Coke. Not so. Certainly hard liquor packs a punch everyone should look out for. But the drink we buy in six packs and the fermented grapes create an effect as well. American beers contain about $4\frac{1}{2}$ per cent alcohol by volume. The alcohol content of wine usually runs somewhere between 12 and 14 per cent. For some, the content is as little as 5 to 6 per cent. And there's a brand highly popular among college students with a content of 10 per cent. These are wines that haven't been fortified. There are sherry and port, the fortified wines, which contain 18 to 21 per cent alcohol. This doesn't sound too potent, when you consider that most hard liquor runs somewhere between 86 and 100 proof. But proof is twice the alcoholic content. Eighty-six proof means that the bourbon, scotch, or what have you is 43 per cent alcohol by volume. So $1\frac{1}{2}$ pints of beer carries the same impact as one $1\frac{1}{4}$ ounce shot glass of hard liquor. It takes about $1\frac{1}{4}$ four-ounce glasses of wine to create the same effect.[3]

Most drugs are a form of poison, and alcohol is no exception. The body quickly neutralizes the poison's effects, though. But the intoxicating effects remain. When somebody swallows liquor, it goes to his stomach and then almost immediately into his bloodstream. Alcohol doesn't have to be digested like food.

Blood carries the alcohol to all bodily tissues, including the brain. As the alcohol is circulating, the body disposes of about 10 per cent of it. Small amounts enter the lungs and get breathed into the atmosphere. This accounts for the odor of whisky on someone's breath. The kidneys also filter some of the intoxicant, making it pass from our systems in urine. But the 90 per cent that remains in the bloodstream is metabolized, or chemically broken down into carbon dioxide, water, and some energy. The average shot glass contains about 100 calories of energy.[4]

A man who weighs about 150 pounds and takes one shot of liquor will almost immediately have 0.03 per cent alcohol concentration in his bloodstream. In other words, for every 100 cubic centimeters of blood, there will be 0.03 gram of alcohol. The body disposes of alcohol at about 0.015 per cent per hour. So it takes this average-sized man about 2 hours to get the alcohol out of his bloodstream after taking a drink. If he continues to drink at the rate his body can oxidize it, he'll feel gently relaxed because of the

TABLE 6-1
Blood Alcohol Levels (Per Cent Alcohol in Blood)

Body Weight	Drinks*											
	1	2	3	4	5	6	7	8	9	10	11	12
100 lb	0.038	0.075	0.113	0.150	0.188	0.225	0.263	0.300	0.338	0.375	0.413	0.450
120 lb	0.031	0.063	0.094	0.125	0.156	0.188	0.219	0.250	0.281	0.313	0.344	0.375
140 lb	0.027	0.054	0.080	0.107	0.134	0.161	0.188	0.214	0.241	0.268	0.295	0.321
160 lb	0.023	0.047	0.070	0.094	0.117	0.141	0.164	0.188	0.211	0.234	0.258	0.281
180 lb	0.021	0.042	0.063	0.083	0.104	0.125	0.146	0.167	0.188	0.208	0.229	0.250
200 lb	0.019	0.038	0.056	0.075	0.094	0.113	0.131	0.150	0.169	0.188	0.206	0.225
220 lb	0.017	0.034	0.051	0.068	0.085	0.102	0.119	0.136	0.153	0.170	0.188	0.205
240 lb	0.016	0.031	0.047	0.063	0.078	0.094	0.109	0.125	0.141	0.156	0.172	0.188
	Under 0.05			0.05–0.10			0.10–0.15			Over 0.15		
	Driving is not seriously impaired			Driving becomes increasingly dangerous			Driving is dangerous			Driving is very dangerous		
				0.08 legally drunk in Utah			Legally drunk in many states			Legally drunk in any state		

* One drink equals 1 ounce of 100-proof liquor or 12 ounces of beer.

Source: Reprinted through the courtesy of the New Jersey Department of Law and Public Safety, Division of Motor Vehicles, Trenton, N.J.

alcohol working on his brain. If he drinks faster, the alcohol in his blood-stream will accumulate, and he'll get drunk. Naturally, the greater the per-centage of alcohol concentration, the greater the effect on bodily func-tions—particularly those connected with the central nervous system. A couple of drinks dull consciousness, remove inhibitions. A couple more, and vision, perception, intelligence, and reasoning become affected. Here is where emotions often take over. A large intake can bring on loss of memory, unconsciousness, even death.[5]

Safe Drinking

Many adults in this country never imbibe. But the vast majority, over 75 per cent, do. Alcohol is a human indulgence that has been with us since the beginning of history. And there are more people indulging today than ever before. Is this shocking? Not necessarily. Alcohol can be a pleasant part of a social situation, a relaxing aid in a hectic world. Despite warnings by prohibi-tionists, it doesn't automatically lead to moral degradation, mental decay, physical incapacitation, or use of drugs like cocaine or heroin. But if you do decide to use liquor it's best to mix a little caution with it. It can make you drunk. And though drunks can be funny, they can be ridiculous spectacles, too. Alcohol can interfere with judgment and reasoning when good judg-ment and good reasoning are called for. And unrestricted drinking can lead to an addiction called alcoholism. Here are a few suggestions that can help maintain, but won't guarantee, safe drinking habits:

1. Drink in moderation. What this means, no one is quite sure. But it definitely doesn't mean letting yourself get "smashed" at parties or drinking yourself to sleep at night or making yourself so incoherent you can barely talk or think.
2. Don't drink at lunch, at least on a daily basis. There are executives, poli-ticians, and college professors who do, of course; and there are execu-tives, politicians, and college professors who have delirium tremens.
3. If it's a mixed drink, measure the alcohol carefully. Don't just tip the bottle and "let it flow."
4. Don't pick up the habit of drinking liquor straight. Although this may seem like the manly way to take it, it's not very wise. Alcohol is absorbed more slowly by the system when it's mixed with soda, water, ginger ale, or the like.
5. Avoid martinis and manhattans. They are great drinks, but their alco-holic content is higher than that of most others, and they probably cause more trouble than most others. If you feel that either of these is your drink, nothing else will do, go easy, And try something a little milder oc-casionally. You might like it as well.
6. Don't gulp drinks. Don't drink on an empty stomach. Alcohol will get into your bloodstream fast enough. Don't give it help.
7. Never take a drink when you're facing a problem. Your mind gets dull; the problem remains. Sometimes it gets bigger. And sometimes the amount you drink gets bigger, too, and you've got another problem.
8. Be ashamed of getting drunk. Let somebody else think it's funny.

9. When you're drinking, talk to somebody. You can't swallow when your lips are moving. And you don't drink too much when you have some-body interesting to listen to either.
10. Never—definitely never—drink alone.
11. Be honest with yourself about your personal drinking habits. This can be a hard thing to do, but it's essential if you want to keep drinking in the proper perspective.[6]

The Alcoholic

If you drink, you fall into one of three categories. There's the normal drinker. This is the fellow who has a beer or two during a ball game, a glass of wine during a holiday dinner, a couple of highballs at an office or neigh-borhood party. He can skip liquor entirely and never miss it. Then there's the alcohol-dependent drinker. This fellow drinks every day, and he drinks more than he'll admit. There are the martinis with lunch, a couple of scotches to calm him down when he gets home, wine with dinner, creme de menthe for dessert, brandy for bedtime. This fellow can cut out liquor with no problem whatsoever—according to him. But doing without it can be a mighty unpleasant experience. Then there's the alcoholic. This fellow has to-tally lost control over his drinking habits. He feels he has to have liquor in order to function, and he doesn't have the will power to turn it down.

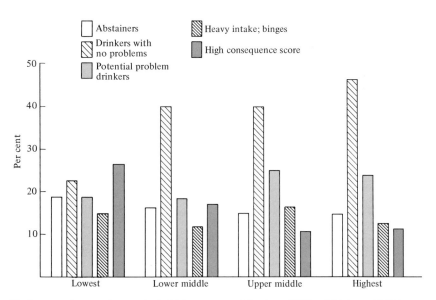

The lowest socioeconomic group had a higher per cent of abstainers (19%) and drinkers with high problem consequences (26%) than any other group.

The per cent of drinkers with no problems was twice as great for the highest socioeconomic group (47%) as for the lowest group (22%).

SOURCE: "Alcohol and Health," U.S. Department of Health, Education, and Welfare (Dec. 1971), p. 33.

FIGURE 6-2. *Prevalence of alcohol-related problems among men in the United States, ages 21–59, by socioeconomic level.*

141

Health Escapes

A lot of people think of alcoholics as skid row derelicts only—the unshaven, unbathed, red-eyed skeletons who beg for the dime for a cup of coffee or the quarter for a bowl of soup. But most alcoholics, about 97 per cent of them, wash daily, wear business suits or sedate dresses, work, and raise families. There are Black alcoholics and White alcoholics, poorly educated ones and well-educated ones, rich ones, poor ones, successful ones, failures. A few have an underlying psychosis, but a few abstainers do, too.

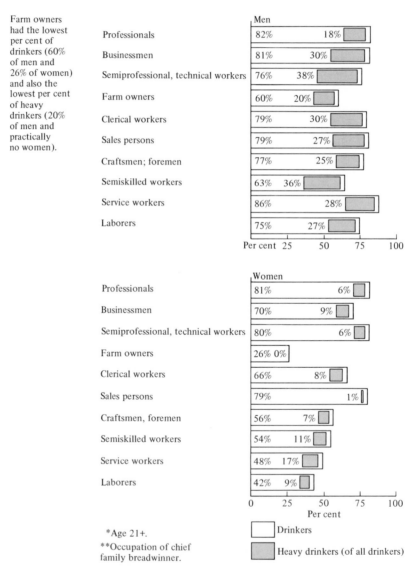

Farm owners had the lowest per cent of drinkers (60% of men and 26% of women) and also the lowest per cent of heavy drinkers (20% of men and practically no women).

Men

Professionals	82%	18%
Businessmen	81%	30%
Semiprofessional, technical workers	76%	38%
Farm owners	60%	20%
Clerical workers	79%	30%
Sales persons	79%	27%
Craftsmen; foremen	77%	25%
Semiskilled workers	63%	36%
Service workers	86%	28%
Laborers	75%	27%

Per cent 25   50   75   100

Women

Professionals	81%	6%
Businessmen	70%	9%
Semiprofessional, technical workers	80%	6%
Farm owners	26%	0%
Clerical workers	66%	8%
Sales persons	79%	1%
Craftsmen, foremen	56%	7%
Semiskilled workers	54%	11%
Service workers	48%	17%
Laborers	42%	9%

0   25   50   75   100
Per cent

*Age 21+.
**Occupation of chief family breadwinner.

☐ Drinkers
▨ Heavy drinkers (of all drinkers)

SOURCE: "Alcohol and Health," U.S. Department of Health, Education, and Welfare (Dec. 1971), p. 28.

FIGURE 6-3. *Per cent of drinkers among adults and heavy drinkers among all drinkers, by occupation and sex.*

142

Some psychologists claim the causes of alcoholism are rooted in the depths of the psyche. Sociologists have seen the environment and pressures of everyday life as causing the problem. And there are physicians who claim that biological defects contribute to the illness. Certainly each of these explanations has merit. But there's one behavior pattern that all alcoholics follow that is an absolute essential for the problem to exist. They drink increasing amounts of liquor on a regular basis for an extended period.[7]

There are lots of these people around. About 10 years ago there were about 5 million alcoholics in the United States. Now there are almost that many alcoholic women. The alcoholics of the 1970s number about 9.6 million.[8] And there are a couple of other numbers in this area that are interesting. There were 555,700 arrests for drunken driving in 1971 and 1,825,500 arrests for drunkenness. True, all of these people weren't alcoholics. But those who weren't had a good start in that direction. The same applies to $33\frac{1}{3}$ per cent of all people arrested in this country each year. The charge is public intoxication. And there's the set between the ages of 16 and 24. Six out of ten of their traffic deaths relate to drinking.[9]

FIGURE 6-4. *Sixty per cent of the traffic deaths for people between the ages 16 and 24 relate to drinking.*

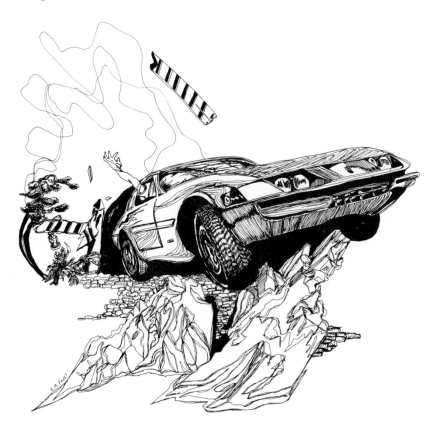

The Cure

One in every 12 to 20 people over the age of 18 is an alcoholic. What to do about it? One simple answer is to pretend you don't have a problem, or ignore the one you admit you have. This might be hard to do when the shivering fits come and the cold sweats and the hallucinations. But the problem might go away quickly with a head-on collision or a terminal case of cirrhosis of the liver. Assuming the alcoholic has a change of heart, though, he should seek medical help. Religious help is a good idea, too. Liquor is too big a problem to face alone.

Medical treatment often consists of putting the person in a sanitarium or hospital for several days so he can "dry out." He's often given a drug called Antabuse. He takes it daily, and it will make him so sick if he swallows liquor he'll think or wish he were dead. Antabuse has produced some miraculous cures, but most alcoholics need broader therapy. There are psychological and social work programs that, when used in conjunction with the doctor's efforts, can improve the chances of rehabilitation.[10]

Alcoholics Anonymous (AA) is a completely free service dedicated to this kind of therapy. The program is based on having alcoholics genuinely admit and accept their problems, on support given by people who have faced this problem and have conquered it, and on total abstinence from liquor in any form. Families can become involved in therapy through Al-Anon and Alateens. Al-Anon holds meetings for spouses and other close relatives of alcoholics. Alateens is for the sons and daughters. Alcoholics Anonymous has recently claimed that 60 per cent of its new members are completely sober after 1 year. This compares favorably with the 5 per cent reported success rate for psychiatric treatment.[11] But statistics of this type are highly questionable. Drinkers have never been known for honesty when reporting their drinking practices.

Some cases of alcoholism produce physical side effects more serious than the drinking itself. There's cirrhosis of the liver, a condition that can kill. Livers enlarge and cease to function effectively after heavy intakes of alcohol. For most people, this condition corrects itself within a few weeks. For people with cirrhosis, the condition can become permanent and progressive. Another alcoholic gastrointestinal disorder is pancreatitis. This can cause severe pain, nausea, even hemorrhaging. And then there are respiratory ailments, cardiac problems, and poor nutrition. One of the greater tragedies, usually not reversible, is brain damage. Here the advanced alcoholic loses intelligence, becomes irritable, forgetful, and loses his ability to concentrate or work.

Chronic medical problems of this type call for something other than psychological counseling, of course. There are shock treatments, intravenous injections, transfusions, operations, administration of tranquilizers and vitamins. But there's no medical cure for alcoholism. Even if the physical side effects disappear, the underlying problem remains.[12]

Drinking Myths

There are thousands of stories that rationalize drinking in one form or another. Here are a few of the more typical ones:

1. *You can't become an alcoholic on beer or wine.*

   Nonsense! The fellows who sleep on park benches and spend Christmas at the Bowery mission usually drink nothing but wine. It's the cheapest way known to get an alcoholic high. And you can get an alcoholic high from beer, too.[13] It may be a little hard on the kidneys, but drink enough of it and you join the bleary-eyed people with the shakes.

2. *Women hardly ever become alcoholics.*

   This may have been true when ladies talked of "limbs," not "legs"; "passing on," not "dying"; "wrong time of the month," not "menstruation." Today, girls wear miniskirts, puff on Virginia Slims, and become drunks. They're not as noticed as the men are, as they do a lot of their drinking at home. They may not have to hold down jobs the way their husbands and boyfriends do. And husbands and boyfriends protect their ladyfolk from the "alcoholic" label. There seems to be something particularly revolting to Americans about a drunken wife or mother. But there are lots of these people, even though they don't make the statistics quite as often as the men do.[14]

3. *If alcohol were less available, there would be fewer alcoholics.*

   America doesn't lack for liquor stores or bars. In some of the larger cities, there are three bars to the block, which stay open on a 24-hour basis. This would seem to invite alcoholism. But in England, where bars are open for 8 hours only, the alcoholism rate is no lower than it is in the United States. Sweden has one of the lowest alcohol consumption rates in the world, but it has a big alcoholism problem. Italians, who drink more alcohol per capita than any group other than the French, have an extremely low incidence of alcoholism. The Greeks and Jews have a low incidence of alcoholism, too. And both of these groups have well-established drinking customs. Apparently, the availability of liquor is a lot less important to the alcoholism problem than how people consume it.[15]

4. *Someone who can hold his liquor can never become an alcoholic.*

   There are people who get high on one or two drinks, and there are people who can drink everybody at the party under the table. The man who feels his liquor quickly often becomes conscious of his drinking and doesn't imbibe too deeply or too often. But the man who can hold more than most sometimes forgets caution. He never shows his drinks, so why worry? His doctor sometimes gets to worrying, though, about his liver, his heart, and his brain.[16]

Tobacco

It was a Y-shaped pipe, and they used to stick a tube up each nostril and inhale. This was the thing to do during ceremonies to bring on good will. The pipe was called "tabaco," and the people who used it were a red-skinned, black-eyed group Columbus called Indians. Columbus was quite taken with their peace pipe, so he brought some burley back to the Queen of Spain. Corncobs, Camels, Marlboros, and White Owls were ready to take their place in Western culture. Tobacco had a lot to do with financing the Revolutionary War, helped build many a Virginia, Carolina, and Kentucky fortune, and now contributes about $1.2 billion to U.S. farm income and about $6.6 billion to manufacture's income.[17]

People use tobacco in several different ways. Some sniff a powdered variety of it called snuff. This was a fairly popular practice in Europe during the seventeenth and eighteenth centuries, but it's never caught on in this country. About ⅕ pound of snuff per year per person is the current rate of consumption for Americans over 15 years old.

People prefer chewing their tobacco to sniffing it. Even though the spittoon is no longer with us, mixtures of tobacco leaves and molasses get masticated at the rate of ½ pound per person per year. This same rate holds for pipe tobacco, even though it's puffed, not chewed. As to cigars, the average American over 15 puffs on 59 per year.[18]

But the cigarette is by far the most popular vehicle for tobacco. This wasn't true prior to World War I. Fellows smoked cigars or pipes or chewed, and women didn't smoke at all. But then came the fight to make the world safe for democracy, and cigarette companies passed out free samples to boys in the service. They did the same during World War II, the Korean War, and the Vietnamese War, giving the American male a good exposure to the habit. As to women, they began asserting their independence in the 1920s. And independence to some meant acting like men. Doughboys did it, veterans did it. Why couldn't women? Also, there were advertising campaigns which associated smoking with female ideals of romance, glamour, sophistication, and independence. Metropolitan Opera stars gave cigarette testimonials. "I protect my voice with Lucky Strikes." Movie stars gave testimonials, too. They smiled as they blew rings from the silver screen. Models smoked

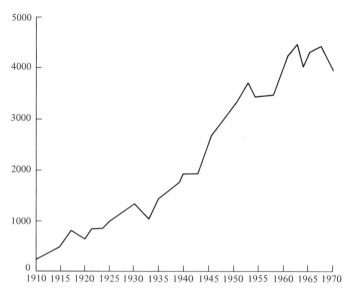

A profile of the growth of cigarette consumption in the United States between 1910 and 1970. These figures include nonsmokers and smokers 15 years old and over. (Compiled from United States Department of Agriculture, Economic Research Service Publications.)

FIGURE 6-5. *Cigarette consumption per person per year.*

FIGURE 6-6. *Girl in a nicotine fog.*

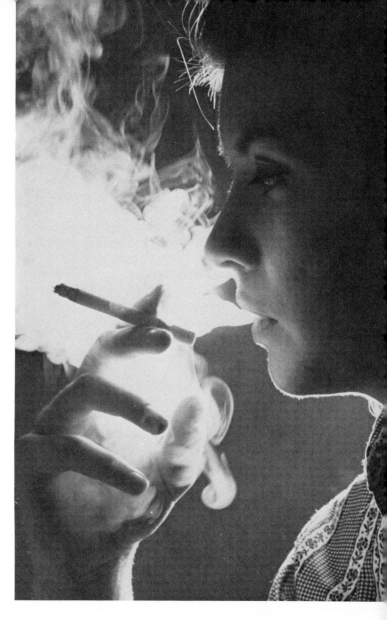

cigarettes on New York's Fifth Avenue while parading in Lucky Strike green. And the slogan "Reach for a Lucky instead of a sweet" implied that girls who smoked would be slender, voluptuous, and desirable.[19]

But women, apparently, aren't convinced as easily as men. In 1970, 31 per cent of the women smoked compared to 42 per cent of the men. In younger age groups, percentages between men and women smokers were much closer. But still the female is predominant in the unhooked generation.[20]

The Smokers

It's the thing to do in some parts of society. The cigarette between the fingers is a symbol of poise, self-confidence, social sophistication. It gives us

147

something to do with our hands. And everybody knows that empty hands make you self-conscious. Some people smoke because they like watching the smoke. People almost never light up in a dark room; and the blind man who smokes is a rarity. Some smoke to be like Mom and Dad. It's a blow for early maturity or teenage independence. And some want to be with the "in-group." You just can't do that unless you smoke. After all, doesn't everyone do it? Some people smoke for stimulation. A cigarette and a cup of coffee in the morning prepare them for the horrible world. Some smoke because they have the habit. They've just "got to have a cigarette" after a certain amount of time has passed. There are people who use cigarettes to fight feelings like distress, anger, and fear. And there are those who fall into the oral gratification category. Something in their mouths gives them a sense of well-being. It's something like a baby's bottle or pacifier.

But whatever the reason for smoking, the habit has to be consciously cultivated. No one who lights up for the first time enjoys it. It can make you dizzy, sick, make you cough. You have to develop a tolerance for tobacco before it stops bothering you. But the human being is a determined and patient animal. He'll teach himself to enjoy smoking no matter how long it takes.[21]

Billboard advertisements show smokers as deeply tanned, rawboned men and deeply tanned, well-rounded young ladies. The man's intelligent, adventurous expression implies that he's just returned from a mining expedition in Montevideo to take over presidency of the New York office. The girl? After her Vassar years, there was a short stint on the stage, which bored her. Then she got involved with volunteer work and graduate school. Are these typical smokers? No. But to be fair, they're not typical nonsmokers, either. Here are some of the findings on people who support the stockholders of R. J. Reynolds, Inc.

The smoking pattern usually starts at an early age, as 15.7 per cent of boys in high school smoke and 13.3 per cent of the girls do. The smoking behavior of boys tends to conform with that of their fathers. And the smoking behavior of girls is like their mothers'. The rate of smoking in Catholic schools is higher than in city public schools. The rate is lowest in suburban schools.

The rate is lower for students who participate in extracurricular activities than for those who don't. This seems logical for athletes. It's hard to run the mile or play basketball when cigarettes have cut your wind. But this statistic doesn't hold for athletes only. Students who play in the band, work on the school newspaper, serve on the student senate, act in the senior play are less likely to smoke than those who do nothing besides go to class.[22]

The average smoker has a lower IQ than the average nonsmoker. This doesn't mean there aren't three-pack-a-day Phi Beta Kappas. When you're playing with numbers, there are a lot of exceptions to the averages. But, putting the exceptions aside, the typical smoker, in addition to having a lower IQ than his clean-breathing counterpart, is a poorer student, comes from a lower social background and a lower economic background. The lowest percentage of smokers, both male and female, is found among college graduates. The highest percentage exists among high school dropouts. There was a study of the freshman class entering the University of Illinois in 1965, com-

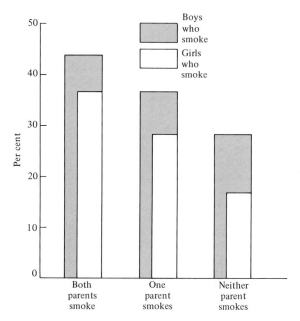

A large majority of teenage smokers come from
homes where one or both parents smoke. (Courtesy
American Cancer Society, Profile 1970.)

FIGURE 6-7. *Smoking habits of teenagers and their parents.*

paring grade point averages to smoking habits. The relationship was almost
perfectly inverse. Of the students with an A average, 17 per cent smoked.
For those with an E average, 59 per cent smoked.[23]

The Statistics

Scare stories abound about the 25-year-old who's dying of lung cancer, the
24-year-old victim of a heart attack who had been chain-smoking since he
was 14, and the teenager who becomes a pulmonary cripple because of the
curse of nicotine. These are exceptional stories, of course. There are smokers who lead healthy, active lives into their 90s. But studies have indicated
that the smoker is taking a bigger gamble with his health than the nonsmoker. Here are some of the findings:

Doctors Doll and Hill, of England, did one of the first studies in this
area. They collected data from 40,000 British physicians over age 35 concerning their smoking habits. Then they let Mother Nature take over for the
next $4\frac{1}{2}$ years. After checking death certificates and autopsy reports, they
concluded that mild smokers were seven times as likely to die of lung cancer
as nonsmokers were. Moderate smokers were 12 times as likely to die of lung
cancer, and heavy smokers were 24 times as likely to die from this disease.[24]
Doctors Hammond and Horn were running a similar study for the American Cancer Society about the same time, and their findings were about the

same.[25] A few years later, Doctor Dorn, of the U.S. Public Health Service, studied the smoking habits of 200,000 veterans over a $2\frac{1}{2}$-year period. He concluded that people who smoked more than a pack a day were 16 times as likely to die of lung cancer as those who didn't smoke and that those who smoked only occasionally were 10 times as likely to die from this affliction.[26] Mr. H. A. Kahn, again of the U.S. Public Health Service, carried on Dr. Dorn's studies for another $8\frac{1}{4}$ years. He decided that Dorn's conclusions had been far too conservative, that risks were considerably higher than Dorn had reported.[27] Dr. E. Cuyler Hammond conducted a study involving more than a million subjects in 1,121 counties in 25 states over a 4-year period. He concluded that death rates from all causes were significantly higher for people who smoked than for those who didn't and that death rates proportionately increased by the number of cigarettes smoked per day. Hammond wasn't just talking about lung cancer. The death rates from coronary heart disease and strokes were twice as high for those who indulged in the tobacco habit as for those who didn't. And death rates were significantly higher for a multitude of other diseases. The death rates from all causes were higher for smokers who began the habit when they were young than for those who took it up in later life. And death rates for ex-cigarette smokers decreased in relation to the time they had given up the habit.[28]

There are about 300,000 premature American deaths each year caused by smoking. This breaks down to about 800 deaths a day, 175 of which are due to cancer, 375 due to diseases of the heart and circulatory system, 250 due to chronic bronchitis, emphysema, peptic ulcers, and a few other related causes.

TABLE 6-2
An American Balance of Hazards to Life, 1966

Excess Deaths from Tobacco	
Lung cancer	41,012
Other cancers (of larynx, bladder)	28,045
Coronary disease	145,956
Other vascular diseases (strokes, etc.)	42,821
All other causes (emphysema, bronchitis, etc.)	43,726
Total Excess Deaths from Tobacco	301,560
*Deaths from Selected Causes**	
All infections	128,180
Tuberculosis	(7,590)
Pneumonia and influenza	(64,230)
All accidents	112,300
Motor vehicle	(53,280)
Diabetes	35,380
Suicide	20,160
Homicide	11,210
Balancing Total	307,230

* Figures in parentheses are included in previous categories.

Source: R. T. Ravenholt, Presented at the World Conference on Smoking and Health, New York City, September 11-13, 1967.

TABLE 6-3
Estimated Years of Life Expectancy at Various Ages for Males in the United States, by Daily Cigarette Consumption

Age	Never Smoked Regularly	Number of Cigarettes Smoked per Day			
		20-24	25-29	30-34	40 and Over
25 years	48.6	44.0	43.1	42.4	40.3
30 years	43.9	39.3	38.4	37.8	35.8
35 years	39.2	34.7	33.8	33.2	31.3
40 years	34.5	30.2	29.3	28.7	26.9
45 years	30.0	25.9	25.0	24.4	23.0
50 years	25.6	21.8	21.0	20.5	19.3
55 years	21.4	17.9	17.4	17.0	16.0
60 years	17.6	14.5	14.1	13.7	13.2
65 years	14.1	11.3	11.2	11.0	10.7

Source: E. C. Hammond, "Life Expectancy of American Men in Relation to Their Smoking Habits," Presented at the World Conference on Smoking and Health, New York City, September 11-13, 1967, 23 pp.

Another way of looking at the statistics is the number of years of life someone gives up for the privilege of enjoying the fine taste of a Winston. Take someone 25 years old. If he smokes less than a half pack of cigarettes a day, his life expectancy is reduced by 4.6 years. It becomes 5.5 years if he smokes a half to a full pack a day, 6.2 years when it's one to two packs a day, and 8.3 years when he's passed the two-pack figure. This decrease in life expectancy of the two-pack-a-day smoker is just about equal to the increase in life expectancy medical technology has provided during the past 50 years. Looking at it from a percentage standpoint, the chance of this 25-year-old man's dying before he's 65 becomes 50 per cent greater when he smokes less than half a pack of cigarettes a day, 70 per cent greater when it's a half to two packs, and 109 per cent greater when he burns more than two packs a day.

Still another way of looking at it is the amount of life lost for each cigarette smoked. The average heavy smoker burns about ¾ million cigarettes in his lifetime. This makes him lose about 8.3 years of life, or 4.4 million minutes. So each cigarette costs this heavy smoker about 6 minutes of living time, or about 1 minute of life for every minute of smoking.[29]

Some feel that the hazards associated with pipes and cigars are relatively minor. And they are minor, if cigarette damage is the standard they're judged by. But they do affect human health to some degree. Between the ages of 45 and 64, the death rate of cigar smokers is 22 per cent higher than that of nonsmokers. For these same ages, the death rate of pipe smokers is 11 per cent higher. Some relationship has been found between pipe and cigar smoking and the incidence of coronary heart disease, peripheral vascular disease, and cancers of the mouth, the pharynx, and the larynx.[30]

Of course, there's the argument that life is meant to be enjoyed. Who cares if you die a little bit early, as long as you enjoy yourself while you're breathing? The only problem with this argument is that smoking does interfere with the enjoyable life for many. Puffing on a cigarette may not make them sad, but it can make the years they spend on earth sickly ones, ones in which they have little energy and a lot of pain. The Life Extension Institute of New York reported over 30 years ago that smokers complained of coughs 300 per cent more often than nonsmokers did, nose trouble 167 per cent more often, palpitations 50 per cent more often, 73 per cent more often for pain over the heart, 100 per cent more often for heartburn, and 76 per cent more often for nervousness.[31] According to the American Cancer Society, men between the ages of 40 and 64 who smoke are hospitalized 50 per cent more often than those who don't smoke.[32]

Looking at the youth group, a British study of people between the ages of 11 and 18 revealed that those who smoked had a higher incidence of respiratory illness, persistant cough, and phlegm than those who didn't. Also, the more the boy or girl smoked, the more likely were these illnesses.[33]

According to a recent national public health survey, workers who smoke cigarettes lose over a third more time from their jobs because of illness than do nonsmokers. It's estimated that there are 77 million work days lost each year that can be attributed to the consumption of tobacco. Smokers spend 88 million days in bed each year because of disability and illness while their nonsmoking friends are at parties, tennis courts, and swimming pools. And there are 306 million days of restricted activity that nonsmokers don't face and smokers do. In this case, the person isn't bedridden, but he has to stay around the house because he just doesn't feel well.[34]

Giving up the Habit

The easiest way to quit, of course, is never to smoke in the first place. Or maybe you don't want to quit. The findings about smoking don't bother you that much; maybe you don't believe them. But if you do have the habit and want to quit, it's not as hard as some make it out to be. About 21 million Americans have successfully gotten rid of the craving for nicotine, and they've done it without crawling walls and swinging from chandeliers. One of the keys to success in this area is concentrating on the benefits around the corner—less illness, more working time, feeling better. That dark brown, fuzzy feeling in the mouth disappears. And so do fatigue and shortness of breath. Also, food tastes better, sleep is sounder, and tensions get smaller. Even the chance of getting cancer decreases, along with death rates from a multitude of causes. If someone has given up smoking for 10 years or longer, his life expectancy becomes almost equal to that for someone who never took his first puff.[35]

But once you're dead, you're dead. The thought of dying often doesn't bother young people, but early disability does. The chance of spending 15 or 20 years with a disease that interferes with the good life, the ability to function well, can be frightening. A way of getting rid of this fear is giving up the habit.

Most people can give up smoking without too much trouble when they really want to. Just wishing that you could or taking a few days without cigarettes to give it a try won't do the trick, though. The person with the tobacco habit has a real craving it takes some grit to overcome. Here are some suggestions from people who have earned their "I Quit" buttons:

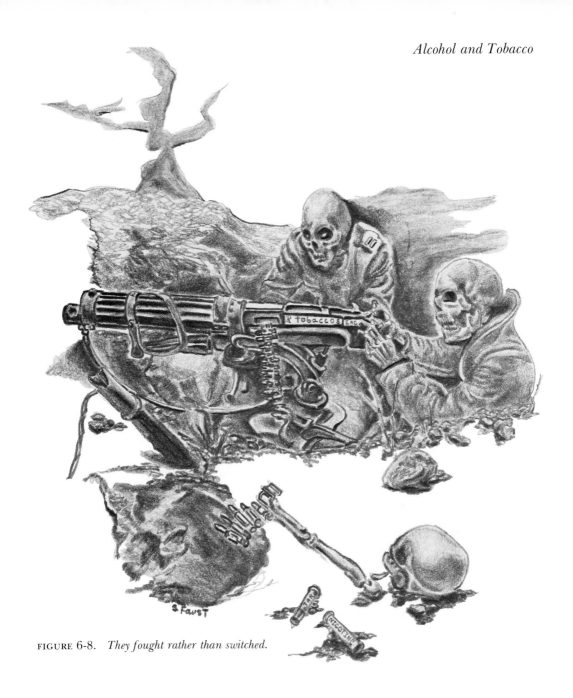

FIGURE 6-8. *They fought rather than switched.*

1. Never look on giving up cigarettes as denial. The smoker has to keep reminding himself that he's adding something to his life—a greater degree of self-confidence, self-fulfillment, and vigor, as well as a longer life span. Otherwise, there will be self-pity. And this can get to be unbearable.

2. Select a day on which you'll quit, and stick to it. No matter how tough things get, make up your mind that you'll never have another puff. And things will get tough for a few weeks. But they'll get better—if you don't give in to the nicotine urge.

153

3. Once you've given up smoking, don't give in to the temptation to "have just one." You'll be back to two packs a day by the end of the week. It's something like being an alcoholic. He can't take that first drink. Even if someone hasn't had a cigarette for 20 years, he's back in habit when he has one drag.

4. Keep cigarettes out of sight. It's better if you keep matches and ashtrays and smoking friends out of sight for a while, too.

5. You can relieve some of the tension you feel by deep breathing and strenuous exercises. It won't relieve all tension, but it relieves more than just sitting in a chair and thinking about your problems.

6. Drink a lot of water. Nibble on candy and nuts, and chew gum. So you gain a few pounds. You can take them off once you've licked your craving.

7. Indulge yourself in every way possible. Make sure the time you've decided to quit is a relatively calm period, that you can sleep late, eat what you like, drink what you like, read what you like, and throw tantrums if you like.

8. Bantron or Nikoban tablets or gum can be helpful. But not everybody can take the tablets. If you have any doubts, check with your physician.

9. Some people would rather cut out cigarettes gradually than all at once. This can work, but beware of it. You can fool yourself into thinking you're making progress and not be progressing at all. This method calls for a definite schedule. Don't smoke between 9 and 10, 11 and 12, 1 and 3. Then increase the nonsmoking periods for 1 hour, $1\frac{1}{2}$ hours, 2 hours. Then smoke only after meals, only in the evenings. Then comes the big day when you just don't smoke.

10. When using gradual withdrawal, it sometimes helps to put as many barriers in the way of enjoying smoking as possible. Wrap cigarettes in individual sheets of paper. This makes them bulky to carry, harder to get at when you want one. If you're right-handed, smoke with your left hand. If you usually put a cigarette in the left corner of your mouth, put it in the right. Never carry enough money to buy a pack of cigarettes. If you run out, you're out. And when you do smoke try holding it to only half a cigarette. This can be as hard on the nerves as quitting altogether.

11. If you want moral support, see your physician or psychologist. Or maybe you'd like a smoker's clinic. Here health professionals give advice on quitting, and people who have licked the problem give quitters encouragement.

12. An excellent time to quit is when you're too sick to enjoy a cigarette. Smoke can taste like moldy hay mixed with fertilizer when you have the flu, a bad cold, or a serious stomach upset. Don't put off quitting until you get sick, of course. But if you are thinking of giving up the habit and sickness strikes, welcome it as an opportunity. Something good can come out of sneezing and a sore throat.

13. If you insist on smoking, lower the danger as much as possible. Try a cigarette the Department of Health, Education, and Welfare rates low on tar and nicotine. Surprisingly, this doesn't increase the amount you smoke. And sometimes you smoke less. Don't smoke a cigarette all the way down. Most of the tar and nicotine are in the last few puffs. These

are the ones which can do the most damage. Take fewer drags on each cigarette. This can be hard. But, with concentration, you can learn to do it. Reduce inhaling. Better yet, don't inhale at all. This is really hard. But it's worth learning. The smoke doesn't do much damage if it doesn't get in the lungs. Smoke fewer cigarettes per day. Pick a time each day when you won't let yourself smoke. Postpone having a cigarette when you really want one. Deliberately run out of cigarettes, and take your time about buying a new pack.

14. Walk through the intensive care unit of a hospital sometime and look at the emphysema victims struggling for breath, victims of thoracic surgery trying to talk without a voice box, amputees who lost their legs from Buerger's disease. Smoking is the primary cause of each of these tragedies. And though the visit might seem a little ghoulish, possibly these people have a story worth paying attention to.[36]

Notes

1. Max Hayman, "The Myth of Social Drinking," *American Journal of Psychiatry,* Vol. 124, No. 5 (November 1967), 39–48.
2. A. E. Bennett, "Compulsive Addictive Personality Problems," *Medical Times,* Vol. 92, No. 5 (May 1964), 433–442.
3. U.S. Department of Health, Education, and Welfare, "Alcohol and Health," DHEW Publication No. (HSM) 72-9099, (December 1971), pp. 6–7.
4. Ibid.
5. Bennett, "Compulsive Addictive Personality Problems."
6. M. Vogel-Sprott, "Alcoholism as Learned Behavior: Some Hypotheses and Research," in *Alcoholism,* ed. by Ruth Fox (New York: Springer, 1967), pp. 46–53.
7. John A. Carpenter, "Issues in Research on Alcohol," in *Alcoholism,* ed. by Ruth Fox (New York: Springer, 1967), pp. 16–23.
8. U.S. Department of Health, Education, and Welfare, "Alcohol and Health," pp. 78–79.
9. Ibid.
10. John Clancy, Richard Vornbrock, and Ellen Vanderhoof, "Treatment of Alcoholics," *Diseases of the Nervous System,* Vol. 26, No. 9 (September 1965), 555–561.
11. U.S. Department of Health, Education, and Welfare, "Alcohol and Health," pp. 78–79.
12. Julian C. Grant, "Treatment of the Alcohol Withdrawal Syndrome," *Journal of the Tennessee Medical Association,* Vol. 61, No. 1 (January 1968), 45–47.
13. Hayman, "The Myth of Social Drinking."
14. Howard Wood and Edward L. Duffy, "Psychological Factors in Alcoholic Women," *American Journal of Psychiatry,* Vol. 123, No. 3 (September 1966), 341–345.
15. U.S. Department of Health, Education, and Welfare, "Alcohol and Health," pp. 23–25.
16. E. A. Martin, "Alcoholic Cerebellar Degeneration: A Report of 3 Cases," *Journal of the Irish Medical Association,* Vol. 56, No. 336 (June 1965), 172–175.
17. Harold S. Diehl, *Tobacco and Your Health: The Smoking Controversy* (New York: McGraw-Hill, 1969), pp. 5–8.
18. Ibid., pp. 9–10.
19. John Gunther, *Taken at the Flood—The Story of Albert Lasker* (New York: Harper, 1960), pp. 169–179.

20. *'74 Cancer Facts & Figures* (New York: American Cancer Society), p. 19.
21. Diehl, *Tobacco and Your Health,* pp. 132–135.
22. Daniel Horn, "Current Smoking Among Teenagers," *Public Health Reports* Vol. 83, No. 6 (June 1968), 458.
23. Dorothy F. Dunn, "Cigarettes and the College Freshman," *Journal of the American Medical Association,* Vol. 199, No. 1 (January 2, 1967), 77–80.
24. R. Doll and A. B. Hill, "Lung Cancer and Other Causes of Death in Relation to Smoking: A Second Report on the Mortality of British Doctors," *British Medical Journal,* Vol. 2 (1956), 1071.
25. E. C. Hammond and Daniel Horn, "Smoking and Death Rates: Report on 44 Months of Follow-up on 187,783 Men," *Journal of the American Medical Association,* Vol. 166 (1958), 1159–1294.
26. H. F. Forn, "Tobacco Consumption and Mortality, from Cancer and Other Diseases," *Public Health Reports,* Vol. 74 (1959), 581.
27. H. A. Kahn, "The Dorn Study of Smoking and Mortality, Among U.S. Veterans: Report on $8\frac{1}{2}$ Years of Observation," *National Cancer Institute Monograph,* No. 19 (January 1966), 1–125.
28. Hammond and Horn, "Smoking and Death Rates."
29. E. C. Hammond, "World Costs of Cigarette Smoking in Disease, Disability, and Death," World Conference on Smoking and Health, New York, September 11–13, 1967.
30. Diehl, *Tobacco and Your Health,* pp. 34–35.
31. "The Effects of Tobacco Smoking," *Proceedings of the Life Extension Institute* (May-June, 1939), 55.
32. U.S. Public Health Service, "Smoking and Illness," *National Clearinghouse for Smoking and Health* (Washington, D.C.: Government Printing Office, 1968).
33. Diehl. *Tobacco and Your Health,* p. 100.
34. U.S. Public Health Service, "Smoking and Illness."
35. Donald T. Fredrickson, "How to Help Your Patient Stop Smoking," *NTRDA Bulletin,* Vol. 55, No. 4 (April 1969), 6–11.
36. Clifton R. Read, "If You Want to Give up Cigarettes" (New York: American Cancer Society, 1968).

7 Quacks and Health Frauds

This isn't the day of the medicine show. It's been replaced by *Marcus Welby, Medical Center,* and *The Doctors.* But around the turn of the century the medicinal hucksters were in their prime. Many of them were quite talented and much better at selling their wares than the current Madison Avenue and CBS groups. There were John Healy and Charles Bigelow, also known as "Doc" Healy and "Texas Charlie." They operated scores of shows for the "benefit of humanity" called the Kickapoo Indian Sagwa. Here there were violent dances, bright beads, maidens, and remedies compounded from wintergreen, yellow birch bark, and sarsaparilla. These were the miraculous medicines the Kickapoos had kept secret since the coming of Columbus. Another of the great shows was put on by "Old Doc" Hamlin, the discoverer of Hamlin's Wizard Oil. And there were Hal the Healer and Brother John and Brother Benjamin, who posed as Quakers. They used "thee" and "thou" and preached the simple wisdom of the Friends and their miraculous remedies.

But the medicine shows weren't the only purveyors of the great cures. There was an organization called Sears, Roebuck, and Company that put out a catalogue. Many pages of this document were filled with advertisements for female pills, a White Star Secret Liquor Cure, and Sears cure for the opium and morphine habit.

This was the golden age of Doctor Hercules Sanche. Doctor Sanche ad-

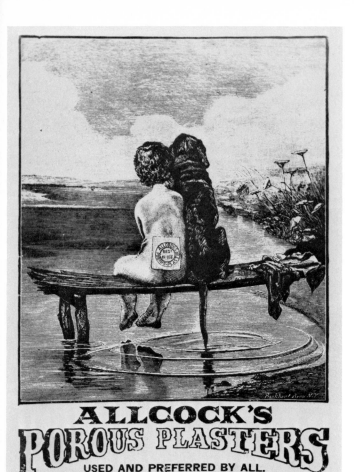

FIGURE 7-1. *Man's best friend.*

ALLCOCK'S
POROUS PLASTERS
USED AND PREFERRED BY ALL.

vertised the Oxydonor in some of America's finest monthly magazines. His machine made the old young, the ugly beautiful, and the weak strong. After all, oxygen is the breath of life, isn't it? Well, the Oxydonor poured life into the body through the pores. Many a woman and more men than were willing to admit it got "revitalized" through these oxygen skin treatments.

But in case this oxygen failed there were lots of brands of celery compound, bitters, vermifuges, alteratives. There were the lung balsams, pectorals, the balms of Gilead. There were the kidney pads, the asthma powders, August flowers, the embrocations, the anodyne cordials. And there were the black draught, the wine of cardui, the Kings of pain, the nervines, the liver regulators, the renovating resolvents, vuchu, cascarine, a lithontriptic, and a cathairon. Add to this Thayer's Slippery Elm Lozenges, and you had cures for all the ills man ever had and preventions for many that might be coming up.[1]

Of course, this is the 1970s, and people are a lot smarter than they were at the turn of the century. Who today would buy Swamp Root, Celebrated Eye Water, or Perry Davis's pain killer? Apparently, without the regulations of the Food and Drug Administration, there would be plenty. P. T. Barnum's adage that a sucker is born every minute didn't go out of vogue with the present generation. Today's quackery costs U.S. citizens about $2 billion a year. And this doesn't include some of the less noticeable forms of quackery that take place within the bounds of certified medicine. Injury, disability, and death come from the 1970s medicine man. Some estimate that his products kill more people than all crimes of violence combined.[2]

Definition of Quackery

What is a quack? Certainly a license to practice medicine, dentistry, podiatry, pharmacy, or the like doesn't guarantee honesty, responsibility, and intelligence. And isn't it possible that Father John's Medicine or Samuel Duffy's Pure Malt really can cure cancer, even though these practitioners operate outside of the "medical trust"? Sure. The AMA, the FDA, the ADA, the APA, and all the colleges in the world don't have a monopoly on creativity, research, and common sense. And these colleges and universities and professional societies turn out their share of quacks, too. A quack is anyone who pretends to have a medical skill he doesn't have in order to promote his personal gain. The M.D. who promises to cure baldness with a worthless salve is just as much a phony as the sidewalk huckster selling the same product. And a phony is a quack, if you're talking about health care.[3] But in fairness to professionals the standards they subscribe to are honorable and extremely demanding. They don't have to stoop to quackery to gain status, and most of them don't.

Of course, the quack is only telling people what they want to hear, giving them hope, dreams, and a certain amount of peace. He sings a siren's song for many a lost sailor. Come to me; end your fears, feelings of inferiority, and pain forever. Surgery, even death, can be whipped—for $5 a bottle, $20 a treatment, a dollar a pill. That's cheap for health, youth, vigor, and immortality.

Some people believe the quack's pitch because of ignorance. They don't realize there's a Food and Drug Administration that monitors and approves legitimate health care products and that there are professional organizations monitoring and endorsing effective health care practitioners. A lot of well-educated people believe quacks, too. Probably fear and gullibility play a bigger role in a quack's following than other factors. Someone afraid of death, of pain, of the unknown is tempted to grab at any hope he's offered.[4]

Then there are the young people, who look on life as a personal possession. Vigor is the way you feel when you're not asleep; pain and suffering are unheard-of strangers. Certainly they have no need of arthritis cures, bone liniment, radio treatments. But teenagers are high on quacks' sucker lists. They want bigger busts, bigger muscles, smaller waistlines. Their skin should have a vibrant look—or is it their hair? In any event, youth is a highly receptive target for mail-order quackery or any other variety.[5]

Types of Quackery

There are all kinds of quackery. There are promises to make you strong, make you charming, make you smart. Whatever man really wants, he can

159

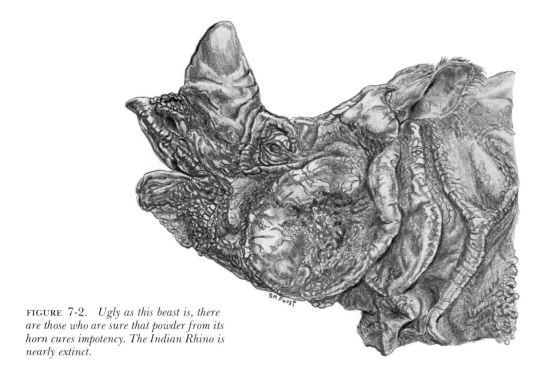

FIGURE 7-2. *Ugly as this beast is, there are those who are sure that powder from its horn cures impotency. The Indian Rhino is nearly extinct.*

find someone who sells it. And quite often the price is ridiculous. Here are some of the more commonly marketed items of the 1970s health phony:

Arthritis Quackery

About 12 million Americans suffer from inflammation of the joints, or arthritis. It's quite painful, sometimes incapacitating, sometimes disfiguring. There's not a lot an ethical physician can do to cure or completely relieve this malady. So the quack has a natural clientele. About half of all arthritis sufferers deal with these hucksters, spending about $\frac{1}{4}$ billion a year on worthless treatments, medicines, and machines. Many claim that they get relief and even get cured, but there's no scientific evidence to back their testimonials. Apparently, what relief they get is psychological. They want to get better, and they don't want to feel they've been taken for fools, so they convince themselves that their pain and swelling have gone away. Also, arthritis symptoms, like the symptoms of any disease, often disappear without any treatment whatsoever. Sometimes quack treatments get credit for the work of Mother Nature.

Most of the 10,000 arthritis quacks in this country deal in nothing but harmless aspirin products and copper bracelets that "suck pain from the bones." There are a few, though, who handle dangerous drugs and treatments.[6] Physicians handle dangerous drugs and treatments, and aspirin, too, but there's a lot of education and scientific research behind their decisions. Anyone with arthritis should see them and them only. If they can't help, no one can.

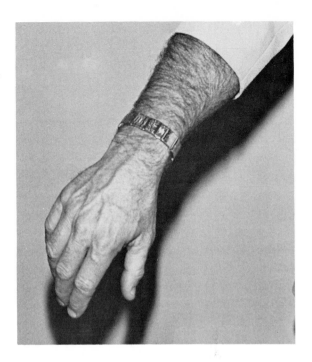

FIGURE 7-3. *The "Super Health Magnetic Bracelet." It supposedly prevents arthritis, cures arthritis, and makes all other arthritic treatment unnecessary.*

Cancer Quackery

Cancer quackery isn't as widely practiced as arthritis quackery. There are more people with arthritis than there are with cancer. Phony treatments in this field, though, bring in about $50 million a year, so you can't look on it as small business. And there are many bogus practitioners in this field with reams of testimonials from grateful patients. These charlatans saved Aunt Suzy and Uncle Horace from their death beds, returned Mary Jo to her five children and beaming husband. Some patients testify in court on their healers' behalf, some picket their state capitals demanding legislation releasing their practitioners from the capitalistic chains of the AMA.

Surely, these patients would know if they still had cancer. There's no wishful thinking strong enough to mask the pain, disfigurement, the feeling of impending death. True, but did they recognize the early stages of cancer? Did the pain in the side, the dizzy spell, the bad cough really signify a malignancy? If a licensed physician diagnosed the case and said that cancer existed, it probably did. But, usually, these "miraculous cures" were diagnosed by the quacks themselves. Charley's hack sounded terrible. He had been on three packs a day for the last 20 years. This is cancer, all right, according to the Doctor of Herbalologicalphysiology who diagnosed the case with soundwave graphs. Three thousand dollars worth of treatment later, Charlie's hack disappeared—and so did his cold. Another miraculous cancer cure took its place in the annals of modern American science.

There's a lot of danger in this kind of racket. Sometimes people really do have cancer, cancer that could be cured if it were diagnosed and treated by ethical medical procedures. But the quack, with his benevolent politician promises, gets in the way of this early treatment. So the cancer grows and reaches a stage where legitimate medicine can't deal with it. Then come suf-

161

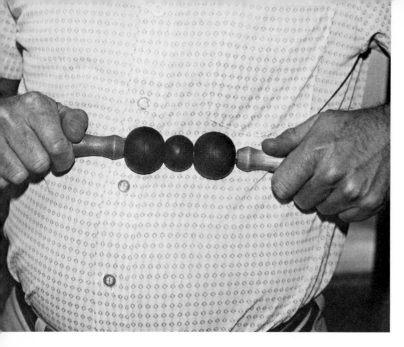

FIGURE 7-4. *The "reducing roller." It makes you grunt and it makes you giggle. In no way does it make you firm.*

fering, death, and one of the quack's failures. But dead people don't write protesting letters, so he doesn't have too much to be concerned with.[7]

Reducing Schemes

Fifty million Americans try to lose weight each year. Every one of them is looking for an easy, quick way to do it. No one wants to believe that to have that lean, hungry look you have to be hungry. Hunger is a painful sensation. It makes you nervous, makes you weak, keeps you from sleeping. Certainly, there ought to be a way of taking pounds off without eliminating the candy bars, the evening highball, the TV snack, and the second helping of potatoes. There isn't, of course. A painless diet makes as much sense as painless exercise, effortless work, and success without a setback. But people keep looking, and quacks lead the search. Some of their more popular items are the following:

VIBRATORS AND MASSAGING DEVICES

Vibrators and massaging devices tickle you, sometimes make you grunt and giggle. They don't take off a bit of weight, and they don't firm up those "flabby spots" with "firm and curvaceous muscle."

REDUCING CREAMS

Reducing creams do the same amount of good as vibrators—none at all. They do sell well, though. After all, it would be great to go to bed looking like a middle-aged salesman and wake up a muscular track star. It's a great dream. People like to buy dreams.

REDUCING PILLS

Doctors prescribe reducing pills sometimes, and they can occasionally be effective. But the kind quacks prescribe are either ineffective or illegal and possibly dangerous. And anyone taking an illegally prescribed drug to reduce needs to have his head treated, not his body.

DIETLESS REDUCING PLANS

There are thousands of dietless reducing plans, hundreds of thousands. Take a dose of castor oil just prior to a big meal. Learn to vomit by tickling your throat. This way you can eat what you like and stay slim and trim and laugh at your friends who turn down the gravy and chocolate pie. This is foolishness, of course. Plans of this type can bring on all kinds of stomach and nervous disorders. And any plan that really does make you lose weight without putting you in a mental institution involves a strict diet, even though the plan may call it something else.[8]

Baldness Cures

Sometimes it's a traveling "baldness clinic" that will make the shiny dome thick with hair, the receding hairline reverse itself—at least, that's what's supposed to take place. These clinics usually operate in hotels or motels, with baldness quacks traveling on to new locations before anyone verifies their promises. Sometimes this business seeks customers through magazine ads, sometimes through newspaper ads. And sometimes there's a warning that they don't have a cure for hereditary baldness. But this warning is

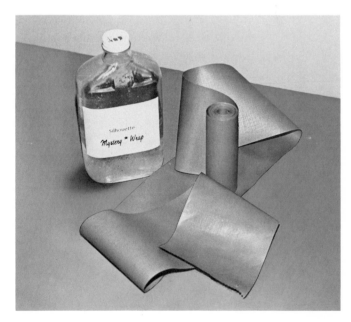

FIGURE 7-5. *The "Silhouette Mystery Wrap." The seller claimed that you could lose weight by wrapping yourself in the fabric material, then pouring the solution between your body and the wrapping. The wrapping strips had actually been cut from window shade material. The solution was a mixture of mineral oil and sodium sulfate.*

always brief and surrounded by implications that they can cure "your" baldness.

Some baldness can be cured, of course. The kind caused by disease, or some local infection, responds to various types of treatment. But the person administering these treatments should be a physician, not some hair tonic salesman, head massage specialist, or someone with a gadget that steams the scalp. Sometimes—unfortunately, most of the time—baldness can't be cured. Physicians will tell you when it can't. Quacks won't.[9]

Breast Development

Some claim *Playboy* started the breast development fad; some blame Jane Mansfield and Marilyn Monroe. But the ideal of the big female bust was popular long before their heyday. There was a time—the Roaring Twenties—when the flat-chested girl reigned as the ideal of gorgeousness. But then came X-rated movies, "bunnies," and topless waitresses. Size 38D was in vogue, and quacks always follow the vogue. Some of their schemes for turning a 32A into the centerfold's Miss January are quite imaginative:

EXERCISES

Exercises improve the posture a little, firm up the tissue supporting the breasts. But they don't do a thing to improve breast size. There are machines, cups, elastic bras, isometric exercises. They don't do harm, except to the pocketbook. They don't do much good, except for the quack.

DEVELOPMENT CREAMS

Some of the development creams contain hormones that should be used under medical supervision only. Those without hormones build breast tissue at the same rate exercise does—not at all. Creams don't require much effort, though, so some women prefer them to straining and flexing.

DIETS

It is complete foolishness to believe that a diet will improve breast development. There's no food in the world that makes breasts grow—that is, without making the whole figure overly voluptuous. Balanced diets make women look and feel better than unbalanced ones do. But there's a limit as to what vitamins, minerals, and proteins can accomplish.

SILICONE IMPLANTS

Silicone implants will increase the breast size. But only licensed physicians should make the injections or perform the operations. There are serious dangers of infection and other health problems associated with this procedure. The Food and Drug Administration condemns it. A lot of plastic surgeons condemn this practice, too.[10]

Beauty Aids

The number of beauty aids is limitless. A lot of them really don't come under the category of quackery. A woman probably does look better with lipstick, fingernail polish, a powdered nose. At least, our culture says she does. Why not indulge the practice? There's no reason for a girl not to cream her face or put her hair in curlers at night, unless her husband objects. If her husband does object, she can point out that cream keeps her skin soft and feminine looking. But his objections to turtle oil, mink oil, orchid pollen, and royal jelly make some sense. There are thousands of "miracle cosmetics" on the market that will supposedly give a middle-aged woman the skin of an 18-year-old, eliminate wrinkles, sagging chins, and baggy eyes. This just isn't so. There's nothing, besides a good diet and good health and cleanliness, that can contribute to skin beauty or that youthful look.[11] Many wish it were otherwise.

Food Quackery

He had bronze skin, heavy shoulders, and a straight, yet natural stature. His smile personified vigor and self-confidence and the excitement of being a healthy human animal. After introducing himself to the lady of the house, he stated that he had a life-building substance for sale—something that could revitalize tired tissue, build energy hard to contain, eliminate any trace of illness, fatigue, depression. What was this miracle product? Food! But this wasn't ordinary food. This was a nutritional wonder the lady's family needed, and now! It would give them an enthralling world, a Shangri-La with carnivals, parades, and picnics. Food quacks were using the door-to-door sales approach long before there were magazines, advertising agencies, and mail-order soliciting. They use the more modern approaches to tout their products now, of course. But many still rely on pushing doorbells. Another old-fashioned technique, which quacks still use widely, is the "nutrition lecture." Here "Doctor" or "Professor" DeFrancisco (he almost always uses a fancy name) warns of how we're killing ourselves with poor nutrition, tells how we can look 10 years younger with proper diet, tells of the fountain of vitality each of us can drink from. Where is it located? In this bottle of Sorghum Extract he's selling for $2 or this Naturopathic Vitamin Emulsion prepared on the Portuguese Island of Ibiza.

Then there are health food stores selling products no more nutritious than you can find at the Safeway. But the labels on the bottles have healthy-sounding names and the proprietor prescribes them as "health foods," so a lot of people buy them. The food fad field is a massive business with an enormous clientele and puts out a huge amount of misleading information. Some of the myths it fosters are the following:

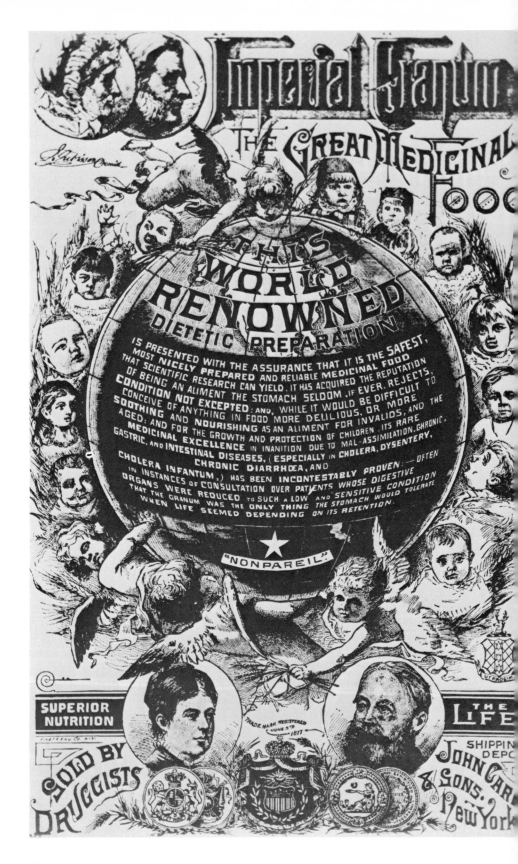

166

1. *You need "organic" or "natural" foods.*

   One of the quacks' favorite claims is that commercial fertilizers drain the organic nutrients from food. If we want the healthy constitutions our grandparents had, we'll have to grow our vegetables with natural fertilizers (manure). This obviously doesn't make sense, as our grandparents' constitutions weren't all that healthy. And it doesn't make sense from an agricultural standpoint, either. Plants can absorb only simple inorganic nutrients from the soil. When you use manure as a fertilizer, bacteria have to break it down into the same simple nutrients used in commercial fertilizers before the plant can get any nourishment. The plant really doesn't know the difference between manure or fertilizer made in the factory. It'll grow the same way for either one.

   The same applies to human absorption of vitamins. Our bodies respond identically to synthetically produced products and vitamins occurring naturally in our food and food supplement products. Salesmen selling these products, though, will swear there's a difference. After all, a vitamin pill is a kind of chemical—everyone knows that's bad. The salesman ignores the fact that all food is a mixture of chemicals, and his "natural vitamin food supplement" is no exception.[12]

2. *Food additives are poisoning us.*

   The term "chemical" has taken on a bad connotation in this day of the naturalist and environmentalist. After all, coloring agents, mold inhibitors, antioxidants, and other food additives can mask inferior quality or even be downright harmful. This is true if some of the additives are used in large doses. But the Food and Drug Administration protects us. It assures that the amounts manufacturers use are completely harmless. Food quacks imply, of course, that the American public is being slowly poisoned, and only the few buying the quacks' products will be saved. They laughed at Noah, too, of course, but the fellow selling organic soybean meal and wheat germ oil builds a funny-looking ark.

3. *The essential food.*

   He's got a new food. Without it you're not going to get a vital nutrient that keeps you peppy and healthy and full of fun. But isn't every key nutrient available on the grocer's shelves? Not according to this huckster. His product has a substance science hasn't come up with yet. Oddly enough, many people believe him—people who should know better.

4. *All illnesses come from a faulty diet.*

   Some illnesses do come from a faulty diet, of course. There are rickets, scurvy, even bad teeth. But you're really not what you eat. A good diet won't make you mentally healthy, or prevent cancer, emphysema, leprosy, or thousands of other sicknesses.

5. *Depletion of the soil depletes food quality.*

   The story goes that we've been growing crops on our land for centuries and these crops drain something from the soil that isn't replaced, so subsequent

FIGURE 7-6. *Yesterday's miracle food.*

167

crops are weaker, less nutritious, less tasty. The story is a complete fable. If there's a mineral lacking in a farmer's soil, he grows a lower quantity of produce, not produce of lower nutritional quality. True, soil deficiency has caused iodine deficiency in some of the things grown. But our salt is artificially iodized, so most of us don't suffer from a lack of it in our systems.

6. *Food is overprocessed.*

Don't we lose some food value by our modern processing methods? Sure. But the food quack exaggerates the amount lost. Old processing methods were destructive to vitamins and some minerals. But modern methods of preserving fruits, vegetables, and meats hardly interfere with nutrition content at all. And the processing makes these foods available on a 12-month basis, not just during certain seasons. Modern man is, or should be, better fed than at any other time in history.[13]

Patent Medicines

There are thousands of patent medicines providing cures for aging, listlessness, impotence, overweight, heart trouble, forgetfulness, bad eyesight. The illegal ones come under the heading of "nostrums," products prepared and usually distributed by quacks. A medicine might bear the name of the quack who made it, or it might carry the name of a research or scientific organization to make it sound reputable. Sometimes they're called "magic potions," sometimes "miracle substances." But these don't have an honest ring, and people in the 1970s avoid them. "Health tonic" is a much more sincere label, and lots of people buy health tonics without question.

There are proprietary and standard drugs, of course, items made by reputable pharmaceutical companies. Physicians use these products, and you

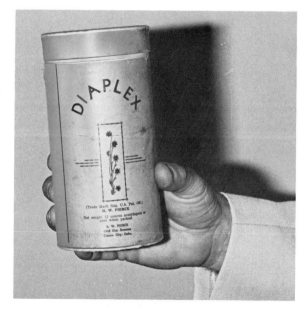

FIGURE 7-7. *"Diaplex." This was made from dried Colorado salt weed. The promoter of the concoction sold it to diabetics, telling them to give up insulin. Diaplex would completely cure their illness if they consumed daily quantities of it with tea.*

FIGURE 7-8. *"B & H Inhalant Powder" consisted of a mixture of borates and silver nitrate crystals. Sniffing a small quantity of it would prevent asthmatic attacks. Sniffing on a regular basis would cure asthma, hay fever, even the common cold, according to the promoter. According to the Food and Drug Administration, the silver nitrate crystals could be extremely harmful.*

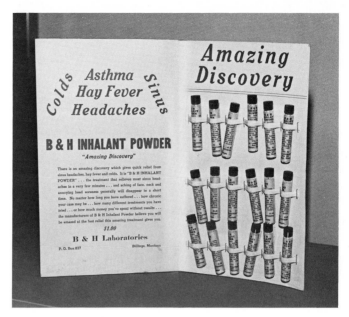

can purchase some of them without prescription on drugstore shelves. The United States Pharmacopoeia or the National Formulary of the American Pharmaceutical Association lists these products. If you're in doubt about a medicine, check with your doctor or druggist.[14]

Therapeutic Devices

The mystical powers of cosmic energy, magnetism, radio waves, the explosive force within the atom can be used to make us new men and women. Gadgets release these "miraculous" powers, and quacks sell or lease the gadgets. They're worthless, of course, but they do have flashing lights, emit eerie sounds, and have elaborate designs that make them appear legitimate. When people are foolish enough to put their money into nonsense of this type, usually no harm is done. So they lost a little money, so they got taken, so what? But sometimes faith and foolishness of this type get in the way of obtaining proper medical attention. The result can be permanent damage, even death.

Gadgets of this type were popular prior to the turn of the century, but there are still an amazing number of them being peddled. They're used by quacks in what appear to be professional surroundings. Some that have recently been in use are the following:

1. *The Theraphone Instrument.* This produces healing through sound waves at frequencies you usually can't hear.

2. *The Plasmatic Therapy Device.* This treats all diseases and conditions of people over 40—there are lots of them—by electricity.

3. *Holder's Electronic-Oscillating Condensator.* This scans the body to locate toxic conditions.

4. *Oscilloclast.* This emits shortwave transmissions and treats over 180

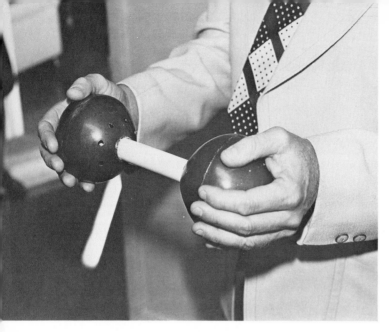

FIGURE 7-9. *The "Z-Ray Applicator" consists of two balls with a tube of "Z-Ray irradiated water" between them. The Z-Ray, says the promoter, strikes the earth at 45° from the northeast. The water it irradiates cures all maladies, prevents all maladies, keeps the user from thinking about maladies. All that is necessary is putting a hand on each ball and letting the Z-Rays from the water surge throughout the body. Price: $75.00.*

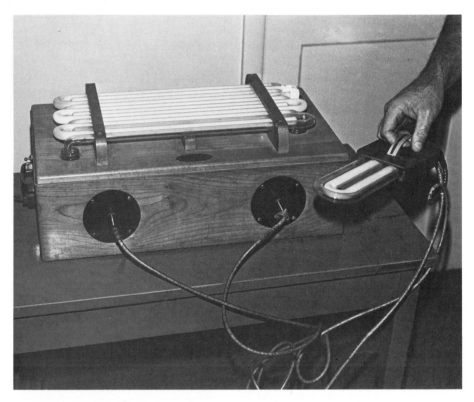

FIGURE 7-10. *The "Color Therm." A chiropractor marketed this device, claiming that all bodily disease came from having kilocycles out of kilter with the rest of the universe. The Color Therm contained several colored neon tubes with a hand applicator. With it, the body could be retuned by exposing it to a complete spectrum of light frequencies.*

diseases and ailments. There's a similar version of the same instrument called the Oscillotron.

5. *The Neurolinometer.* This diagnoses abnormal bodily functions through "nerve interferences."

Again, this stuff didn't emerge during the Spanish-American War. It's peddled and used today. And there are many more innovative devices on the drawing boards for next year, the next decade, and the next century.[15]

Spotting the Quack

He's got a long mustache, shifty eyes, hands that he rubs together constantly. Or is it his brightly colored shirt and cheap, striped suit that give the quack away? After all, you can spot a phony at first glance. Who said that? Or who said, "It takes one to know one"? The truth is that all of us are a little bit phony. Pure sincerity, like the honest man, exists in some philosopher's imagination. We laugh when we think a joke is horrible. We agree with the boss a little more often than we should, and we tell our wives they have great taste in hats and really know how to make great meatloaf. A little phoniness is an admirable trait, in a way. And, if not admirable, it's at least common. So a quack certainly can't be recognized as being different from the crowd. It's his method of operation that sets him apart from the legitimate physician. Some of his more common tactics involve

1. Downgrading of what he calls the "medical monopoly."
2. Claim that he's persecuted by jealous physicians.
3. Use of fear tactics concerning health.
4. Lots of case histories and testimonials of cures.
5. Contempt for immunization, surgery, and X-rays.
6. Guarantee of a quick and sure cure.
7. Claim that the cure was given to him through a divine power.
8. Treatment based on a secret formula or a newly developed machine.[16]

Interpreting Health Information

It's sometimes easier to spot a quack than a quack claim. A phony individual may not have overly phony manners or an insincere way of speaking, but there is the whole person to judge. With health information, there are words only that help you make up your mind, and words can be misleading and confusing. After all, there are our cultural backgrounds to contend with. Quacks prey on these, and when it's only the quack's words that we read or hear we tend to accept them when they jibe with what we believe. What we believe, of course, isn't always the way things are—even if we are part of the "educated elite." College students, college graduates, and college professors believe a lot of old wives' tales about health, just as a lot of old wives do.[17]

But old wives' tales aren't a strong enough argument for a good health sales package. Superstition has to be authenticated by a modern superstition called statistics. Or maybe the statistics can stand by themselves. In this day of the computer and space flight, the numbers game has taken on an almost biblical significance. "Seven out of ten doctors recommend Milk of Magnum laxative." Sometimes the fellow making this statement is wearing a white coat and has a stethoscope around his neck. But otherwise the statement isn't amplified. Did the doctors recommend that you take this laxative on a regular basis—whenever you feel like it—whenever you're constipated—after you've had a thorough physical? What kinds of doctors are we talking about—chiropractors, naturopaths, M.D.'s, Ph.D.'s? How was the sample taken? Was every physician in the United States contacted? Was it a random sample of 10 per cent, 5 per cent? Or did it consist of ten doctors selected arbitrarily? This being the case, selections could be repeated over and over until a group of ten was found having seven who really did prefer Milk of Magnum laxative.

Statistics can be used to explain a finding, to shade the truth, to downright lie. Quacks are excellent liars and excellent statisticians. For that matter, so are the advertisers of some legitimately made products. "Mouthwash doesn't have to taste bad to do the job. Pinko, with methosulfachloraphene, kills bad breath on contact. Your mouth feels fresher for hours." What in the heck is methosulfachloraphene? It sounds scientific, but this has nothing to do with how effective it is. And as to "doing the job," does this mean that you can forget bad breath and bad taste problems? Certainly, this wouldn't apply to people with sour stomachs or badly decayed teeth or people who eat a lot of garlic. Liars, exaggerators, and statisticians have all kinds of approaches.[18]

Testimonials

And don't forget testimonials. Any self-respecting quack has thousands of them. "My arthritis was so bad I couldn't stand up. Then I heard about Doctor Clean's Linament. It's been a new world, I'll tell you. Two weeks ago I walked to town. Last week I worked in my garden. Tonight I'm going to a dance." People who give these testimonials often mean well; they often think they've been cured or helped. But the scientific authenticity is nonexistent. Lots of the patients would have gotten well without any treatment whatsoever. Some had never been sick. The American Medical Association considers testimonials, of any type, completely unethical and discourages physicians from using them. A recent United States Post Office investigation showed that 75 per cent of the people giving printed testimonials were dead. A good number of them died from the diseases they claimed they were cured of.[19]

Meaningful Health Information

Isn't there anyone you can believe? Not completely. No one, no organization has a strong enough title, a clean enough reputation, or a comprehensive enough background to make its words divine. No regulation or law makes thinking unnecessary. There is the physician, though, and the organization to which most physicians belong, the AMA. Certainly, the AMA's health information isn't perfect; and, at times, it may not be completely honest. But it's one of the more reliable and scientific sources of information we have. There are also governmental agencies, state, local, and federal, whose main job it is to evaluate health care products and practitioners and warn against fraud and malpractice. Their information is pretty reliable, even though many people don't have much faith in anything connected with the government these days. Then there are private agencies like the Ford Foundation, Ralph Nader's group, and Good Housekeeping, which publish a lot of material pertaining to health. It's usually quite sincere, and it's usually backed by lots of investigation.[20]

Of course, despite the information you get and try to follow, it's still easy to get confused. It's an ever-changing market, this health care field, and certainly one that's extensive. It takes in some highly specialized items, which grow hair, prevent leg cramps, strengthen fingernails. And there are remedies in general that deal with overall loginess, the "blahs," hyperactivity, and paranoid distrust of mankind. You can eat these products, inhale them, spray them, sniff them, drink them, rub them. They come in purple, red, blue, and orange. And they're big and small, round, rectangular, octangular, hexagonal, and pea-shaped. You can buy them in tubes and bottles and cans, boxed, frozen, or dehydrated. No question about it, the health care field is a vitamin jungle, a pharmacy of mazes, mirrors, and illusions.[21] The following guides won't completely solve this puzzle, but they can give it a recognizable shape and form:

1. Never take a drug without a physician's advice. This includes aspirin, cold tablets, and laxatives. This might up your medical bill slightly, but it's money well spent.
2. Buy products that have government approval and carry some seal of acceptance by an approved organization.
3. Buy health products from reputable pharmacies and medical supply houses only. Door-to-door salesmen, health food stores, and people giving lectures on nutrition don't come under the category of "reputable."
4. Always read the labels on any health product you buy. You may not totally understand the contents, but you can get enough of an idea to make a comparison with a similar brand.
5. If you're in doubt about a health product's value, check the research findings of consumer organizations or testing and rating services.
6. Never buy a product that's a guaranteed cure for anything. Be it a specific health problem or the hodgepodge of all illnesses, there is no "surefire" cure.
7. Look out for lots of testimonials and lots of razzle-dazzle advertising. The good-quality products don't need this kind of promotion and usually don't have it.[22]

Selecting a Doctor

You really do have a choice in selecting a doctor, assuming you don't live in a ghetto or some rural community. In the latter case, physicians have become so scarce that ones in these areas can get by with surliness, incompetency, and outrageous fees. Not that most physicians practicing under these conditions deliver this kind of care. The vast majority of doctors, no matter what the circumstances, do the best job they can. But some do better jobs than others. It's up to the patient, or potential patient, to figure out who can give the best type of treatment. Probably as soon as you arrive in a given location you should select a general practitioner or internist to act as your family physician. If you need treatment by a specialist, he will recognize it and recommend someone appropriate. But the selection of this internist, general practitioner, or some other specialist you think you need shouldn't be done casually. If there's more than one physician you can use, and if you really have a choice, then make it intelligently. Here are some guidelines:

1. He must have a license to practice medicine in his state. This license is almost always displayed on his office wall.
2. He should be a member of his local professional society and participate in a national program or two, also. Sometimes doctors are excluded from medical society membership for nonprofessional reasons. Sometimes the exclusion has to do with malpractice.
3. He should be a member of the staff of an accredited hospital. Without this membership, physicians can't have patients admitted for treatment without the cooperation of other physicians on the staff.
4. He should seek professional growth through self-education, postgraduate studies, seminars, and the like. Granted, this is hard to check on. But sometimes the information is available.
5. He should have a good reputation in the community. This includes both professional and personal reputation. The professional, of course, is more important; but a doctor known for bad debts, drunken brawls, and wife swapping may not be one you want.
6. He should have a clean and neat office and equipment that seems modern. The office doesn't have to be flashy, but a sloppy desk and waiting room don't create the best impression of work habits and organization.
7. He should have had the kind of residency that provides specialized training in the illness you're having treated. Preferably, he should have passed his board examination and be a diplomate in this area as well.
8. He ought to have the type of personality you want in a doctor. For most people, this means pleasing, wholesome, genuine. Others prefer the rugged individual type. But, in any event, be sure he's the kind of person you can form healthy relationships with and a person you don't mind telling your innermost problems.[23]

The Fight Against Quackery

Isn't anyone doing anything to run these hucksters out of town, to protect our citizenry from the selfish, venal peddlers of misery, incompetence, and false hope? Yes, there are all kinds of organizations working on the problem. But they're a long way from corraling all of the charlatans. There's the Food and Drug Administration, which sets the standards for purity and safety and proper labeling of all drugs and food products that move across state lines.

FIGURE 7-11.

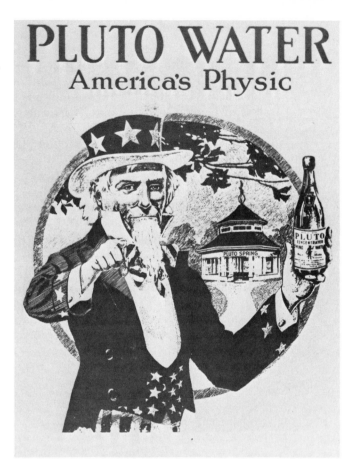

There are innumerable state, county, and city agencies involved in quackery suppression. And the United States Postal Service is strong on preventing and prosecuting mail-order fraud. Also, there are several privately financed organizations fighting the quackery business. There are the better business bureaus, the chambers of commerce, and the Bureau of Investigation of the American Medical Association. These don't have any legal power to regulate or prosecute, but they can bring offenders to the attention of the public and the courts.[24] But, despite these efforts, quackery persists and at times flourishes. Why?

Some blame the quack. This dirty scoundrel may not be too skilled at curing disease or increasing life span, but he certainly knows the tricks of advertising and salesmanship. How can you stop a fellow with a pleasant smile, a clever patter, and big promises? Also, the modern quack has a good knowledge of the legal system and tries not to get too far outside the law. And he usually succeeds. Possibly, there's no way of convicting him. What he did may have been somewhat illegal, but proving it is another thing. And remember the pleasant smile and the disarming manner, and don't forget the profits he's made. There should be more than enough to hire a good lawyer. And if he does get convicted, it's usually just a fine or short jail sentence that he has to deal with. Once he's free, he can change locations and begin his lucrative practice again.

Some blame the courts. Why aren't there stiffer penalties against quackery? And why aren't they enforced?

Some blame our health care system itself. It is cumbersome; it is expensive; it is difficult to get the kind of treatment you'd like without waiting. And, at times, it's a little cold. Maybe the doctor is busy and doesn't have time to explain or listen the way he should. Maybe the nurse brushes by the waiting patient with a formal nod rather than a smile. Maybe the receptionist is more worried about the patient's ability to pay than what his complaint is. Professionals tend to look on health care as a business. And that's exactly what it is. But, possibly, they make it a more callous and self-centered business than it has any right to be.

And there are those who blame the individual for the quackery problem. How can anyone be so stupid as to buy a baldness cure, breast expander, muscle-building wheat germ? Possibly, it's not stupidity at all. Some, maybe all, know that they're being taken. Maybe they want to buy a dream, a hope, or what appears to be a harmless escape from a disappointing and painful world. But the escape isn't always harmless, and the costs can run pretty high.[25] There are other ways to escape that are a lot cheaper and not nearly so dangerous.

Notes

1. Eric Jameson, *The Natural History of Quackery* (Springfield, Ill.: Thomas, 1961).

2. Harry E. Neal, *The Protectors* (New York: Messner, 1968), pp. 66–80.

3. C. J. S. Thompson, *The Quacks of Old London* (Philadelphia: Lippincott, 1971), pp. 19–23.

4. J. H. Young, "The Persistence of Medical Quackery in America," *American Science,* Vol. 60 (May-June 1972), 318–326.

5. James H. Young, *The Medical Messiahs* (Princeton, N.J.: Princeton University Press, 1967), pp. 282–296.

6. L. A. Healy, "Mexicali Treatment of Rheumatoid Arthritis," *Arthritis and Rheumatism,* Vol. 16 (May-June, 1973), 426–427.

7. L. F. Saylor, "California's Cancer Quackery Law," *California Medicine,* Vol. 107 (January 1970), 94–95.

8. Bernard Idson, *Antiobesity Drug Manufacture* (Park Ridge, N.J.: Noyes Data Corporation, 1970).

9. Agnes F. Savill, *The Hair and Scalp* (Baltimore: Williams and Wilkins, 1966), pp. 44–66.

10. Colette Dowling, *The Skin Game* (Philadelphia: Lippincott, 1970), pp. 152–169.

11. Ibid., pp. 13–127.

12. T. Rosebury, "Zen Diets," *Journal of the American Medical Association,* Vol. 218 (December 13, 1971), 1703.

13. H. Bouck, "The Allure of Food Cults and Nutrition Quackery," *Journal of the American Diet Association,* Vol. 57 (October 1970), 316–320.

14. Adelaide Hecktlinger, *The Great Patent Medicine* (New York: Grosset and Dunlap, 1970), pp. 217–234.

15. T. E. Byers, "A Look at Medical Devices," *Proceedings of the Rudolph Virchow Medical Society in the City of New York,* Vol. 24 (1965), 8–14.

16. D. E. Rogers, "Identification of Mountebank Healing Artists," *Journal of School Health,* Vol. 43 (May 1973), 281–283.

17. John Q. Anderson, *Texas Folk Medicine* (Austin, Texas: Encino Press, 1970), pp. 3–91.

18. Sidney Shindell, *Statistics, Science and Sense* (Pittsburgh: University of Pittsburgh Press, 1964), pp. 1–51.

19. "Quackery Persists," *Journal of the American Medical Association,* Vol. 201 (August 21, 1972), 914.

20. *AMA: New and Non–official drugs* (Philadelphia: Lippincott, 1959).

21. *AMA Drug Evaluations* (Chicago: AMA Press, 1971).

22. Harry F. Dowling, *Medicines for Man* (New York: Knopf, 1970), pp. 213–267.

23. Worthington Hooker, *Physician and Patient* (New York: Arno Press, 1972), pp. 172–200.

24. Young, *Medical Messiahs,* pp. 158–191, 390–408.

25. F. B. Hodges, "Public Health Report: The Laetrile Hoax," *California Medicine,* Vol. 118 (June 1973), 78.

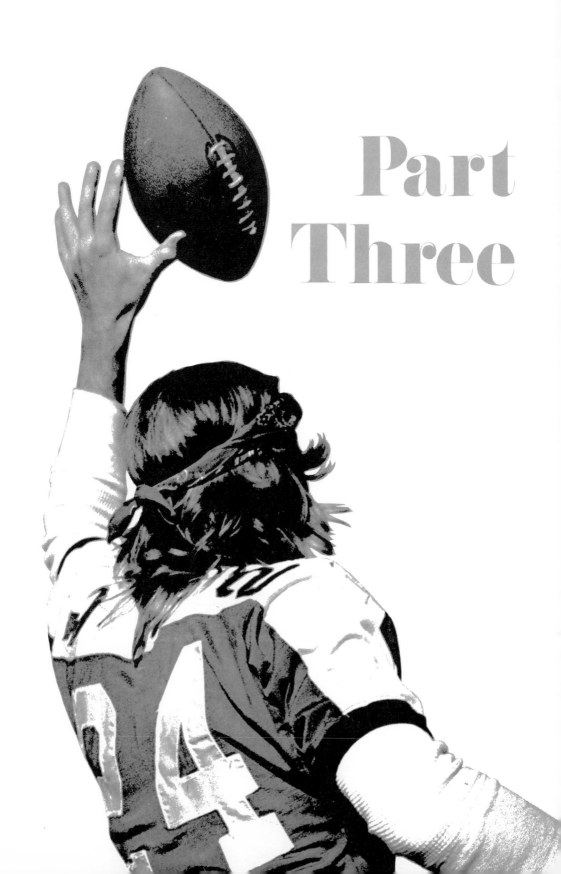

Part Three

Physical
Health

8 Effective Nutrition and Diet

She had the all-American breakfast—a cup of black coffee and a cigarette. She was trying to lose a little weight, and she never really liked breakfast anyway. Around 10 o'clock, though, she got to feeling a little weak. This called for a Coca-Cola and, of course, another cigarette. After all, you need something to pick you up, and this did pick her up. After a few minutes' rest, she felt just fine. By noon, though, she felt starved. What she wouldn't give for a malt, some french fries, and a two-decker hamburger. But she was strong-willed. A lettuce and tomato sandwich was all she needed and was all she got. There was another cigarette, of course. This helped to hold down the appetite and keep that pale, thin appearance. By dinnertime she was nearly ready to cry. Her hands trembled a little, and she had to take a nap before she could get up the energy to shower and change. But was that dinner great! Mashed potatoes, chicken, gravy, creamed onions, and chocolate cake for dessert. She had a second piece of the chocolate cake. Why not? She'd earned it, hadn't she? After all, she'd been dieting all day.

Americans are a well-fed group and a poorly fed group. They eat sensibly, and they eat foolishly. They're well nourished, and they suffer from malnutrition. These statements are common sense, of course. Eating habits vary tremendously—in accordance with food preferences we've learned at home, our economic status, which part of the country we're living in, and food likes and dislikes we've picked up for a thousand unknown reasons.

These preferences in eating habits can contribute to a healthy and vigorous life, a sense of well-being, the impression of strength and vitality. They can make us feel listless, irritable, make us too fat or too skinny, make us look weak or bloated. Poor eating habits can make us ill, produce brain damage, can kill us.

Eating Habits

But certainly Americans have made progress in this area. Twenty years ago, 10 years ago, we didn't have the knowledge we have today about space travel, heart transplants, and food. We know more about vitamins, burning of calories, and the functions of carbohydrates than we ever have. Hasn't this knowledge paid off in better eating habits? Unfortunately, no. The Ameri-

FIGURE 8-1. *It tastes great, but fare like this isn't recommended for a steady diet.*

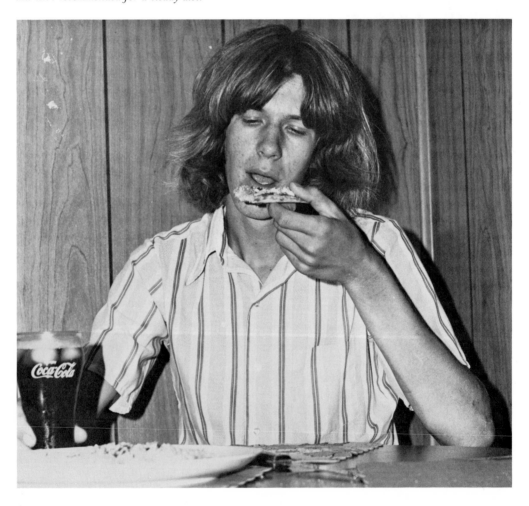

can diet today, according to a recent federal survey, is worse than it was 20 years ago. We've increased our consumption of cake, buns, cream puffs, and other bakery products, except bread. We've upped our consumption of soft drinks, fruit ades, and punches. And we've decreased our consumption of milk, fruits and vegetables, and cereals and flour. About one-fifth of our household diets provide less than two-thirds of one or more of the nutrients we need.

The American teenager has particularly bad eating habits. His diet tends to be low in vitamin A and vitamin C and calcium. Many teenage girls have dietary deficiencies in iron. And a lot of teenagers skip meals, whereas those who don't often don't eat enough fruits and vegetables.[1]

Diet Constituents

This may not sound like a serious situation, and quite often it's not serious. We can become too preoccupied with food, relate all moods, ills, vigor to what we eat. This, of course, is nonsense. Nutrition isn't that precise a discipline, and the human body's demands aren't that specific. But, in the long run, we have to have a balanced diet in order to be healthy or even survive. And although there is a lot of disagreement on what a balanced diet is, authorities agree that it has to include reasonable proportions of the six basic diet constituents: carbohydrates, fats, protein, vitamins, minerals, and water.[2]

Carbohydrates

Carbohydrates supply over 50 per cent of the calories in most American diets. They, along with fats, are what give us big stomachs, double chins, pearlike shapes. They are energy foods, though. Too few of them in the diet can make you feel weak and nervous and tired. Limit them for an extended period of time, and the system suffers a poisoning effect called "acidosis" or "ketosis."

Carbon, hydrogen, and oxygen are what carbohydrates are made of. The elements combine in varying amounts to form sugars or starches, fuel for the body. Most carbohydrates are plant products, but a notable exception is milk sugar, or lactose, which comes from animals.

There are three basic types of carbohydrates: monosaccharides (simple sugars), disaccharides (double sugars), and polysaccharides (many sugar groups per molecule). We can absorb simple sugars directly through the walls of our intestinal tracts, but our digestive systems have to break down the polysaccharides and disaccharides to simple sugars before the absorption can take place. The liver converts these sugars to glucose, which can be utilized by body tissues. If the liver makes more glucose than the body can use, the glucose is converted to glycogen, a form of animal starch, which is stored until needed.

Foods with lots of carbohydrates in them include rice, corn, most grains, potatoes, and anything that tastes sweet, like candy, syrup, and preserves. When we eat too many of these foods, we get more carbohydrates in our systems than our bodies can burn, and the excess is converted to fat. So we start to spread. Of course, everyone is going to eat some carbohydrates and should. But it's a good idea to select foods high in carbohydrate content on the basis of vitamins and minerals they also contain. Whole grain cereals, starchy vegetables, and fruits are examples of foods of this type.[3]

Fats

Fats occur in foods such as whole milk, cheese, olives, nuts, and meat. Margarine, shortening, and butter are almost pure fat. Cooking oils are fats with such low melting points they're liquids at normal ambient temperature.

Fats have a much greater energy content than carbohydrates. The latter yield 4.1 calories per gram, whereas the yield for fats is 9.3. And they not only give us this energy when we eat them, but they also serve as a reservoir for an energy supply to be used at a later time. They play a key role in absorption of fat-soluble vitamins into the blood and are important in the structure of cellular membranes and nerve sheaths.[4]

Protein

Protein is the stuff we and all other animals are made of. Our bodies manufacture this protoplasmic material from building blocks called amino acids. Many kinds of animals get a lot of these acids from eating plants. But the human animal is one that satisfies more of his protein needs by eating other animals. The cow, the hog, and the lamb provide a large part of this essential to the human diet.

Plants synthesize amino acids from nitrogen they've taken from the soil and air. Animals eat the plants and develop a form of protein of their own. So, in a sense, all proteins originate in the plant kingdom. But many proteins don't contain the essential amino acids that animal proteins do. For a healthy diet, at least a third of protein consumption should be of the animal variety.

About 10 to 12 per cent of our diets should consist of protein. Milk contains a lot of this component, and so does liver. Other good sources are beef, fish, poultry, certain types of vegetables like beans and peas, and cheese and eggs. Cottage cheese is a good protein food when you're on a diet. Its carbohydrate and fat content is low, and it's not too expensive.[5]

Vitamins

There were a lot of rats that died before the turn of the century. Scientists had fed them on diets of highly purified carbohydrates, fats, proteins, and minerals. Obviously, the diets were lacking something. It wasn't until 1911 that this something got named by Casimir Funk, a Polish biochemist. He isolated a substance from unpolished rice that prevented beriberi. He called it "vitamine." It was actually a misnomer, based on Funk's incorrect theory that rice compounds contained "amines," chemical substances vital to life. But the name was appealing, and even though the theory was later disproven, the term "vitamin" is still with us.[6]

Vitamins are chemically unrelated substances, which are loosely grouped into a category. They usually don't act alone, but are part of an over-all enzyme system. They're often divided into two groups, those that dissolve in water and those that dissolve in fat. The fat-soluble type are vitamins A, D, E, and K. Most others fall into the water-soluble category.[7]

VITAMIN FUNCTIONS

There are probably more vitamins than there are letters of the alphabet, but only a few have to be considered when planning a balanced diet. There's vitamin A, which builds resistance to bodily infection and improves night vision. There's vitamin C, or ascorbic acid, which prevents scurvy, or mild forms of this disease such as bleeding gums. Vitamin D, the "sunshine vi-tamin," is essential to the body's utilization of calcium and phosphorus. Without enough of it, teeth won't form properly, and children develop bone deformities, restlessness, and potbellies—symptoms of rickets.

There are three important B complex vitamins—thiamine, niacin, and riboflavin. Thiamine (vitamin B_1) plays a key part in the utilization of carbohydrates, maintenance of the appetite, and functioning of the intes-tines. Lack of it can cause beriberi. Riboflavin (vitamin B_2 or G) contributes to the growth process and keeps the mucous membranes functioning ef-ficiently. Niacin prevents pellagra. This is a disease that used to be prevalent among the poor in the South. It brings on skin eruptions, diarrhea, loss of weight, mental depression, and a sore tongue. A steady diet of hominy grits and molasses was the cause of the Southern malady, but the addition of fresh fruits and vegetables has pretty well eliminated the problem.[8]

Some people worry about getting pellagra themselves or worry about rickets or scurvy or beriberi, so they take vitamin pills to assure that they stay in the pink of health. This is nonsense. Any diet that takes in a variety of foods sold in any grocery store will supply all the vitamins you need. They're widely distributed among plant and animal foods, and it's pretty hard not to get enough of them. Sometimes we go on weight-loss diets, though. Taking vitamin pills at this time isn't a bad idea. And sometimes we get sick and run-down and aren't eating as we should. A vitamin supplement can help us to get well and stay that way. But usually you can find all the vitamins you need in milk, egg yolks, lettuce, liver, spinach, green beans, carrots, squash, apricots, and peaches. Meat, fish, and poultry are excellent sources of thia-mine. So are pork, milk, and cereals. Milk, liver, lean meats, carrots, beets, eggs, and peanuts provide riboflavin, and similar types of foods are rich in niacin. There's lots of vitamin C in citrus fruits. And vitamin D comes from the ultraviolet rays of the sun.[9]

VITAMIN EXCESS

Can you get too many vitamins? Yes. Too much vitamin D can make your bones too hard and brittle, and too much vitamin A can stunt a child's bone growth. That's why the FDA has limited the potency of vitamin A and D supplements. But the body rids itself of water-soluble vitamins it doesn't need, so it's almost impossible to get an overdose of vitamin B or C.[10]

185

TABLE 8-1
Fat-Soluble Vitamins

	Deficiency Symptoms	Toxicity Symptoms	Important Sources	Characteristics
Vitamin A (retinol) (carotene precursor)	Night and glare blindness Inflammation of the eye Rough, scaly skin Dry mucous membranes, causing a general lowered resistance to microbe invasion Poor tooth formation	Anorexia Fatigue Weight loss Irritability Skin lesions Joint and bone pains Spleen and liver enlargement Loss of hair Increased intracranial pressure	Liver and liver sausage Butter, cream, whole milk Egg yolks Green and yellow vegetables Yellow fruits Ripe tomatoes Fortified margarine Fish liver oils	Mineral oil interferes with absorption Stable to acid and alkali Destroyed by rancidity Stable to heat by the usual cooking methods but slowly destroyed by exposure to air, heat, drying Stored in the liver Bile is necessary for absorption
Vitamin D (calciferol)	Soft bones Bowed legs Poor teeth Lowered amount of calcium and phosphorus in the blood Poor posture	Anorexia Fatigue Weight loss Nausea and vomiting Diarrhea and polyuria Weakness Headache Renal damage Calcification in the soft tissues of the heart, blood vessels, lungs, stomach, renal tubules	Vitamin D milk Small amounts in butter, egg yolk, liver, saltwater fish Fish liver oils	Stable to heat and oxidation Destroyed by rancidity Skin synthesis by activity of ultraviolet light on cholesterol Stored in the liver Enhances absorption of calcium and phosphorus

Vitamin		Food Sources	Characteristics
Vitamin E (tocopherol)		Vegetable oils Green leafy vege- tables Margarine Egg yolk Milk fat Nuts Wheat germ oil	Stable to light and heat, except deep-fat frying Destroyed by rancidity Destroyed by ultraviolet irradiation Is a strong antioxidant Synthesis in the intestine
Vitamin K	Prolonged clotting time of the blood Hemorrhagic disease in newborn Hyperbilirubinemia In infants: Jaundice Kernicterus Mild hemolytic anemia	Green leafy vege- tables Liver Cauliflower Cabbage	Easily destroyed by light, alkali Synthesis in the intestine Mineral oil interferes

Source: Phyllis Sullivan Howe, *Basic Nutrition in Health and Disease* (Philadelphia: Saunders, 1971), p. 83.

TABLE 8-2
Minerals

	Function	Deficiency Symptoms	Sources
Calcium	Development of strong bones and teeth Help muscles contract and relax normally Utilization of iron Normal blood clotting Maintenance of body neutrality Normal action of heart muscle	Rickets Porous bones Bowed legs Stunted growth Slow clotting of blood Poor tooth formation Tetany	Milk, cheese Mustard, turnip greens Clams, oysters Broccoli, cauliflower, cabbage Molasses Small amount in egg, carrot, celery, orange, grapefruit, figs, and bread made with milk
Phosphorus	Development of bones and teeth Multiplication of cells Activation of some enzymes and vitamins Maintenance of body neutrality Participates in carbohydrate metabolism	Rickets Porous bones Bowed legs Stunted growth Poor tooth formation	Milk Cheese Meat Egg yolk Fish Nuts Whole grain cereals Legumes
Iron	Constituent of hemoglobin, which carries oxygen to the tissues	Nutritional anemia Pallor Weight loss Fatigue Weakness Retarded growth	Red meats, specially liver Green vegetables Yellow fruits Prunes Raisins Legumes Whole grain and enriched cereals Molasses Egg yolk Potatoes

Mineral	Function	Deficiency Symptoms	Sources
Iodine	Constituent of thyroxine, which is a regulator of metabolism	Enlarged thyroid gland Low metabolic rate Stunted growth Retarded mental growth	Iodized salt Seafoods Foods grown in non-goiterous regions
Sodium	Constituent of extracellular fluid Maintenance of body neutrality Osmotic pressure Muscle and nerve irritability	Muscle cramps Weakness Headache Nausea Anorexia Vascular collapse	Sodium chloride (table salt) Sodium bicarbonate (baking powder, baking soda) Monosodium glutamate (Accent) Milk, cheese Meat, egg white
Fluorine	Resistance to dental caries Deposition of bone calcium		Water supply containing 1 ppm Small amount in many foods
Potassium	Acid-base balance Carbohydrate metabolism Conduction of nerve impulses Contraction of muscle fibers	Apathy Muscular weakness Poor gastrointestinal tone Respiratory muscle failure Tachycardia Cardiac arrest	Whole grains Meat Legumes Some fruit and vegetables

Source: Phyllis Sullivan Howe, *Basic Nutrition in Health and Disease* (Philadelphia: Saunders, 1971), p. 83.

Minerals

About 4 per cent of what we're made up of is inorganic minerals. In most of us there's enough iron to make a nail, enough sodium to fill a salt shaker. These minerals regulate our metabolism. There are 14 of them we need for nutrition, but only three are likely to be lacking in the American diet—calcium, iron, and iodine. When these elements are present in the foods we eat, the other 11 elements are usually present, also.

Calcium, which is plentiful in milk and shellfish, plays a key role in the growth and development of bones and teeth. It's also essential to the clotting of blood and helps to regulate the heart beat. Adequate intake during a lifetime helps prevent osteoporosis, a major bone problem of the old.

Phosphorus is prevalent in many foods, particularly those that contain calcium. Usually, if a person has an adequate calcium intake, there's an adequate phosphorus intake as well. Like calcium, phosphorus contributes to the bony development of the body. It also plays a key role in carbohydrate and fat metabolism.

Iron is plentiful in liver and other meats. We don't require much of it, only about 18 milligrams a day. But often we don't get as much as we should. Iron deficiency anemia is quite common. And iron plays an essential part in blood and blood-forming organs. Without it, our red blood cells couldn't transport oxygen.

Iodine is artificially added to common table salt and is a natural constituent of seafood. The thyroid gland needs it to manufacture thyroxine.

Another element found in common table salt is sodium. This, along with potassium, helps maintain the body's water balance.

Like vitamins, minerals are found in all types of common foods. A good variety of them provide all the minerals we need, and no artificial supplements are necessary.[11]

The Balanced Diet

All of us have different nutritional needs. A sedate great-grandmother in a nursing home obviously doesn't burn as much energy as a marathon runner. The girl who's bedridden with a broken leg won't want to eat the same things as her cheerleading sister. Our food requirements vary with our age, sex, size, and physical activity. Someone might have too many or too few hormones or enzymes or a biological quirk that keeps him from using nutrients in the same way most other people do. There's the diabetic who can't properly metabolize sugar. And there are people who have a tendency to be fat, even though most overweight people don't have genetic problems of this type. A well-balanced diet for one person isn't necessarily a well-balanced diet for someone else. But, in most cases, we should eat reasonable amounts of the following four food groups: milk and milk products; meat, eggs, and foods generally high in protein; fruits and vegetables; breads and cereals. Select foods from these four groups in the right proportion, and you'll get all the fats, vitamins, proteins, carbohydrates, and minerals you need.

A simple way to eat wisely is to eat a wide variety of common foods.

TABLE 8-3
A Recommended Daily Food Pattern

Foundation Foods

1. Milk group:	3 or more glasses* milk—children
	4 or more glasses milk—teenagers
	2 or more glasses milk—adults
	3 or more glasses milk—pregnant women
	4 or more glasses milk—nursing mothers
	Cheese, ice cream, and other milk-made foods can supply part of the milk
2. Meat group:	2 or more servings†
	Lean meats, fish, poultry, eggs, cheese, with dry beans, dry peas, nuts, as alternates
3. Vegetable-fruit group:	4 or more servings‡
	A dark green or deep yellow vegetable at least every other day
	Citrus fruit or other vitamin C-rich sources daily
	Other fruits and vegetables
4. Bread-cereals group:	4 or more servings§
	Enriched, whole grain, or restored

Foundation Foods form the nucleus for good daily meals. Use more than the minimum choices offered—in quantity and quality—to insure nutritional adequacy.

Additional Foods

Add fats, sweets, unenriched cereals, and flavorings within the limits of individual calorie needs to round out meals in food nutrients and in variety, flavor, and satiety value.

Provide vitamin D during the growth cycle (childhood, pregnancy, lactation) to supply 400 IU daily. This amount is furnished by 1 quart of vitamin D milk.

* 1 glass milk: 1 cup; 8 oz (½ pt).
† Meats: approximately 3 oz, cooked.
‡ Vegetables, cooked: ½ cup. Fruits, raw: units, as one medium-sized orange.
§ Bread: 1 slice. Cooked cereal: ⅔ cup. Ready-to-eat cereal: 1 oz, about 1 cup.

Source: Ethel Martin, *Nutrition in Action* (New York: Holt, Rinehart and Winston, 1965), p. 182.

Don't eat just one kind of meat and avoid a certain kind of vegetable. Eat a little of everything, and broaden your food tastes as much as possible. The odds are you'll solve any nutritional problem that might arise.[12]

Weight Control

When we eat food, our bodies burn it in a chemical reaction that brings on heat and energy. This is where the "calorie" enters the picture. This is the amount of heat that's needed to raise 1 gram of water 1 degree Centigrade in temperature. This is a very small unit of heat, so nutritionists use the "kilocalorie," a thousand times greater. But the term "calorie" has become the one that's commonly used, the "kilo-" having been dropped.[13]

Everything being equal, which it never is, the more calories in the food we eat, the heavier we get. Foods vary tremendously in the number of calories they contain. A given weight of candy bar has more calories than the same weight of boiled eggs. There are more calories in a cup of chocolate milk than a cup of black coffee. So a person who eats a lot of calorie-rich

TABLE 8-4
The Calorie Content in Some Favorite Foods and Drinks

Breakfast	Calories	Drinks	Calories
1 scrambled egg	110	Whole milk, 1 cup	160
2 slices fried bacon	100	Nonfat milk, 1 cup	90
Ham, slice, lean and fat	245	Malted milk, 1 cup	280
1 wheat pancake	60	Cocoa, 1 cup	235
1 waffle	210	Orange juice, frozen, 1 cup	
Grapefruit, ½ whole	55	diluted	110
Cantaloupe, ½ melon	60	Apple juice, 1 cup	120
Corn flakes, 1 oz	110	Grape juice, canned, 1 cup	165
Oatmeal, 1 cup	130	Yoghurt, 1 cup	120
White bread, 1 slice	60	Cola drink, 1 cup	95
Butter, 1 pat	50	Ginger ale, 1 cup	70
Jam, 1 tablespoon	55	Beer, 1 cup	100

Lunch or Dinner	Calories	Snacks	Calories
Tomato soup, 1 cup	90	Cheddar cheese, 1-inch cube	70
Spaghetti, meatballs, and		Bologna, 1 slice	85
tomato sauce, 1 cup	335	Peanut butter, 1 tablespoon	95
Pork chop, 1 slice lean	130	Peanuts, roasted, 1 cup	840
Roast beef, 1 slice lean	125	10 potato chips	115
Hamburger, meat only, 3 oz	245	Raisins, dried, 1 cup	460
1 frankfurter, cooked	155	1 apple	70
Chicken, ½ breast	155	1 banana	85
Mashed potatoes, buttered,		1 orange, navel	60
1 cup	185	1 peach	35
Pizza, 1 section	185	Watermelon, 1 wedge	115
Cottage cheese, creamed,		Popcorn, 1 cup	65
1 cup	240	2 graham crackers	55
Custard, 1 cup	285	1 doughnut, cake type	125
Angelfood cake, 1 section	110	Candy, milk chocolate, 1 oz	150
Iced chocolate cake,		Marshmallows, 1 oz	150
1 section	445	Pretzels, 5 small sticks	20
Apple pie, 1 section	345	1 fig bar	55
Ice cream, 1 cup	285	1 cookie, 3-inch	120
Sherbet, orange, 1 cup	260	Cornstarch pudding, 1 cup	275

Source: Nutritive Value of Foods, Home and Garden Bulletin No. 72, rev. ed. Washington, D.C.: U.S. Department of Agriculture, September 1964.

food, or even a lot of food containing a modest number of calories, is running the risk of building his calorie intake beyond his capacity to utilize them. So the nutrients get stored in the form of fat, and the waistline begins to grow.

There's a healthy weight each of us should maintain. Sex, height, and bone structure, in most cases, determine what this weight should be. And, if we exceed it by up to 20 per cent, we're considered "overweight." We become "obese" when we're more than 20 per cent heavier than the ideal. Of course, there's the football player or wrestler who's overweight because of his excess of muscle. But most overweight and obese people are just plain fat.[14]

WEIGHT PSYCHOLOGY

A lot of people think of the fat person as jolly, rolypoly, and self-confident. In most cases, this just isn't so. The majority of overweight people are anxious people who are using food as some kind of tranquilizer. Sometimes their food anxieties developed in their childhood. If they were good children, they got candy and popcorn and fruit. If they were bad, they were sent to bed without dessert.

There are people who look on food as a love substitute, some kind of consolation prize in life. A boy has a case of acne and can't get a date, so he takes up chocolate sundaes. Some people look on foods as defensive or offensive weapons. They armor themselves against a hostile world by eating so much they can't be pushed around. But they refuse to think of themselves as overweight; they're really bursting with health and strength. A lot of the problem of weight control is psychosomatic. There aren't any pills, drugs, or exercise machines that will effortlessly "remove pounds of unsightly fat." There's no way of maintaining an ideal weight that isn't tied to individual will power and a healthy attitude toward life.[15]

LOSING WEIGHT

It's really simple. If you take in more calories than you burn, you gain weight. When your output is greater than your intake, you lose weight. Nothing could be more basic—or more tedious. A diet can test the soul of the noblest of Christians.

The first step is figuring out how many calories you burn. These vary with how old you are, your sex, weight, job, and hobbies. The male student who spends his spare time reading and watching TV probably burns around 2,500 calories a day. If he goes out for football, he'll use 5,000 calories on the day of a game or tough practice session. The female student uses around 2,100 calories a day, assuming she doesn't have an outside job. If she pays for her tuition by waiting on tables, she can burn 3,000 calories or more. These are estimates, of course. They vary with the situation and the individual.

The next step is figuring out how many calories you're taking in. One pound of protein or carbohydrates will yield 1,814 calories, whereas 1 pound of fat yields 4,082. Equal amounts of carbohydrates and proteins yield the same number of calories whereas an equal amount of fat yields $2\frac{1}{4}$ times as many. Using this concept as a general guide and checking the information in a calorie chart can give you a pretty good idea of how many calories go down your throat each day. If this seems to be less than calories you're burning, the pounds should start disappearing. If your weight doesn't go down, and losing weight is what you want, lower the calorie intake a little, increase your activities, or do both.[16]

For a simple guideline to this diet, check what your desirable weight should be from the weight chart (Table 8-5). Multiply this weight by 13 if you lead a slow and kind of lazy life. Multiply by 15 if you're fairly active, by 17 if you're the "make way for me" type. This will give you the number of

TABLE 8-5
Desirable Weights
(Weight in Pounds According to Frame, in Indoor Clothing)

Men of Ages 25 and Over	*Height (with Shoes on) 1-Inch Heels*		*Small Frame*	*Medium Frame*	*Large Frame*
	Feet	*Inches*			
	5	2	112-120	118-129	126-141
	5	3	115-123	121-133	129-141
	5	4	118-126	124-136	132-148
	5	5	121-129	127-139	135-152
	5	6	124-133	130-143	138-156
	5	7	128-137	134-147	142-161
	5	8	132-141	138-152	147-166
	5	9	136-145	142-156	151-170
	5	10	140-150	146-160	155-174
	5	11	144-154	150-165	159-179
	6	0	148-158	154-170	164-184
	6	1	152-162	158-175	168-189
	6	2	156-167	162-180	173-194
	6	3	160-171	167-185	178-199
	6	4	164-175	172-190	182-204

Women of Ages 25 and Over	*Height (with Shoes on) 2-Inch Heels*		*Small Frame*	*Medium Frame*	*Large Frame*
	Feet	*Inches*			
	4	10	92-98	96-107	104-119
	4	11	94-101	98-110	106-122
	5	0	96-104	101-113	109-125
	5	1	99-107	104-116	112-128
	5	2	102-119	107-119	115-131
	5	3	105-113	110-122	118-134
	5	4	108-116	113-126	121-138
	5	5	111-119	116-130	125-142
	5	6	114-123	120-135	129-146
	5	7	118-127	124-139	133-150
	5	8	122-131	128-143	137-154
	5	9	126-135	132-147	141-158
	5	10	130-140	136-151	145-163
	5	11	134-144	140-155	149-168
	6	0	138-148	144-159	153-173

For girls between 18 and 25, subtract 1 pound for each year under 25.

Source: Four Steps to Weight Control (Metropolitan Life Insurance Company, August 1967).

calories you should swallow daily to maintain this ideal weight. If you want to lose weight, cut the calories by 20 per cent to 25 per cent.[17]

A lot of people don't like to count calories, so they use the fraction system for losing weight. What they do is eat what they want three times a day, but eat only half or three-fourths or one-fourth of what they'd normally consume. This is an excellent diet for people who eat out a lot or have an active social life. You can't always refuse rich desserts or tell your hostess not to serve you mashed potatoes and fried chicken. But you don't have to take second helpings, and you can take small portions the first time around.[18]

Another diet, yet, that takes the pounds off fast is restricting what you eat to meat, dairy products, fruits and vegetables, and cereal grains. You can't have snacks, alcoholic beverages, desserts, gravy, butter, mayonnaise, and the like.[19] The big trouble with a diet of this type is that it gets boring. And there's a temptation to go on a "calorie binge" the minute you come off it. When you lose weight quickly, you often gain it back just as quickly when the diet is over.

STICKING TO A DIET

Here are some ideas that make sticking to that diet a little easier:

1. Drink a lot of water. Drink it before meals, during meals, after meals, anytime you feel hungry. While it won't completely kill your hunger, it gives you that "full" feeling.
2. Don't get too good a look or too deep a smell of tasty foods. Overcoming temptation can build will power, but giving in to it builds big waistlines.
3. Eat slowly. Rushing through your meal makes it seem like you haven't had much, no matter how big the meal was.
4. Don't let the hunger pangs get ravenous. Give in to them every so often and nibble on some low-calorie, high-bulk foods. There are raw carrots, lettuce, and celery that you can eat freely. The same applies to cucumbers, onions, pickles, salad greens, parsley, and green peppers. And you can drink all the coffee and tea you like, as long as it doesn't have any sugar or cream in it. If you feel you have to have some sugar, try the natural kind—apples or honeydew melon or watermelon. And if you crave bread, try a slice of melba toast or a couple of rye wafers.
5. Go light on salt. It helps you retain water and makes weight loss difficult.
6. Keep a positive attitude. Ninety per cent of accomplishing anything is knowing you can do it. Losing weight is no exception.
7. Weigh yourself twice a week. Don't do it every day. This can get too discouraging. You don't lose weight on a steady basis, and some days you even gain a little. A twice-a-week weighing will give you an honest picture of your progress and keep the frustration at a minimum. Always weigh at the same time of the day, using the same scale, wearing the same amount of clothes.[20]

EXERCISE

There's an argument that exercise in no way helps you to lose weight. After all, you have to walk for 1 hour and 37 minutes to burn off the calories in a milk shake—or ride a bicycle for 61 minutes or swim for 45. Who has that kind of time or energy? And while you're doing all this exercise, you're building an appetite that makes you want more milk shakes, chicken dinners, and pizzas. This argument implies that you have to burn your calories all at once. This just isn't so. Few people are going to take a 97-minute walk or a 26-minute run. But you can take a 15-minute walk or a 5- or 10-minute run and make a dent in that potbelly. If you do this regularly, the effects of the exercise accumulate. And as to building appetite, this doesn't

TABLE 8-6
Burning off Those Extra Calories

Food	Calories	Walking*	Riding bicycle†	Swimming‡	Running§	Reclining‖
Apple, large	101	19	12	9	5	78
Bacon, 2 strips	96	18	12	9	5	74
Banana, small	88	17	11	8	4	68
Beer, 1 glass	114	22	14	10	6	88
Bread and butter	78	15	10	7	4	60
Cake, 2-layer, $\frac{1}{12}$	356	68	43	32	18	274
Carbonated beverage, 1 glass	106	20	13	9	5	82
Carrot, raw	42	8	5	4	2	32
Cereal, dry, $\frac{1}{2}$ cup with milk, sugar	200	38	24	18	10	154
Cheese, cheddar, 1 oz	111	21	14	10	6	85
Chicken, fried, $\frac{1}{2}$ breast	232	45	28	21	12	178
Cookie, plain	15	3	2	1	1	12
Cookie, chocolate chip	51	10	6	5	3	39
Doughnut	151	29	18	13	8	116
Egg, fried	110	21	13	10	6	85
Halibut steak, $\frac{1}{4}$ lb	205	39	25	18	11	158
Ham, 2 slices	167	32	20	15	9	128
Ice cream, $\frac{1}{6}$ qt	193	37	24	17	10	148
Ice cream soda	255	49	31	23	13	196
Malted milk shake	502	97	61	45	26	386
Milk, 1 glass	166	32	20	15	9	128
Milk, skim, 1 glass	81	16	10	7	4	62
Orange, medium	68	13	8	6	4	52
Orange juice, 1 glass	120	23	15	11	6	92
Pancake with syrup	124	24	15	11	6	95
Peach, medium	46	9	6	4	2	35
Pie, apple, $\frac{1}{6}$	377	73	46	34	19	290
Pizza, cheese, $\frac{1}{8}$	180	35	22	16	9	138
Pork chop, loin	314	60	38	28	16	242
Potato chips, 1 serving	108	21	13	10	6	83
Club sandwich	590	113	72	53	30	454
Hamburger sandwich	350	67	43	31	18	269
Tuna salad sandwich	278	53	34	25	14	214
Sherbet, $\frac{1}{6}$ qt	177	34	22	16	9	136
Shrimp, french fried	180	35	22	16	9	138
Spaghetti, 1 serving	396	76	48	35	20	305
Steak, T-bone	235	45	29	21	12	181
Strawberry shortcake	400	77	49	36	21	308

* Energy cost of walking for 150-pound individual = 5.2 calories per minute at 3.5 mph.
† Energy cost of riding bicycle = 8.2 calories per minute.
‡ Energy cost of swimming = 11.2 calories per minute.
§ Energy cost of running = 19.4 calories per minute.
‖ Energy cost of reclining = 1.3 calories per minute.

Source: F. Konishi, "Food Energy Equivalents of Various Activities," *Journal of the American Dietetic Association*, Vol. 46 (1965), 186.

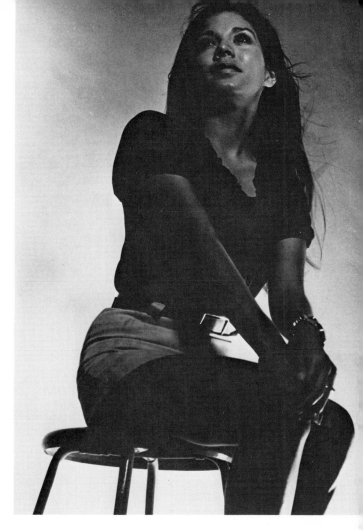

FIGURE 8-2. *A winner in the exercise and diet contest.*

hold over an extended period. Hunger increases at the beginning of any exercise program, but the appetite quickly adjusts. You eat no more food, or often less, than you did before the exercise program started. Also, exercise helps to redistribute body weight, gives your skin a firm and healthy appearance.

Most people don't go on diets to avoid coronaries or strokes. They want to look better, and they're convinced that taking off a few pounds will help—which it can. But in most cases, exercise, even a small amount of it, will have more effect on the double chin, sagging belly, and rounded shoulders than counting calories will. People get discouraged on weight-loss diets because they find themselves looking worse, not better. There are the sickly pallor, hanging skin, hollow eyes to contend with. And there are friends who ask how you're feeling, parents who want you to see a doctor. Exercise won't completely overcome these problems, but it can keep them at a minimum and give you the morale to stay on that diet a little longer.[21]

Food for the Heart

Most people don't worry about their hearts until they get in their 40s, or at least their 30s. After all, of the 600,000 people who died from coronaries last year, most of these were over 65. Many begin thinking about heart problems when social security checks arrive. This can be a mistake, a very painful, even a deadly one. Nikolai Anichkov, a Russian pathologist, pointed this out

TABLE 8-7
Cholesterol Content of Foods

Food	Mg per 100 g	Food	Mg per 100 g
Beef, heart	140	cod	46
kidney	350	crab	125
liver	250	haddock	64
roast, chuck	55	halibut	33
rump	58	herring	75
round steak	68	lobster	200
tallow	56	mackerel	80
tripe	150	oysters	161
Brain, calf	1810	perch	63
Caviar	290	pike	71
Cheese, American process	87	salmon	55
Bleu	157	sardine	70
Cheddar	98	scallops	166
Cream	140	shrimp	161
Cottage cheese		sole	20
creamed	15	trout	57
dry	1	tuna	57
Emmentaler	130	Lamb, chops	66
Gouda	33	Lard	95
Limburger	92	Pork, chops	55
Mozzarella		ham	42
(part skim)	61	tenderloin and Canadian	
Parmesan	74	bacon	57
Roquefort	73	Sweetbreads (thymus)	280
Swiss	91	Turkey, dark	96
Chicken, dark	76	light	61
light	54	Veal, brains	1810
Duck	70	flesh	71
Fish, carp	490	kidney	350
clams	118	liver	350

Food	Mg per Serving	Food	Mg per Serving
Butter, 1 tsp	10	Mayonnaise, 1 tbsp	15
Cereal	0	Milk, 1 cup whole	35
Cream, 1 tbsp	18	1 cup skim	1
Egg, 1 yolk	240	1 cup fortified	
1 white	0	skim (less than 0.5%	
Fruits	0	butterfat)	6
Ice cream, ½ cup	30–45	Peanut butter	0
Ice milk, ½ cup	17	Sherbet, ½ cup	3
Margarine, vegetable fat	0	Vegetables	0
65% animal fat	70	Vegetable oils	0

Source: Phyllis Sullivan Howe, *Basic Nutrition in Health and Disease* (Philadelphia: Saunders, 1971), p. 358.

in 1913. He fed some rabbits diets heavy in cholesterol and animal fat and found they developed atherosclerosis. This is a condition that leads to hardening of the arteries, which in turn leads to coronary problems. Other researchers have duplicated Anichkov's findings in other animals, as well as in humans. They found that people living in countries where a lot of saturated fats were consumed (apparently, unsaturated fats don't increase blood cholesterol levels) have a higher rate of heart disease than those from countries that go light on the fats. The average person in Finland gets 22 per cent of his calories from saturated fats, and Finish people have a heart disease rate of 120 per thousand. Americans get 17 per cent of their calories from saturated fats, and their heart disease rate is 80 per thousand. The Japanese have a heart disease rate of only 20 per thousand, and only 3 per cent of their calories are in this saturated fat category. This is merely circumstantial evidence, of course, and in no way proves that fatty diets or fat people are more prone to having heart trouble than people who stay slender and go easy on the cholesterol. There are many factors that contribute to heart disease, such as smoking, stress, lack of exercise, hypertension, and obesity. Diet seems to affect this crippling and killing problem, though, and it's best to give it some thought before trouble develops.[22]

Diet During Pregnancy

Many doctors used to recommend that women not gain more than 14 pounds during pregnancy. They felt this made the delivery easier on both mother and child and helped both to recover quickly from birth trauma. But the National Research Council has begun to question this advice. The United States ranked twelfth among 40 countries in the number of children who die at birth. Could the restricted diets of America's future mothers have something to do with this? The Council now recommends that weight gain during pregnancy be increased to an average of 24 pounds. They emphasize that severe weight-reduction programs should be avoided by all pregnant women, particularly teenagers and those who are underweight to begin with.[23]

Also, some recent studies have shown that pregnant women with seriously deficient diets pass on malnutrition to their unborn children. In some cases, the babies literally starve to death in the womb. And infants from low-income families normally weigh 12 to 15 per cent less than those from families that have a more nutritious diet. Even the organs of these lower-income-family infants seem stunted. Apparently, no one has a greater stake in the nutrition field than the girl who's about to give birth.[24]

Nutrition Myths

This is the day of antipollution devices on cars; the court case against the industrialist who pollutes streams; and the "back to nature cereal" that hasn't had all the vitamins and minerals removed by some money-hungry manufacturer. It's kind of an occult, spiritual movement, this ecology thing. It has the militancy of old-time religion, the fervor of profootball's final quarter. In this ugly, technically monstrous, self-seeking, capitalistic machine we live in, can't we find a bucolic piece of grandma's apple pie and buttermilk? It is a tempting dream, an all-encompassing one, substituting the entrepreneural country store for the supermarket, the small farm for organization-man bureaucracy, the gentle rhythm of Old Dobbin for the frantic dashes and jam-ups of the speedway, lemonade in the front parlor for the cigarette and six-pack at the drive-in movie. And one of the key elements of this dream is natural, tasty, truly healthful food, in place of the imitation, flavorless, vitaminless, mineralless mush we cram down our throats during late breakfasts and 15-minute lunch hours.

Although this kind of thinking is great for bringing on relaxation and sleep, it has a couple of shortcomings in the reality area. Grandmother wasn't really as hard working, as noble, as worry free, as healthy, or nearly as good a cook as romantics portray her. Sassafras tea was her spring tonic, and it's been shown that this produces cancer in the small intestines of rats, so you can't buy it anymore. Butter, if it wasn't rancid, tasted pretty good, but was a lot higher in saturated fats than the artificial stuff we use. The raw milk she served carried the risk of tuberculosis, undulant fever, and staphylococcal food poisoning.[25]

There are an unlimited number of theories, claims, and half-truths associated with nutrition. "You are what you eat," "Look younger—live longer," "Healthy food for a healthy mind," "Food for sexual growth." Diet has been guaranteed to cure old age, baldness, impotence, timidity, bad breath, and just plain ugliness. But the truth is that nutrition is a mighty loose science. No one knows exactly what happens to things we swallow into our bodies. And no one is quite sure what effect any one element will have on muscular development, neural efficiency, bowel habits, and mental health. There are lots of foods that are good for us, possibly certain ones that meet our individual needs better than others. But no one has figured out a way to deal with such a complex problem. So it's best to eat a wide variety of foods that you enjoy, that you know are generally healthful, and avoid fad diets that make you "master of your universe," "the tiger of Middlewest U."[26]

There are health food zealots who are sure that black strap molasses prevents cancer, cures varicose veins, ulcers, and arthritis. And there are zealots who are strong on rose hip or acerola-berry jam. This gives them their vitamin C. And others go for wheat germ, vitamin E, apple cider vinegar, and yoghurt. These things don't have a thing to do with improving your health, you say? You must be a member of the "medical trust."

And there's the "organic" food fad with its phobia against chemicals. Devotees of this cult are convinced that chemical pesticides and chemical fertilizers are slowly poisoning the American public. So they bring on high crop yields and keep food prices from inflating out of price range? Who cares? We're better off to pay extra for the fruits and vegetables fertilized with animal manure, according to them. These have the "natural" vitamins, the kind you don't find in foods fertilized with potash, phosphates, and inorganic nitrates. This just isn't so. Organic elements in the soil have to be broken down into inorganic elements before they can enter the plants. It doesn't make a bit of difference whether the organic substances are natural or synthetic. Mother Nature treats them the same, and the plant doesn't know the difference.

There have been some ridiculous fears of chemicals that have brought on unfortunate effects. There are some communities in the Midwest that won a battle against companies making table salt. They had found that the salt was treated with iodine, and they successfully forced the producers to eliminate this "artificial chemical treatment." Now several people in these communities suffer from thyroid problems and have disfiguring goiters because of iodine deficiencies in their diets. There are communities that have fought hard against the "poisoning effects" of fluoride in drinking water. Those that won have young people with an unusually high number of cavities in their teeth.[27]

The ecology movement has its place. It's made us conscious of some tragic abuses of our environment and some dangers we face in the destruction of beauty, health, even life. But any philosophy carried to extreme can do more harm than good. The same applies to nutrition. We should be aware of the benefits of a balanced and sensible diet, but food prices are high enough these days. There's no reason to pay extra for "health" foods or dietary supplements. They're of dubious value, if not worthless.

Notes

1. Anne Burgess, *Malnutrition and Food Habits* (New York: Macmillan, 1962), pp. 3–19.
2. Albert T. Simeons, *Food: Facts, Foibles and Fables* (New York: Funk and Wagnalls, 1968), pp. 105–141.
3. Frank Dickens, *Carbohydrate Metabolism and Its Disorders* (New York: Academic Press, 1968).
4. Lester M. Morrison, *The Low–Fat Way to Health and Longer Life* (Englewood Cliffs, N.J.: Prentice-Hall, 1959), pp. 13–25.
5. K. F. Mattel, "The Functional Requirements of Proteins for Foods," *Journal of the American Oil Chemists Society*, Vol. 48 (September 1971), 477–480.
6. Stanley F. Dyke, *The Chemistry of Vitamins* (New York: Interscience, 1965).
7. H. F. De Luca and J. W. Suttie, *The Fat–Soluble Vitamins* (Madison, Wis.: University of Wisconsin Press, 1970).
8. William H. Sebrell, *The Vitamins* (New York: Academic Press, 1967), pp. 1–7.
9. Marie V. Krause, *Food, Nutrition and Diet Therapy* (Philadelphia: Saunders, 1961), pp. 108–117.
10. V. Reddy, et al., "Urinary Excretion of Lysosomal Enzymes in Hypovitaminosis and Hypervitaminosis A in Children," *International Journal of Vitamin and Nutrition Research*, Vol. 41 (1971), 321–326.
11. Isadore Zipkin, *Biological Mineralization* (New York; Wiley, 1973).
12. W. Merty, "Human Requirements: Basic and Optimal," *Annals of the New York Academy of Sciences*, Vol. 199 (June 28, 1972), 191–201.
13. P. Webb, "Metabolism Heat Balance Data for 24-Hour Periods," *International Journal of Biometeorology*, Vol. 15 (December 1971), 151–155.
14. Joseph I. Goodman, *Diet and Live* (Cleveland: World Publishers, 1966), pp. 153–160.
15. E. E. Abramson, "Anxiety, Fear and Eating," *Journal of Abnormal Psychology*, Vol. 79 (June 1972), 317–321.

16. Goodman, *Diet and Live,* pp. 139–192.
17. Dorothea Turner, *Handbook of Diet Therapy* (Chicago: University of Chicago Press, 1970), pp. 12–19.
18. Ibid., pp. 3–11.
19. Clara-Beth Young Bond, et al., *Low Fat Cholesterol Diet* (Garden City, N.Y.: Doubleday, 1971), pp. 8–24.
20. L. S. Levitz, "Behavior Therapy in Treating Obesity," *Journal of the American Dietetic Association,* Vol. 52 (January 1973), 22–26.
21. M. M. Kenrick, "Exercise and Weight Reduction in Obesity," *Archives of Physical Medicine and Rehabilitation,* Vol. 53 (July 1972), 323–327.
22. V. F. Froelieber, Jr., "The Dietary Prevention of Atherosclerosis," *Alabama Journal of Medical Sciences,* Vol. 9 (April 1972), 137–142.
23. H. N. Jacobson, "Nutrition and Pregnancy," *Journal of the American Dietetic Association,* Vol. 60 (January 1972), 26–29.
24. J. Smibert, "Weight Reduction and Pregnancy," *Medical Journal of Australia,* Vol. 1 (March 4, 1972), 494.
25. Gerald N. Wogan, *Mycotoxins in Foodstuffs* (Cambridge, Mass.: MIT Press, 1964).
26. Earl W. McHenry, *Foods Without Fads* (Philadelphia: Lippincott, 1960), pp. 14–21.
27. A. J. Snider, "Beware of Back-to-Nature Fads," *Science Digest,* Vol. 72 (September 1972), 48.

9

Building a Healthy Body

We're a bunch of soft, weak men and wheezing, shapeless women, we Americans. We look 10 years older than we are, often feel 20 years older, and think and dream with early senile inefficiency. Run? The average woman, in low heels or high, couldn't make it half the length of a city block. The average man might finish the block, but it would take him the rest of the morning to recover from the ordeal. The same applies to climbing a few flights of stairs or swimming a few hundred yards. Americans, young or old, male or female, Black or White, are in terrible physical condition.

This comment doesn't apply, of course, to Jim Ryun, Johnny Bench, and Roger Staubach. Today's athletes are in far better condition than their gladiator ancestors were or yesterday's rugged individuals. But they represent only a minute fraction of the fat, fatigued, and headachy Americans. The majority of us enter athletic contests in Walter Mitty dreams only, exercise by turning the TV set to Sunday's pro football contest or walking to the refrigerator for a beer and sandwich.

Youth, of course, is the exception. When you're 18, you can run marathons, rip telephone books, get by on 2 hours' sleep. To some extent, this is true. There's no exercise program in the world that completely compensates for aging, can make someone who's 48 look and feel like he's 28. Youth is as precious a gift as we ever get—something that can make the world a brass band parade, a pheasant picnic. But to get the most out of being young you

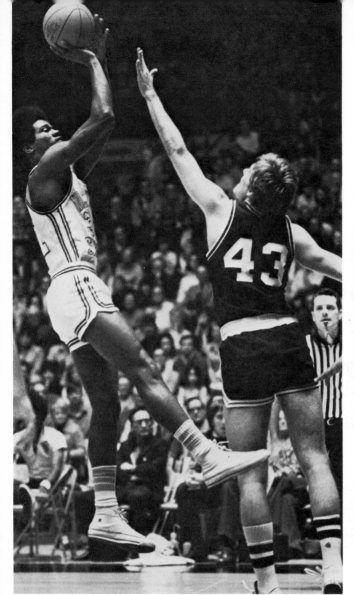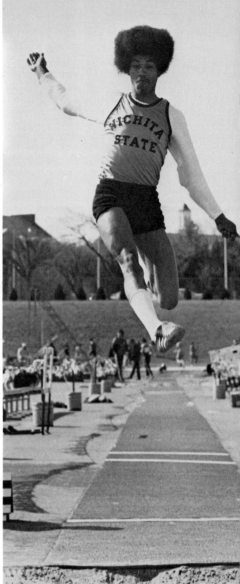

FIGURE 9-1. *Today's gladiators.*

have to feel young. There are teenagers who look, think, and act as though they're in their 40s. There are people in their 20s starting to slow down because of the strains of that "jungle world." This is a shame. There's a kind of fun and excitement that only young people can experience. And when they pass it by, they never get a second chance. The teenager has to work at being his age, just as the middle-aged professor does.[1]

Being Fit

What is physical fitness? There's no precise definition of it, no exact way of measuring it. Being in condition to some is the ability to climb a flight of stairs without getting out of breath. To others, it's running the mile in less than 4 minutes. Another way of looking at it involves our ability to produce energy. Everything we do requires energy, of course. And we get the energy from food and oxygen. The food you can store. Eat more than you need, which too many of us do, and your body stores the excess for a later day. But it doesn't work this way with oxygen. We have to breathe every minute of our lives in order to keep the oxygen flowing into our systems. When we stop breathing, life is over.

For people who aren't poverty stricken, there's not much of a problem in getting the food. And oxygen in the air is free and plentiful. The problem comes when we have to get the oxygen to the parts of our bodies where the food gets burned. Without the oxygen, energy isn't produced.

For most of us, most of the time, this energy production is no problem. We can talk, think, read, or watch TV or a movie with no concern whatever. But when our activities get more vigorous, we have our own private energy crisis. Each of us has his maximum energy capacity—the maximum amount of energy his body can produce by getting oxygen to his tissues. The difference between this maximum capacity and normal energy requirements is the measure of physical fitness. People in the best condition have the widest spread. People with the flabby bellies and the wheezing coughs have the thinnest spread. Sometimes the minimum energy requirement and maximum capacity are identical.[2]

Hypokinetic Diseases

Physiologists have measured the maximum amount of oxygen a person can take into his body. This is called "aerobic capacity" and is used as an indicator of overall physical fitness. People with a high aerobic capacity can engage in vigorous physical activity like cycling, running, and swimming without a lot of fatigue. They are the physically fit group, the ones with the healthy hearts, healthy lungs, and well-toned muscles. They're not the typical American. Yet most Americans who want to can join their group.

People have been talking and writing about the values of exercise for centuries. They were sure it had something to do with a longer and more vigorous life. But it wasn't until 1961 that these ideas were totally investigated and documented. Doctors Wilhelm Raab and Hans Kraus published a study called "Hypokinetic Diseases." "Hypokinetic" means too little movement, so the term refers to people who don't get enough exercise. Raab and Kraus compared the incidence of various disorders, such as overweight, chronic fatigue, backache, headache, chronic anxiety, high blood pressure, coronary artery disease, muscular weakness and atrophy, shortness of breath, atherosclerosis, and accelerated degenerative aging between the sedentary and those who were physically active. The physically active people were better on all counts. And there have been several studies since 1961 that confirm these findings.[3]

Exercise Benefits

Of course, exercise can't prevent or alleviate diseases. It won't eliminate the common cold or tuberculosis, prevent leprosy. But it does build physical reserves and improve the efficiency of bodily functions. Here's how exercise works in certain ways to give us better lives.

Tension

This is the day of the office jungle, the overcrowded freeway, and no-fault divorce. Our predecessors in the caves fought off lions and tigers with clubs, which got their adrenalin to flow freely. But the modern cave man has to adhere to the new social code of being "cool." Your fortune gets wiped out in the stock market—laugh and buy a round of drinks for your friends. After all, it way only money. Your wife starts an affair with the next door neighbor—show savoir-faire. After all, these are the 1970s. And as to flunking out of school, getting pregnant out of wedlock, or losing your job, these should be taken with a grin. Who wants a boring and uneventful life? Although this cool attitude has a lot to be said for it, it's not the best way to work off our feelings. Mentally we may be 1970 sophisticates, but our bodies are still back in the stone ages, warding off wild beasts. Our tensions build the same as our ancestors' did, but we can't work them off by fighting tigers and swinging from vines. So we come up with unresolved stress, which brings on constricted arterioles, high blood pressure, and a fast heart rate. This keeps us from relaxing, brings on ulcers, insomnia, and all kinds of cardiovascular and digestive problems.

Some try to solve modern man's psychological dilemma with double martinis, fifths of scotch, sleeping pills, and heroin. These kinds of solutions can bring on bigger problems yet. A healthier way to get rid of tension is through exercise. It does work, it does bring on relaxation, and it doesn't bring on guilt feelings and police raids.

Childhood Development

Exercise plays a key role in children's healthy growth and development. Some grow without much exercise, of course, and they seem to survive just fine. But their nervous systems, hearts, lungs, muscles, and bones don't get the movement and oxygen supply they should, which can bring on trouble in later life. Exercise, of course, is important at any age, but middle-aged and older people who weren't physically fit when they were developing are more likely to have hypokinetic disorders than those who have been in condition.

Appearance

Exercise does build strength, good muscle tone, a healthy appearance. Advertisements for muscle-building courses claim that 97-pound weaklings can have Mr. America bodies with 15-minute daily workouts. Girls with flat chests, skinny legs, and double chins can go into competition with Raquel

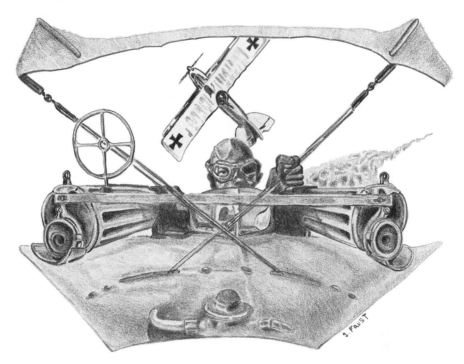

FIGURE 9-2. *Would the Red Baron's nerves have held up in the 1970s?*

Welch. This is obviously ridiculous, but exercise does help us get the most out of what we have. There's no way in the world of turning a 140-pound accountant into a linebacker for the Chicago Bears. But he can develop or maintain firm muscle tone, correct posture, a flat stomach, and a vital attitude. The same applies to the 160-pound nurse and the 95-pound hairdresser.

Also, unexercised muscles get smaller and weaker. Take someone with a broken leg. After he's had it immobilized for a few weeks, atrophy sets in, and it becomes smaller than his other leg. Muscles waste away. Even his bones and joints begin to deteriorate. It takes awhile for him to build the strength to walk again after the cast comes off. Astronauts face the same kind of problem when they spend much time in a weightless environment. Their muscles get weak and begin to deteriorate if they don't perform some kind of artificial exercise.

Obesity

Exercise can control obesity. Enemies of physical activity say that it can't. After all, you have to walk $11\frac{1}{6}$ hours to lose a pound of fat, they say, swim $5\frac{1}{2}$ hours, or bicycle for $7\frac{1}{2}$ hours. Who has that kind of time? Who cares that much about a little flab, anyway? That kind of argument assumes the exercise will be done in one painfully long ordeal. Actually, the loss takes place whether the exercise takes a few hours or a year. You can bicycle steadily for $7\frac{1}{2}$ hours to lose the pound or do it for half an hour at a time. In the latter case, the pound vanishes after 15 days. Keep this up steadily for a year, and you have 26 fewer pounds to carry on your frame. Also, the fatter you are the more calories you burn in any physical activity. A 200-pound handball player needs a third more energy than his 150-pound opponent.

Of course, if losing weight is the main objective, physical activity won't substitute for limiting the intake of food. Professional football players, weight lifters, and wrestlers certainly aren't skinny. But exercise can help to burn off some body fat. There's a popular notion among the armchair set that the more you exercise the bigger your appetite becomes, so why bother to exercise? This notion is only partially true. Granted, when your body burns more energy your hunger increases, and usually your food intake does, too. But increased exercise increases efficiency in utilizing the food we absorb. Once our bodies adjust to the new energy expenditure, our appetites often decrease rather than increase.[4]

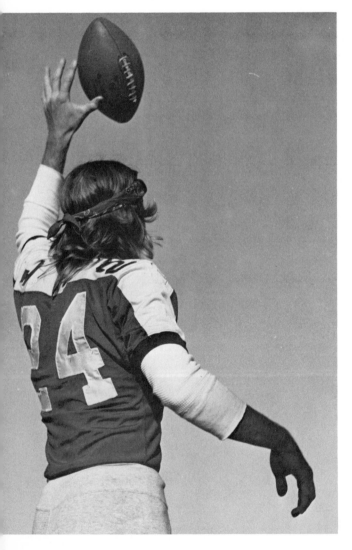

FIGURE 9-3. *The Saturday Super Bowl.*

Manufactured Exercise

Getting in shape can be fun. There are handball, squash, a swimming pool. All you have to do is get a little expertise in an individual sport, and you'll have more exercise than you need. Or, better yet, try a team sport. Go out for football or lacrosse. Or are we talking foolishness? A mighty small number of people, no matter what their ages, have the talent and background to make third string, let alone the varsity, in almost any collegiate sport. Sometimes intramurals are offered, and these are great, if you like this kind of thing. Few artificial exercise programs will give you the workout that 30 minutes of basketball will. But even intramural sports aren't everyone's idea of the best way to spend a Saturday afternoon. The same applies to individual contests like cross-country running or tennis. It takes a lot of time and effort and sometimes money to get good at them. Playing these sports each day can put you in excellent condition, but quite often you can't find the time, facilities, the companions to play them more than once a week. Exercise can be fun and should be fun—whenever possible. But sometimes the fun and the exercise have to go separate ways. Incidentally, don't look on pastimes like golf, bowling, or splashing in a pool as a physical workout. They're great ways to spend leisure time and create relaxation and good fellowship. But they don't do much for the cardiovascular system or the muscles.

So most of us looking for a daily workout will have to manufacture one. This can be a problem, because artificial exercise can be grim. And then there's the problem of just what kind of exercise to get. Should you build a body beautiful, be the envy of the bikini and surfboard set? Or do you just want to get your blood to flowing, get a better sense of well-being and vitality? Probably the latter is the better choice. Not that there's anything wrong with looking great in a pair of trunks or a bikini, but most muscle-building programs demand almost monastic dedication and tremendous amounts of time, and don't do much to improve health. When you build thick, knotty muscles, you spread your blood vessels without adding new ones. So it's harder for your tissues to get oxygen from these vessels and dispose of their wastes. You lose endurance, begin to feel tired more often than you should, and all physical activity begins to bore you. What some call "stamina training" brings a different result.[5]

Aerobics

Major Kenneth H. Cooper, an Air Force physician, summarized some of the key concepts of stamina training in a book called *Aerobics*. "Aerobic" means "with oxygen," and, in the sense that Cooper uses it, it refers to extended exercise, creating oxygen demands by the body that our systems learn to satisfy. Cooper contrasts this with "anaerobic" exercise, in which the bodily demands exceed the oxygen supply produced, creating an "oxygen debt."

The body cells have to have oxygen in order to extract energy from food and store it as adenosine triphosphate (ATP). ATP, upon being broken down, releases energy for the functioning of all our organs and systems, for

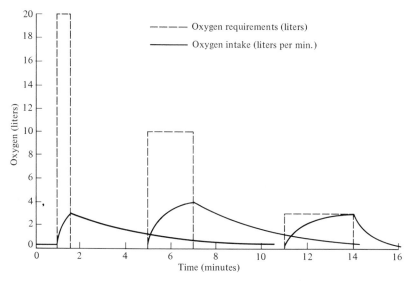

The oxygen requirement, oxygen intake, oxygen deficit, and oxygen debt during three periods of exercise of different intensities. The rectangles represent oxygen requirements for each exercise; their areas are equal to the corresponding sums of oxygen intake, during both the exercises and the recovery periods. The parts of the rectangles above the curve represent oxygen deficit and are equal to the excess oxygen consumption during recovery, or oxygen debt.

SOURCE: John Fulton Farguhar, *Howell's Textbook of Physiology* (Philadelphia: W. B. Saunders, 1946), p. 213.

FIGURE 9-4. *The role of oxygen in physical exertion.*

the transportation of matter in and out of our cells, for the synthesis of our biological chemicals and the maintenance of body heat. Oxygen may not be the only key to life, but it's hard to think of something more essential.

There are times when we don't get the oxygen we need for a given activity—for instance, when we sprint, bicycle quickly up a hill, or swim as fast as we can for a lap or two. At times like this we have to get our energy anaerobically, or without oxygen. This creates an oxygen debt. Sugar and lactic acid fill this sudden energy need, but they can't do it for long. And when we get our energy this way, we pay for it with fatigue. But when we have a large aerobic capacity, we can support intense activity for an extended period without having to draw on our anaerobic processes.

The way to build this aerobic capacity is by sustained exercise that builds the heart rate to 150 beats per minute or more. The training benefits don't begin until about 5 minutes after the exercise is started, but they continue for the duration of the exercise from that point forward. If the exercise isn't vigorous enough, this 150-beat-per-minute heart rate has to be continued a lot longer than 5 minutes before any physical training benefits take place.

Of course, someone exercising will never be able to figure out what his heart rate is, so Cooper took exercises that he knew demanded oxygen aerobically and measured them for the oxygen they required. Then he translated these measurements into points. The more vigorous exercises,

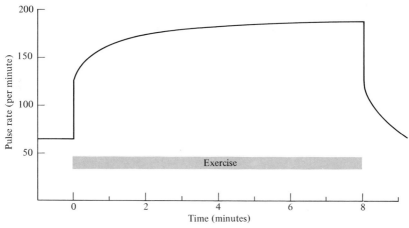

SOURCE: Roy J. Shephard, *Alive Man* (Springfield, Ill.: Charles C. Thomas, 1972) p. 52.

FIGURE 9-5. *A typical heart rate response to a period of submaximal exercise.*

requiring the most oxygen to produce needed energy, received the most points, and those requiring less oxygen received fewer points.

Here are some exercises worth 5 points each:

1. Running a mile in less than 8 minutes.
2. Swimming 600 yards in 15 minutes or less.
3. Cycling 5 miles in under 20 minutes.
4. Running in place for $12\frac{1}{2}$ minutes.
5. Playing handball for 35 minutes.

Do any of these once a day, 6 days a week, and you accumulate 30 points, the amount Cooper says is necessary to maintain a minimum aerobic training effect. Of course, you can mix these exercises. You can run twice a week, swim twice a week, take a day of cycling, and have a game of handball. Or you might want to earn more than 5 points in a day by exceeding the minimums Cooper suggests. Possibly you can run 2 miles in 16 minutes or less or swim 1200 yards in half an hour. This way you don't have to exercise each day. But you do have to exercise a minimum of 4 days each week and amass a minimum of 5 points on any given exercise day.[6]

Too Much Exercise

Of course, you have to build your endurance gradually to meet these training standards. If you're really out of shape, it takes 3 or 4 months, or longer, before you can run a mile in less than 8 minutes. And there is such a thing as more exercise than you're in condition to take. There's the fellow who hasn't done a thing more strenuous for the last few months than open a Coke or beer bottle who goes out to play an afternoon of touch football. It

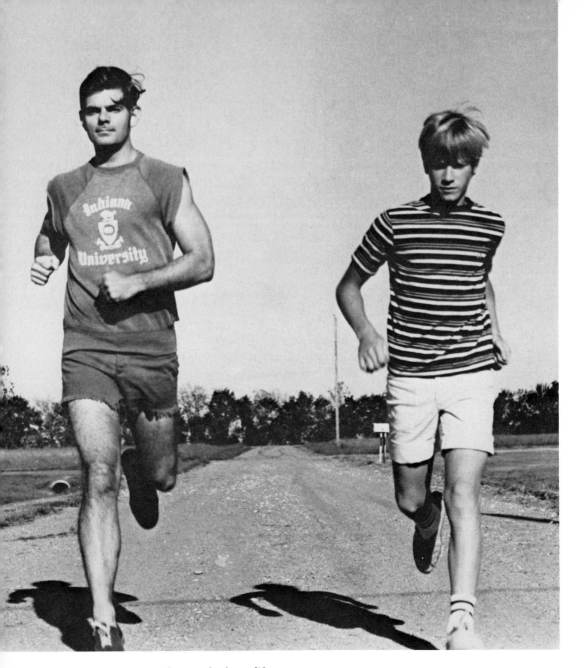

FIGURE 9-6. *A stride toward a better life.*

takes days before he stops wincing when he gets out of bed or walks up a flight of stairs. Good physical fitness comes from regular exercise, not sporadic spurts.

And even if you exercise on a daily basis you can overexert. This breaks down physical fitness rather than builds it, and you have to reduce your activities while you're recovering. And if you work out while you're fatigued you're much more prone to injury or illness. You should always start training gradually, be satisfied with slow but steady progress. Here are a few signs that call for reexamination of the strenuousness of any physical fitness program.

1. Continuous fatigue, even extending into the day following the workout.
2. Problems with sleeping. Exercise should improve rest, not hinder it.
3. Pulse rate that doesn't return to 120 beats a minute, or less, within 2 minutes after the exercise is over.
4. Staleness. Exercise suddenly seems like some tedious and boring chore. All exercise enthusiasts face this problem at one time or another. Probably the best thing to do is to vary the exercise routine so that it seems interesting and challenging. Don't let staleness be a reason for stopping conditioning altogether.

It's a good idea to have a physician check you over before starting any new training program. Probably you're healthy; and, if you're not, you probably don't have a condition that exercise could harm. But it pays to be sure about things like this if for no other reason than to eliminate worry.[7]

Fitness Fads

There are a lot of fitness fads that are popular, always have been. After all, who can pass up the opportunity to build a beautiful, strong, and healthy body in anywhere from 10 seconds to 5 minutes a day? Or is it a special food or a certain gadget that gives you the Sophia Loren or Mark Spitz body without working at it? Most of these fads do little if any good, and some are costly. Isometrics—muscle tension without movement—is a good example. It's true that you can build a little strength with this kind of program, firm up a few flabby muscles. But this does nothing to improve endurance, joint flexibility, or circulation.

As to health-building foods, a balanced diet is a must for physical fitness. But a healthy diet can be composed of foods on grocery store shelves. There's no need for oils, tonics, or "natural" food substances. And spot-reducing exercises are completely useless. There's no way fat can be burned off a given part of the body without getting the whole body involved in the process.

There are some gadgets that can be useful. Weights and springs can build bulging muscles and a lot of strength. Stationary bicycles and treadmills can build up endurance. But these gadgets aren't necessary for a good conditioning program. Push-ups, chin-ups, and sit-ups can bring on excellent muscle tone, though admittedly won't produce the glamorous, rippling triceps and biceps that weights will. And as for endurance, there's no machine invented that can build it as well as jogging or even running in place. It doesn't cost a penny to get in shape, even though advertising firms sometimes imply otherwise.[8]

Calisthenics

Calisthenics are the exercises that supposedly build muscle tone, healthy appearance, and good posture. They don't build endurance the way aerobic exercises do, and they don't make you lose much weight. But, within reason, they do accomplish a specific purpose. They can't change the basic shape of us, make us handsome when we're homely, beautiful when we're plain. But neither can clothes, cosmetics, or hairdos. These things help us look the best we can, though, so we should give some thought to them.

Isometrics

Isometric exercises became very popular during the 1950s and 1960s. There were two Germans, Th. Hettinger and E. A. Mueller, who claimed that a 6-second-a-day isometric exercise increased muscle strength more than 5 per cent a week and 50 per cent in 10 weeks. The exercise involved muscular contractions to the utmost of the individual's ability with no movement. Isometrics could bring on amazing results, they said, in a short period. But other investigators weren't amazed. They found that isometric enthusiasts experienced a slight increase in strength and muscle tone, but nothing to really rave about. Certainly, these exercises are simple and don't consume a lot of time. And they do bring on better conditioning than no exercise at all. But they don't bring on the beautiful bodies that some devotees claim they do.

Some isometric practitioners pit various parts of their bodies against each other. They try to raise one arm while the other arm holds it down. They put their hands together in front of their bodies and try to push from side to side. But no movement takes place. Work at a dozen or more of these exercises involving various parts of the body—the neck, the stomach, the legs, shoulders, wrists, and arms—and you'll theoretically look trim and athletic. Each calls for a 6- to 15-second maximum effort, and your exercising is over for the day. Some think they can get a more flexible routine by using a door frame, a broomstick, or a desk or chair. Some get even fancier by using barbells with weights too heavy to lift or spring dynamometers. But the principle is still the same—the body doesn't move; the muscles just flex. It's something like pushing a car that's stuck in the mud.[9]

Isotonics

Isotonic exercises follow an unlimited number of patterns. There are sit-ups, push-ups, chin-ups, touching the toes, even flexing the fingers. One of the more popular programs in this category is the 5BX (five basic exercises) plan for physical fitness developed by the Royal Canadian Air Force in the early 1960s. These exercises were primarily for men, but there was a companion ten-exercise program for women called the XBX. These were a graded series of relatively simple exercises that supposedly could be completed in 11 minutes a day. Over half of the 5BX time was devoted to running in place, which is really aerobic exercise rather than calisthenics. But other parts of the program consisted of sit-ups, pull-ups, and "squat thrusts." Squat thrusts

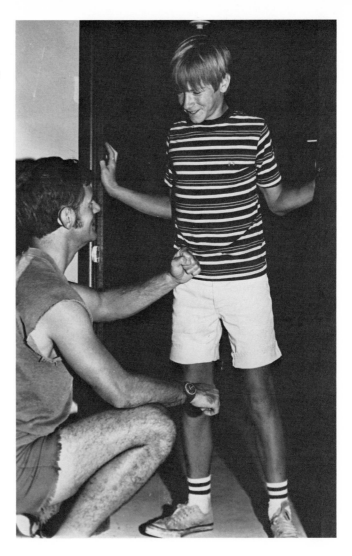

FIGURE 9-7. *Push the house down.*

were carried out by bending the knees and placing the hands on the floor, kicking the legs to the rear so that the body was in a push-up position, then returning to the squat and erect positions. Men in reasonable physical shape should be able to do three pull-ups and 14 sit-ups. And they should complete four squat thrusts in 10 seconds. Women, according to XBX standards, should do eight modified pull-ups (heels remain on the floor while the body is pulled to a chest-high chinning bar from a leaning-back position) and ten sit-ups and have 10 seconds to complete three squat thrusts. These programs were meant to eliminate "desk-bound flabbiness," and to some extent they accomplish their purpose. But calisthenics, at best, supplement stamina training. They don't replace it. And, like all other forms of solitary exercise, it takes a lot of motivation and will power to keep going.[10]

Recreation

What's so wonderful about being healthy if we have to spend every spare minute jogging, doing push-ups, flexing biceps? Nothing is good about it. If healthy bodies belong to fanatics only, they're not worth having. The concept of general or total fitness applies to somebody's being able to function efficiently. When you're bored, efficiency just isn't going to be there. So any conditioning program should provide for recreation. There are golf, bowling, archery, and bridge. But you shouldn't look on them as exercise. They're worth doing—for some people—because they're fun. The same applies to certain kinds of intercollegiate sports, collecting stamps, or going to the beach. A lot of people in this "get to the top," "martini for lunch," "easy down payment plan" world have forgotten how to have a good time. It's something that won't come automatically when you have free time. You should develop a positive attitude about recreation, an organized plan for enjoying life. How much time do you have for recreation, or how much time do you want to spend? What kind of person are you? Do you relax better with people or enjoy getting away by yourself? How much is this recreation going to cost, and can you afford it? If you can't afford it, is it worth saving for? Is the pastime you've got in mind something you're really looking forward to? If not, what else seems exciting? Answers to questions like these can provide a lifetime of fun. And, in most cases, if you're not having fun it's your own fault.[11]

Relaxation

Sometimes, though, we get so tense that we need to relax more than have fun. Fun is a form of relaxation, of course. But every so often, probably daily, you should concentrate on completely letting go. Bowling, golf, or even smiling calls for a certain amount of tension. People who hang onto tensions compile an impressive list of failures and disappointments.

Some people claim they can't relax, but this is nonsense. You don't need pills to do it, and you don't need liquid aids, either. A long, slow walk in a quiet neighborhood or, better yet, in the woods or country can do wonders. If you want relaxation faster, tense specific areas in various parts of the body, then concentrate on relaxing them. Another technique that helps is leaning forward in a chair, closing your eyes, then rotating your head in a slow circle. If you're doing close work, shut your eyes every so often, then open them and look from side to side and up and down. Stand up and stretch. Relaxation techniques take only a few seconds a day and make you feel better, make you a much more efficient and self-confident person, and help you get a lot more pleasure out of life.[12]

Fatigue

It happens to all of us. There are days when we just don't want to face the sun, when the simplest tasks become some major effort we'd like to put off, when things that are usually fun seem boring and tedious. Some call this the "Monday morning blues." But no matter what it's called, it really gets in the way of a good life.

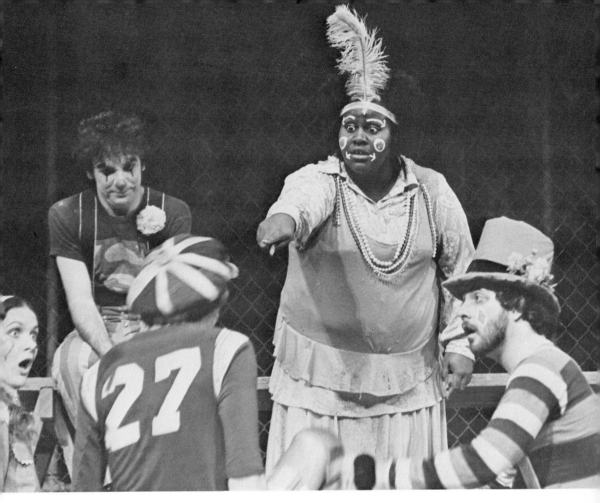

FIGURE 9-8. *Having fun.*

Physical Fatigue

There are several types of fatigue. One of the most common is physical, the kind brought on by exertion. There's a certain level of carbon dioxide and lactic acid in our blood that produces this exhausted feeling. Suddenly we know it's time to rest or have a change of pace. This is a natural feeling, and it's cured by a good night's sleep or an afternoon nap.

Pathological Fatigue

But there's no quick cure for pathological fatigue. This is the kind associated with illness. It can be an early warning sign that all is not right with your physical health. There can be a certain amount of muscular weakness and pain associated with this kind of fatigue. It usually comes on suddenly and is quite severe. It's best to see a physician when these kind of symptoms strike. Another kind of pathological fatigue is the type that hangs on when you're getting over the flu or a cold. This is a kind of bodily defense mechanism that warns you to take it easy for a while, or you might have a relapse.

217

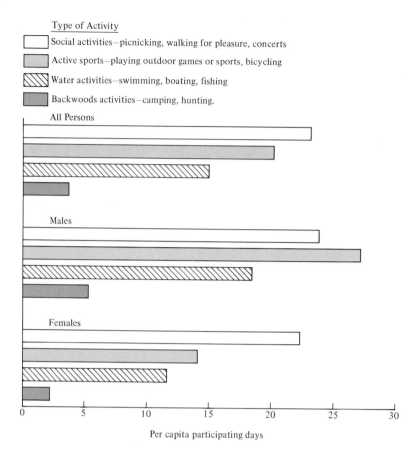

Type of Activity

☐ Social activities—picnicking, walking for pleasure, concerts

▨ Active sports—playing outdoor games or sports, bicycling

▧ Water activities—swimming, boating, fishing

▨ Backwoods activities—camping, hunting.

Per capita participating days

SOURCE: U.S. Department of the Interior, Bureau of Outdoor Recreation, *The 1970 Survey of Outdoor Recreation Activities, Preliminary Report,* 1972.

FIGURE 9-9. *Participation in outdoor recreation by sex, 1970.*

Psychological Fatigue

Then there's psychological fatigue, the kind brought on by those days when you flunk your midterm, can't find your car in the parking lot, find you've lost your key when you finally do find your car. Everyone has "those days." By evening you feel pretty wrung out. Usually this is a transitory feeling. A day or so later the world doesn't seem so grim, and energy and pep have come back to normal levels. But sometimes this kind of fatigue persists. You feel tired constantly; the doctor can't find anything wrong with you, and you've hardly moved, let alone exerted yourself. This can mean you're in the middle of an emotional battle—with yourself. There are people who resort to headaches, bad backs, and asthma when they can't get the world straightened out in their heads. Then there are people who just plain feel tired all the time. It usually takes professional help to solve these problems.[13]

Sleep

We spend a third of our lives in a comatose state. Usually we do this in bed. If we haven't spent enough time in the prone position, we have a tendency to fall asleep when reading a book, watching television, or, worst of all, sitting in class. We need these periods to withdraw from the world, recuperate from tension and fatigue, and let our body cells, run down by activity, restore themselves. Sleep—the right amount of it—is essential for a productive and healthy life.

The amount of sleep each person requires varies. Some can get by nicely on 7 hours; some need 9. Patterns of sleep are individual things, too. Some get their best rest by the "early to bed, early to rise" routine. Others can't unwind until after midnight. And there are some who like to sleep in spurts, 3 to 5 hours at a time, but do this a couple of times a day. The only way to determine which pattern is best for you is to experiment a little and find the one that makes you feel the best. If you hate to face that alarm clock in the morning, daydream for hours when you first get in bed, you might be using a pattern that isn't for you.

Insomnia

Lack of sleep can seriously interfere with the way we perceive and think. There have been several experiments in which people were kept awake for long periods. Most of them began hearing and seeing things that weren't there. Also, they had a tendency to become paranoid, feeling that people were talking about them and plotting against them. Although most of us will never have to experience such extreme sleep deprivation, we can lose a certain amount of efficiency and a sense of well-being through a minor sleep loss.

"Insomnia" is the label we give to the tossing and turning problem. Considering the number of sleeping pills sold, both prescription and nonprescription, there are many million Americans bothered with this problem. It's not really serious if it doesn't strike too often. All of us have an occasional night when we're too keyed up to give way to the sandman. Or maybe we're just too tired to sleep. But the next night, or the one after that, we sleep a little longer and a little deeper and make up the sleep we've missed.

If the insomnia persists, there's probably something wrong with our life style. Dietary habits can affect our sleeping routine, and so can exercise. Violent exercise before bedtime can keep you from falling asleep for several hours. So can green peppers and pizza. Some people try a few shots of whiskey so they'll fall asleep right away. This is a life-style pattern that leads not only to sleeping problems but also to some serious problems when we're awake. And there are some people who save frustrations, worries, and anger to review the minute they get in bed. Obviously, this doesn't lead to a restful night. Life styles can usually be changed once we identify the problem areas. If we can't identify the problem areas, then insomnia will probably persist. We should seek help.[14]

Sleep Brain Waves

The physiological process of sleep is still pretty much of a mystery. But there has been a lot of research on sleep brain wave patterns. Here the subject is connected to an electroencephalograph shortly before he drifts off, and the instrument records the electrical energy patterns in his head. Analysis of these patterns has indicated that there are two kinds of sleep. During one phase we have rapid eye movements called "Rems." It's during these Rem sleeping periods that dreaming occurs. The other kind of sleep, the non-Rem type, has four distinctive stages. The first stage, sometimes called "alpha rhythm," is when we're completely relaxed but still awake. Relaxation slowly deepens, and sleep begins during this first stage, becoming much more complete during the second, third, and fourth stages. During the second stage, the eyes slowly roll from side to side, but the sleep is still quite deep. Temperature decreases, and so does blood pressure. During the third phase, the pulse becomes much slower. The sleep during this stage is quite deep and calm. The deepest sleep takes place during the fourth stage. This period is brief and is when nightmares and sleepwalking probably take place. After completing stage four, we go back through stages three and two, reenter the Rem stage, where we probably have another dream. Then comes another cycle of deeper and lighter sleep stages, the overall pattern repeating itself three or four times a night. And the longer we sleep, the longer our Rem periods become, and the more vivid are the dreams.[15]

Posture

Stand straight and tall, throw your chest out, pull your shoulders back, keep your head high. It's the finest exercise known to build good health. Nonsense! The good posture concept has been stressed for centuries, probably because people were impressed with straight soldiers and stiff-necked politicians. Certainly, a slouching posture can indicate poor health. But it's not what causes poor health. It may mean that the person is fatigued, slightly deformed, or completely unsure of himself. Or it can mean that the person has adopted a posture that's comfortable to him. The way we stand and sit is an individual thing, just as the way we dress and the way we speak. And if our posture doesn't express us as individuals, it's not natural, and the posture is poor. Imitating statues is fatiguing, and it looks silly. True, it doesn't hurt to think of standing tall occasionally, imagining that hooks from the ceiling are pulling at your ears. These thoughts can straighten you a little, momentarily improve your appearance. But preoccupation with this kind of attitude is unnatural and unhealthy.[16]

Elimination Habits

Many are sure that there's something wrong with them when they don't have a bowel movement on a daily basis. This just isn't so. Like posture, elimination habits vary with the individual, and a good routine for one person isn't necessarily good for another. If you're feeling healthy, aren't uncomfortable, and don't seem to be constipated, you probably have an elimination pattern that is effective. Whatever your routine is, though, it probably fails occasionally, and you get to feeling logy. Usually this situation will correct itself. But if it persists you should see a physician.

Some people get in the habit of using laxatives instead of depending on natural elimination processes. This can bring on further problems. Regular exercise and a diet heavy in fruits, vegetables, and liquids can help to maintain a healthy elimination routine. And it's a good idea to identify your elimination pattern, then establish definite times for the bowel movements that comply with this pattern.[17]

Foot Care

Over two-thirds of the people in the United States born with normal feet have foot trouble before they reach middle age. This is partly because we wear shoes that don't fit, partly because we wear socks that are too small, partly because we trim our toenails incorrectly. Shoes that are too short, too narrow, that don't conform to the shape of our feet, can bring on corns, bunions, calluses, and ingrown toenails. Tight-fitting socks can contribute to these problems, too. When you buy shoes, take your time. Always try them on, even though you think you know what your shoe size should be. Designated lengths and widths vary slightly, particularly with shoes made by different manufacturers. And be sure to try on both shoes of the pair. The shape and size of both your feet aren't exactly the same. Although a new shoe on your right foot may be perfectly comfortable, the one on your left can create problems.

Be sure to stand and walk in shoes before you buy them. Feet spread and become longer when we put body weight on them. If the shoes aren't comfortable, seem to be rubbing or creating unwanted pressure, don't decide that you can "break them in." Feet get broken in right along with the shoes.

As to trimming toenails, never cut them too short. Cut straight across. Cutting into the corners of the toes can bring on ingrown toenails.

Since our feet are enclosed in shoes much of the time, air often doesn't get to them the way it should. This creates a breeding ground for various kinds of infections, such as athlete's foot, and can cause a bad odor. If you wash your feet daily, completely dry them, preferably powder them, you shouldn't have trouble in this area. Also, put on clean hosiery each day and wear different shoes each day to let them dry between wearings.

Each of our feet has 26 bones, bound together by ligaments, cushioned by sacs of fluid called bursae. The foot has two arches, one of which is just back of the toes and runs crosswise, called the metatarsal arch. The other, the longitudinal arch, runs from the heel to the toes. When this longitudinal arch breaks down, we get a condition known as "flat feet" or "fallen arches." Flat feet can be painful and can interfere with the ability to stand or move. But many people with flat feet have no handicap whatsoever. And just because someone has a high arch is no guarantee his arch is strong. In fact, an arch can be too high. This can bring on pain and movement problems as well.[18]

Dental Health

Tooth and gum problems have plagued man since his life span extended beyond 20 years. Shakespeare referred to toothaches; the first Queen Elizabeth endured them; and George Washington suffered through extractions and primitive dentures. Cures for this malady have been quite innovative and sometimes so distasteful that the fellow with the toothache forgot about them. Filling the hollow of the tooth with excretions from a raven was one cure. Another was biting off the head of a live mouse, and another yet involved filling the aching mouth with cold water and sitting on a hot stove. Obviously, man's oral cavity was a nightmare of pain before modern dentistry came along. Still, many people today suffer with their teeth and gums. There are parts of the world where dental care isn't available, where people are so poor they can't afford it. And even in the United States a large percentage don't get the dental care they need and don't practice good oral hygiene.

Men entering the military service are a fairly healthy group, certainly much younger and healthier than the average American. Yet for every 100 putting on a uniform, 20 need dentures, 80 need extractions, and 25 need bridges. These 100 young men also need 450 fillings.

Pain is just part of the bad tooth and gum problem. There's also bad breath, which can be a joke to anyone who doesn't have it, a lowered resistance to infection, the aggravation of other bodily infections, and poor appearance. Our teeth are one of the most important factors in how we look. Straight, clean-looking teeth give the impression of vitality and health. Teeth that are stained, dull, or need brushing make the person seem lazy or sickly. Dental disease can lead to premature wrinkles, facial deformities, and an early appearance of aging.

The loss of teeth is the loss of youth, many people think. Yet, in most cases, there's no reason to lose teeth, even if you live into your 90s. Following good dental hygiene habits and seeing your dentist regularly can almost assure that you'll never wear dentures. And though this can't assure a youthful appearance, or no dental-related problems, it can help in this area.[19]

Dental Structure

Teeth are rugged structures. They survive fires, crushing blows, and hundreds of pounds of pressure. They won't survive the invasion of bacteria, though. And two sets of teeth are all a man gets.

Our first set of teeth are called "primary," or "deciduous," teeth. They start forming around the sixth week of prenatal life. By the time we're $2\frac{1}{2}$, we have our full complement of 20 primary teeth. These are smaller than our permanent teeth, which is fine, since our jaws are smaller at that time, too.

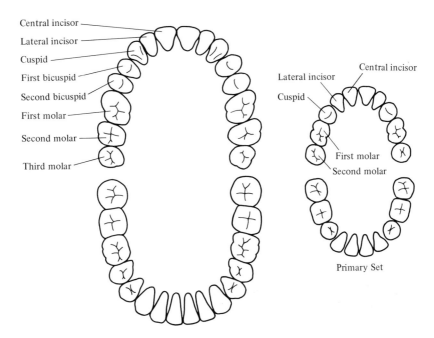

FIGURE 9-10. *Human teeth.*

Although our permanent teeth don't begin to show themselves until we're 6 years old or older, they begin calcifying shortly after birth. By the time we're 17 to 21 years old, we have 16 teeth in each jaw, or a total of 32. The last four teeth to emerge are the third molars, or "wisdom teeth." We also have second molars and first molars, which are probably the most important teeth in our mouths. Located in the center of the jaw, they do the heavy work of chewing. For biting, we have four sharp front teeth in our top and bottom jaws called incisors. Next to them on each side stands a cuspid, sometimes called an "eyetooth." Then come the first and second bicuspids to link up with the molars.

We can see only about a third of our teeth. Two-thirds, the roots, lie below the gum line. The front teeth, the incisors, usually have just one root, while the others have two or three. The crown of the tooth, the part that shows, is covered with enamel. It's the hardest substance in the body and makes the tooth surface extremely rugged. The roots are also covered with a tough material called cementum. This isn't as hard as enamel, but it provides excellent protection against foreign particles and bacteria. Softer yet, but still harder than bone, is dentin, which forms the body of the tooth. And inside this body is a pulp chamber containing blood vessels and nerves. These blood vessels and nerves extend to the top of each root through narrow channels called root canals. The nerves are extremely sensitive, so if there's a break in the enamel and the dentin gets exposed the tooth becomes sensitive to hot and cold temperatures and sweets. If decay goes deeper than the dentin, we have a toothache.

There's a thin, soft tissue beneath the gum line called the periodontal membrane. This surrounds the teeth, holds them in place, and acts as a

223

shock absorber. It's somewhat resilient, so our teeth move slightly when we grind them or chew.[20]

Tooth Decay

Other than the cold, cavities are the most common ailment human beings have. In order for them to form, there have to be teeth, of course, and also sugar, and also a certain kind of bacteria. The bacteria breed in a filmy substance covering our teeth called plaque. You can get rid of a lot of this plaque by brushing, but you never get rid of all of it; so you don't get rid of all the bacteria. The bacteria absorb the simple sugars formed by the breakdown of food in our mouths. And they get energy by converting this sugar to acid. Usually our saliva has enough buffers in it to neutralize this acid and prevent tooth decay. But occasionally saliva doesn't perform the job it should, and the acid takes over. It starts by eroding the tooth enamel, usually without notice. There's no warning pain until the bacteria reach the dentin. If this condition isn't treated, the cavity can work its way to the tooth pulp and sometimes to the tissues surrounding the root. Abscesses form, and pus creates a gumline infection that causes pain and sometimes serious illness.

ORAL HYGIENE

So what to do? Obviously, if you're having toothaches or other dental trouble, see a dentist as quickly as possible. But you shouldn't wait for pain before making a dental appointment. Appointments should be scheduled on a periodic basis, preferably twice a year. Here teeth get cleaned and X-rayed to identify dental trouble before it becomes serious.

But the dentist, no matter how good he is, can't make up for poor personal hygiene. The ideal is to brush teeth immediately after meals or even after a minor snack. It takes only a few moments for bacteria to transform sugar to erosive acid. So removing them before they can do any damage is a sure way to prevent cavities. But this ideal is hard to conform to. You can

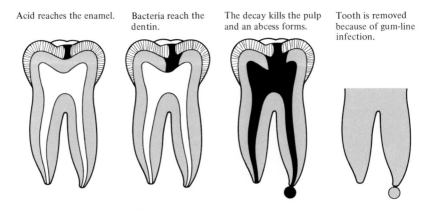

Acid reaches the enamel.   Bacteria reach the dentin.   The decay kills the pulp and an abcess forms.   Tooth is removed because of gum-line infection.

FIGURE 9-11.   *Untreated tooth decay.*

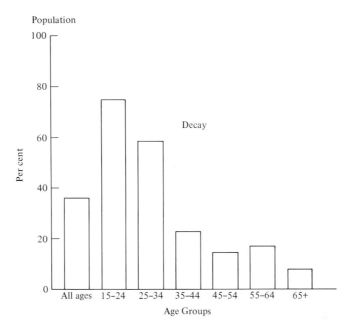

Population

SOURCE: Pauline F. Steel, *Dental Hygiene* (Philadelphia: Lea and Febiger, 1970) p. 27.

FIGURE 9-12. *Incidence of caries in the United States, by age group.*

brush your teeth after having a hot dog or drinking a Coke at a football game, but how many people are really going to do it? How many people will brush after eating popcorn or candy at a movie, or even bother to carry a toothbrush with them when they leave the house? A good compromise is to brush at least twice a day—immediately after breakfast and just before going to bed. It takes plaque about 10 hours to form, and this twice-a-day brushing keeps it pretty well under control. To keep plaque from forming between teeth, you should use dental floss twice a day, too.

DIET

Diet is another factor that affects tooth decay, particularly during the prenatal period and the first 8 years of life. Pregnant women's and young children's diets should be rich in vitamins A, C, and D, as well as calcium and phosphorus. These contribute to normal and strong tooth structure. And though adult teeth are fully calcified and don't require calcium to stay healthy, the bones holding these teeth in place do. Adult dental health calls for enough protein for tissue replacement and reasonable amounts of vitamins B and C.

You can also reduce cavities by reducing intakes of sugar. Foods like candy, cake, soft drinks, and canned fruits contain just what mouth bacteria thrive on.[21]

225

FLUORIDE

There are fluoride toothpastes, fluoride tablets, and fluoridated water. Fluoride hardens the enamel of teeth when they're developing and makes them more resistant to the acid produced by bacteria. Probably the most reliable way of getting the right amount of fluoride is to live in a community that has the chemical placed in its water supply. This way you don't have to think about it. Two-thirds of the major cities in the United States, including New York and Chicago, provide this service for their residents. But water fluoridation is controversial. Some feel that this is a medical remedy, and medical remedies should be taken only when we're sick. Also, they say, fluoridation is primarily of benefit to the very young. So fluoridating the drinking supply, while benefiting one age group, endangers the health of the overall population.

There are 44 national health and health-related organizations that don't agree with this argument, though, and endorse the fluoridation of drinking water. This practice has been shown to reduce children's cavities by 45 to 70 per cent.[22]

Periodontal Disease

Most people don't lose their teeth from cavities. Be you middle aged, elderly, or still in high school, if your teeth are coming out, it's probably periodontal disease that's causing it. About two-thirds of the people between 18 and 24 in the United States have some form of gum (periodontal) problem. And there are 5 million of them who won't have a tooth in their heads by the time they're 35. Diseased gums will be all that remain.

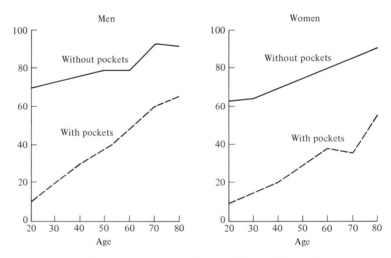

Per cent of men and women with periodontal disease, with and without pockets, by age, among adults in the United States.

SOURCE: Pauline F. Steel, *Dental Hygiene* (Philadelphia: Lea and Febiger, 1970) p. 27.

FIGURE 9-13. *Per cent of men and women with periodontal disease, with and without pockets, by age, among adults in the United States.*

TABLE 9-1
Dimensions of Dental Hygiene
(Diagrammatic outline of the disease process in periodontal disorders and dental caries and levels of prevention)

Periodontal Disease		Dental Caries	
Levels of Prevention	*Process*	*Process*	*Levels of Prevention*
	Tissue susceptible to breakdown ↓	Tooth susceptible to caries ↓	
Primary prevention (reversible periodontal changes)	Oral structures disposing to accumulation of oral debris ↓	Carbohydrate intake and other nutritional factors ↓	
	Dental plaque ↓	Dental plaque present on the tooth surface ↓	Primary prevention
	Calculus ↓		
	Inflammatory changes (reversible) ↓	Enzyme system that facilitates breakdown of starches to sugars ↓	
Secondary prevention (irreversible changes and moderate destruction)	Soft tissue breakdown ↓	Initial cavitation ↓	Secondary prevention
	Bone resorption ↓	Advanced cavitation ↓	
	Loss of tooth support ↓	Invasion of pulp ↓	
	Increased difficulty in eliminating local irritants ↓	Systemic invasion ↓ Tooth loss ↓	Tertiary prevention
Tertiary prevention (advanced disease and destruction)	Increasing tissue and bone loss ↓	Drifting and malposition of other teeth	
	Tooth loss		

Source: Pauline F. Steel, *Dental Hygiene* (Philadelphia: Lea and Febiger, 1970), p. 18.

Periodontal disease doesn't always cause tooth loss, though; at least, not for a while. There can be bleeding, poisoning of the system, which creates a general rundown feeling, problems with chewing, and halitosis.

TARTAR

The problem usually starts with plaque. This accumulates on the teeth and hardens into what's called tartar or calculus. The ideal, of course, is to remove all plaque by brushing so that this can't happen. But we can't brush as efficiently or as often as we like. So the tartar forms at the base of our teeth and in between them and irritates the gums. Tartar itself isn't an irritant, but it has sharp edges that make the gums pull away from the teeth and

227

leave pockets. Bacteria accumulate in these pockets, and bacteria irritate the gums and make the gums pull farther away from the teeth, which makes it easier for more tartar to form, and so on. This chain of events continues for an extended period until a person gets a condition called gingivitis—inflammation of the gums. This is the first stage in the periodontal disease growth pattern.

GUM DETERIORATION

Plaque isn't the only cause of gingivitis. There's a mouth disease called Vincent's infection, sometimes known as "trench mouth." This, along with the tartar, inflames the gums, ulcerates them, makes them red and sore. They bleed a lot and give off a repugnant odor. Also, a bad bite, or "malocclusion," can contribute to the gingivitis problem. This brings on stresses, strains, unnecessary pressure on the teeth, and, therefore, unnecessary pressure on the gums.

Some people don't know that they have gingivitis. Their gums bleed a little, seem a little red. But they don't suffer a lot of pain, so it's probably best to ignore it. Some realize they do have gingivitis but decide to ignore it anyway. After all, the bad breath problem can be covered with a mouthwash or a mint, and that's the real problem, isn't it? No, it's not. If you don't visit your dentist regularly to have the tartar removed and have gingivitis problems treated, the gums will recede more and more from the teeth, and underlying tissues will start to deteriorate. Periodontal disease then enters its second stage, called periodontitis. Here the teeth become loose, pockets that developed in the gums fill with pus, and the pus destroys the supportive bone structure. Inflammation begins to spread. If it spreads far enough and long enough, the periodontitis becomes pyorrhea, the most serious stage of periodontal disease. Without immediate treatment for this condition, all teeth will be lost.

It's a lot easier to prevent periodontal disease than cure it. Brushing your teeth at least twice a day and using dental floss after each brushing are a good start. You can also use electric toothbrushes, water-pressure devices, toothpicks, and rubber or plastic gum massagers. But these won't substitute for visiting your dentist on a regular basis and having the tartar removed from the gum line. You won't get rid of it in any other way.[23]

MOUTHWASH

Should you use a mouthwash? It won't do any harm, and it might solve a temporary bad breath problem. But it won't substitute for brushing. Of course, TV and radio commercials imply that without a mouthwash you'll never have a date who kisses you good-night or a close friend who tells you what your real problem is. This is nonsense. Stomach trouble can cause bad breath. But, if your stomach isn't upset, the key to keeping breath fresh is keeping decaying food particles out of the mouth. This can be done only by regular brushing and regular visits to the dentist.[24]

Notes

1. Herbert A. deVries, *Physiology of Exercise* (Dubuque, Ia.: William C. Brown Co., 1973), pp. 174–182.
2. Robert Hockey, *Physical Fitness: The Pathway to Healthful Living* (Saint Louis: Mosby, 1973), pp. 3–23.
3. Roy Ald, *Physical Fitness After 35* (New York: Essandess, 1967), pp. 9–12.
4. Peter Karpovich, *Physiology of Muscular Activity* (Philadelphia: Saunders, 1971), pp. 65–74.
5. Frank Vitale, *Individualized Fitness Programs* (Englewood Cliffs, N.J.: Prentice-Hall, 1973).
6. Kenneth H. Cooper, *Aerobics* (New York: Lippincott, 1968), pp. 31–43.
7. Pernow Bengt and Saltin Bengt, *Muscle Metabolism During Exercise* (New York: Plenum Press, 1971), pp. 87–97.
8. Rodahl Kare, *Be Fit for Life* (New York: Harper and Row, 1966), pp. 44–56, 93–104, 134–159.
9. Curtis Mitchell, *Put Yourself in Shape* (Garden City, N.Y.: Doubleday, 1965).
10. I. G. Edmonds, *Isometric and Isotonic Exercises for Men and Women* (Derby, Conn.: Monarch Books, 1964).
11. Richard Kraus, *Recreation Today* (New York: Appleton-Century-Crofts, 1966), pp. 94–126.
12. Josephine L. Rathbone, *Relaxation* (Philadelphia: Lea and Febiger, 1969), pp. 2–33, 77–103.
13. Ernst Limonson, *Physiology of Work Capacity and Fatigue* (Springfield, Ill.: Thomas, 1971), pp. 211–236, 241–242.
14. W. P. Congress, *Sleep Deprivation: Aspects of Human Efficiency* (London: English Universities Press, 1972), pp. 177–195.
15. Ernest Hartmann, *Sleep and Dreaming*, Vol. VII, No. 2 (Boston: Little, Brown, 1970), pp. 277–290.
16. Justus J. Schifferes, *Healthier Living* (New York: Wiley, 1970), pp. 122–123.
17. George B. Jerzy Glass, *Introduction to Gastrointestinal Physiology* (Englewood Cliffs, N.J.: Prentice-Hall, 1968), pp. 170–174.
18. Dudley J. Morton, *The Human Foot* (New York: Columbia University Press, 1948), pp. 153–159, 219–233.
19. Wilma E. Motley, *Ethics, Jurisprudence, and History of the Dental Hygienist* (Philadelphia: Lea and Febiger, 1972), pp. 106–120, 298–304.
20. Russel W. Bunting, *Oral Hygiene* (Philadelphia: Lea and Febiger, 1954), pp. 56–96.
21. Sydney Garfield, *Teeth, Teeth, Teeth: A Treatise on Teeth* (New York: Simon and Schuster, 1971).
22. L. F. Swejda, "Fluorides in Community Programs," *Journal of Public Health Dentistry*, Vol. 32 (Spring 1972), 110–118.
23. Robert A. Cobby, Hamilton Robinson, and Donald A. Kerr, *Color Atlas of Oral Pathology* (Philadelphia: Lippincott, 1971), pp. 55–90.
24. Bunting, *Oral Hygiene*, pp. 249–250.

10 Components of a Healthy Body

Some claim it's the most beautiful, the most complex, the most creative structure of engineering ever developed, this human body. Leonardo da Vinci and Michelangelo drew pictures of it. They carved statues of it, too, just as the Greeks, the Romans, and the Americans did. And watching girls at the beach or ones in miniskirts is an American hobby. For most, the human body is an artistic masterpiece, far beyond anything Rembrandt or Picasso could come up with.

There have been a few, though, who looked on the human body as sinful, disgusting. They flagellated it, they mutilated it, covered it so that no one could be tempted by fleshly sins. And there were fewer yet who wanted to understand this human body, know its parts, its functions, and life-sustaining mysteries. After all, they felt, life does seem to be what this world is about. Without it, there's no movement, no impressions, no appreciation of beauty, no speech, no sound, no growth, no love. Life, though it's not always pleasant, is a miracle that makes most other miracles seem insignificant. And because the human body contained the secrets of human life, they decided to analyze it. They didn't find what this life secret was, of course, but they discovered another dimension of beauty and understanding that is worth looking into. It can give a better appreciation of the functions and structure of the human animal, of why we look, we think, and act as we do.

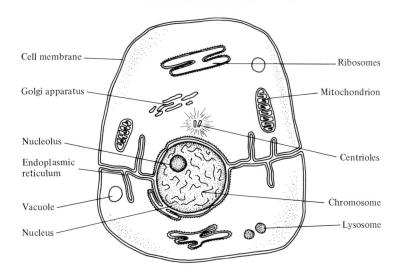

Cell membrane —

Golgi apparatus —

Nucleolus —

Endoplasmic reticulum —

Vacuole —

Nucleus —

— Ribosomes

— Mitochondrion

— Centrioles

— Chromosome

— Lysosome

FIGURE 10-1. *A typical cell.*

The Cell

We're made of hydrogen, carbon, sulfur, nitrogen, oxygen, and phosphorus, we humans. Dogs could claim the same, of course. And so could trees and anteaters, if they could speak. Rocks, dirt, and water are also made of these things in various combinations. But objects that aren't alive lack something, which trees and anteaters and humans have, called protoplasm. This is a life-sustaining substance that no one understands, that can't be made in a test tube. Protoplasm looks like an egg white and feels like slippery oil.

Cells are minute specks of protoplasm, and are the basic units of life itself. Each has its own characteristics, and cells work together in highly intricate ways to form tissues and organs and people. About 100 trillion cells make up each human being. And when you consider that each of the cells is a living unit in itself, the human body gets to be a pretty complex mechanism. Most evolutionary theorists feel many more millions of years went into the development of the cell than into the development of the human from the cell.

Each of the different types of cells in our bodies carries out a different role. There are blood cells, which transport gases; nerve cells, which transmit messages about the environment; male and female sex cells, which reproduce the species; muscle cells, which contract; bone cells, which become stiff and strong. But despite the differences, cells have some important similarities. All of them live, all of them grow, and most reproduce. And most have two major parts—the nucleus and the cytoplasm.

Cytoplasm is a jellylike mass containing various complicated proteins. A few of the more typical proteinaceous structures are mitochondria, the Golgi apparatus, the centrioles, and the fibrils. The nucleus controls the events that take place in this complicated mass, such as digestion, respiration, excretion, and secretion. And the nucleus, the cell's governor, contains some elements of its own. There is a round, minute body called the nucleolus and small, irregular masses called chromatin granules.[1]

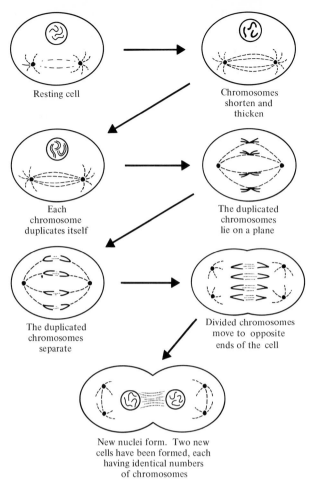

Chromosomes
shorten and
thicken

Each
chromosome
duplicates itself

The duplicated
chromosomes
lie on a plane

The duplicated
chromosomes
separate

Divided chromosomes
move to opposite
ends of the cell

New nuclei form. Two new
cells have been formed, each
having identical numbers
of chromosomes

FIGURE 10-2. *Mitosis—the production of two genetically identical cells.*

Mitosis

Most cells can reproduce themselves simply by dividing. So one cell becomes two cells, two become four, four become eight, etc. That's how we grow, how the life process is maintained. This phenomenon, mitosis, begins when the centriole, a small body just outside the nucleus, divides. The chromatin, which looks like a lot of scattered granules when the cell is at rest, arranges itself into definite threads. These threads then become chromosomes, which are made up of chromatin particles. These particles are groups of genes. And genes are the units that transfer traits from parent cells to daughter cells. They're the things that give us brown eyes, red hair, and 32 teeth. They're the basis of inheritance. So, during mitosis, each gene must divide into two daughter genes. The other parts of the cell divide, too. This is what makes a fertilized human egg grow into a fetus, a baby, a grown person. It explains how skin cells grow to cover an open wound, how bone cells mend a fracture, how injured organs return to normal function.

The two new daughter cells each have half of the original cell wall, half of the cytoplasm, half of the nucleus, and half of everything else that made up the parent. So daughter cells are small. And, like all living things, they have to grow before they can function efficiently and reproduce themselves when their time comes.[2]

This growth requires food. This shouldn't present much of a problem, since the liquid cells are bathed in contains the food materials they need. But there's a protective wall surrounding each of the cells called a membrane. This wall could keep cells from getting their nourishment if it were some type of solid barrier. But the membrane is permeable to food particles, which can pass through the wall to the cell's digestive system. Also, cells, like other organisms, have waste products. These have to work their way through the membrane in the opposite direction. And the membrane keeps proteins and other life-sustaining substances confined and keeps undesirable substances out. So the cell wall is semipermeable—it isn't permeable to some molecules and is permeable to others.[3]

Bodily Systems

There are specialized types of cells in our bodies that combine to form tissues. And the tissues combine into organs, and the organs group together to form what are called systems. The systems are grouped according to the key bodily functions they carry out. There's been a little disagreement on just what a key bodily function is. Some divide the human body into nine bodily systems, some into ten, others into eleven.[4] But all agree that our bodies are balanced systems with parts arranged in regular patterns and interacting according to a specific set of rules. Here is one of the more commonly accepted subdivisions.

The Skeletal System

Bones, over 200 of them, form the framework for the rest of our bodies. Muscles hang on them; so do skin and toenails. Without bones, we'd be shapeless masses of rubbery stuff, something like squid or jellyfish. To do their job, bones have to be hard, like brick or cement. But this hardness doesn't mean that our bones are inanimate. There are live cells in bones, and they have their own nerves and their own blood systems.

Bones are hollow, and in their center is marrow. There's red marrow, which manufactures most of our red blood cells, and there's a yellow variety, which is primarily fat. Bones are surrounded by a membrane called the periosteum. This contains nerves that let us know when we get kicked in the shins or bumped on our arms. The periosteum helps to repair bones after they've been fractured and helps with bone production when we're growing.

Put all human bones together, and you've got a human skeleton. This can be divided into two main groups. There's the axial skeleton, which comprises our trunks and the bony framework of our heads. And there's the appendicular skeleton, which provides the framework for arms and legs.

The skull, the framework of the head, in turn subdivides into two parts. There is the cranium, a rounded box surrounding the brain, and the bony frame of the face.[5]

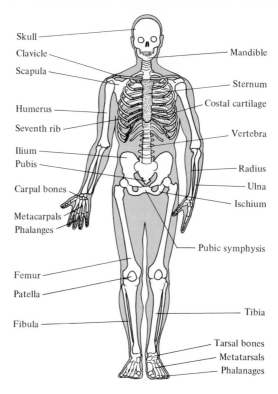

Skull

Clavicle

Scapula

Humerus

Seventh rib

Ilium

Pubis

Carpal bones

Metacarpals

Phalanges

Femur

Patella

Fibula

Mandible

Sternum

Costal cartilage

Vertebra

Radius

Ulna

Ischium

Pubic symphysis

Tibia

Tarsal bones

Metatarsals

Phalanages

FIGURE 10-3. *The skeleton.*

Ligaments and Joints

The points where bones meet each other are called joints. A capsule containing a thick, slippery fluid surrounding each of these joints provides lubrication for ease of movement. Bones, of course, would slip out of joint constantly if something didn't keep them in place. And this something is called ligaments. They're strong, fibrous cords on the sides of the various joints. Sometimes they're on just two sides of the joint, letting it move freely in one direction but not in the other. Sometimes they let the joint hardly move at all, and sometimes they let the joint turn in almost any direction, like those in the spine and the hips and the shoulders. They let us bend forward, backward, sideways, even rotate parts such as our necks and wrists.[6]

The Muscular System

Muscles connected to our bones move the parts of our bodies the directions our ligaments allow. For instance, there's one major muscle in the front of the knee joint with several behind it. Contract the front muscle, and the lower leg moves forward. Contract the muscles behind the joint, and back comes the leg again. The same applies to muscles that move the ankles. Ankle ligaments let the ankle joints move from side to side as well as forward and backward.

Muscles almost never act alone. As in the knee joints, a muscle or muscle group gets paired against other muscles. This is called antagonism. In order for the leg, the arm, the head, the big toe to move, one set of muscles must

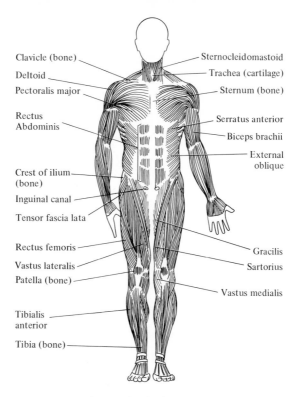

FIGURE 10-4. *The chief muscles of the body.*

relax while the others contract. This provides for all kinds of flexibility in movement and lets us swing baseball bats, ride bicycles, or do most things that come into our heads. Actually without antagonism we'd never be able to stand or move. Gravity would keep us pinned flat to the ground.

We have a lot of muscles that aren't associated with our skeletal systems. There are muscles in our stomachs, intestines, and other internal organs that contract much more slowly and rhythmically than those connected to our bones. We don't have much control over muscles of this type, so they're often referred to as involuntary muscles. And the muscles in our hearts, though they're involuntary, also, have such distinct properties and structure that they're put in a category by themselves.

Muscles come in all shapes and sizes. There are fat ones and thin ones, long and short. The smallest skeletal muscle of the body is the stapedius in the middle ear. This is only a few millimeters long. But the sartorius in the thigh is almost 2 feet long. The biceps, which lifts the lower arm, and the gastrocnemius, which holds down the foot, are cigar-shaped. There's no end to the structural variations. But, despite the differences, muscles work together to create a unified force that keeps us functioning, moving, reacting, and creating.[7]

The Circulatory System

Our muscles and bones and ligaments aren't dead tissue. They consist of living cells; and, like all living matter, the cells have to get a continuous supply

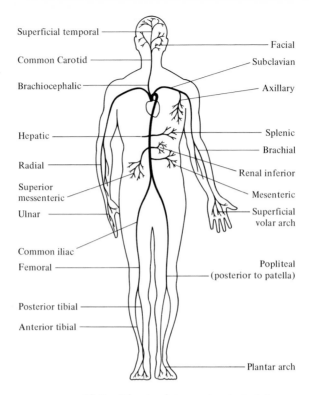

FIGURE 10-5. *The circulatory system (arteries).*

of nourishment. This is the circulatory system's job. Blood carries this nourishment, oxygen, to all parts of our bodies and takes waste material away.

The blood is a tissue in its own right. There's about 5 quarts of it in most of us. And almost half of it is cells. They're specific types of cells, of course, unlike cells in other bodily tissues.

The half of the blood that doesn't consist of cells is called plasma. This contains proteins and minerals and other soluble substances. One of the proteins is fibrinogen, which makes the blood clot when we cut ourselves. Without this, of course, we'd all bleed to death.

THE HEART

Blood has to be constantly on the move in order to do us much good. Motionless blood could never transport oxygen to where it's needed and take waste products from tissues that have to get rid of them. So a pump, the heart, is necessary to keep this blood circulating. The heart really consists of two pumps, side by side, each of which has two chambers. The left pump pushes blood to our brains, our toes, our fingertips. The pump on the right side forces blood into the lungs, where it absorbs oxygen and releases carbon dioxide.

The blood's journey starts as it leaves the lungs and enters the left atrium, the chamber at the top of the heart. It then pours into the left ventricle, a pumping chamber just beneath the atrium. When the ventricle contracts, blood leaves the heart and travels through the body's arteries, ar-

236

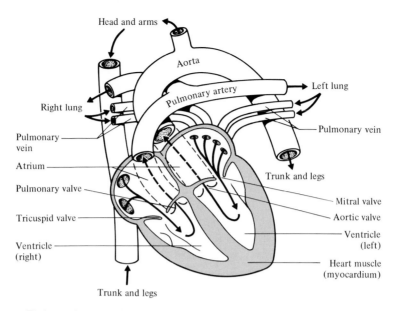

The human heart, like the heart in all mammals, has four chambers. Two of these chambers (one atrium and one ventricle) perform systemic circulation. The two remaining chambers carry out pulmonary circulation. There is a wall between the chambers (the septum), which prevents oxygenated blood from mixing with deoxygenated blood. Valves between the atria and ventricles prevent backward flow when the heart contracts.

FIGURE 10-6. *The heart.*

terioles, and capillaries. Blood returns to the heart through our veins, which have valves to prevent backward flow. At this point, the blood has lost its oxygen and is carrying waste products the cells have cast off. So, upon reaching the heart, it enters the right atrium, which quickly contracts and forces it into the right ventricle. Contraction of the ventricle sends the blood pulsating through the pulmonary artery to the lungs. Here the blood gets rid of its waste products and absorbs oxygen before entering the left atrium to begin the cycle once more.

A solid wall called the septum separates the left ventricle from the right ventricle and the left atrium from the right atrium. Also, there are heart valves that keep the blood moving out of the atria to the ventricles from backing up. Blood can flow in one direction only; it can't return. And there are outlet valves in the ventricles that keep blood from flowing back into the heart once it has entered the arteries.

THE LYMPHATIC SYSTEM

There's an accessory circulation system that keeps protein molecules, dead bacteria, dead tissue debris, and the like from accumulating. It's called the lymphatic system and has capillaries next to blood capillaries. Blood capillaries, of course, are porous, but the pores are extremely small. Large particles can never get through them into the bloodstream. The lymphatic capillaries are much more porous yet. Large particles can get through them to be carried by lymph fluid along lymphatic vessels to our necks. Here these vessels empty into our neck veins.

There are several points in the lymphatic system where these large par-

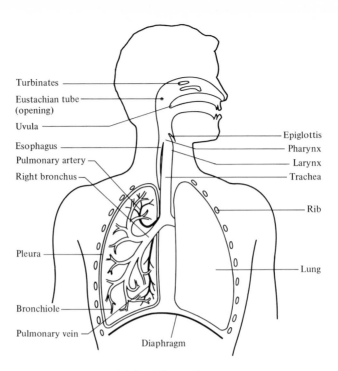

Turbinates

Eustachian tube (opening)

Uvula

Esophagus

Pulmonary artery

Right bronchus

Pleura

Bronchiole

Pulmonary vein

Epiglottis

Pharynx

Larynx

Trachea

Rib

Lung

Diaphragm

FIGURE 10-7. *The respiratory system.*

ticles get filtered out. These are called lymph nodes. At these points, special cells surround and digest harmful bacteria.[8]

The Respiratory System

Respiration is the process of breathing in and breathing out. Our rib muscles play a key role in this process, working with another muscle called the diaphragm. The diaphragm forms a dome between the abdomen and the chest. During inhalation, the diaphragm and rib muscles contract, enlarging the chest cavity. The lungs are quite elastic, so they expand right along with the chest wall. This creates a partial vacuum in the lung air sacs. Air rushes in to bring the lung pressure back to that of the atmosphere. During exhalation, the diaphragm and rib muscles relax, forcing the chest cavity and lungs to contract. This raises the pressure in the lung tissue and forces air outward.

While respiration is going on, blood continuously flows along the lungs. There's a very thin membrane separating this blood from breathed air. The membrane is porous to gases, so oxygen from the air passes freely to the blood, which carries it to the cells, where it combines chemically with foods. This releases energy we need to keep our bodies functioning. Blood going back to our lungs carries carbon dioxide, a waste product released by our cells. This, like oxygen, passes through the porous membranes in the lungs, where it is released back into the air.[9]

The Excretory System

Our bodies can't use everything we take in. We breathe in air, but certainly we don't use all of it. Carbon dioxide and other waste products have to be

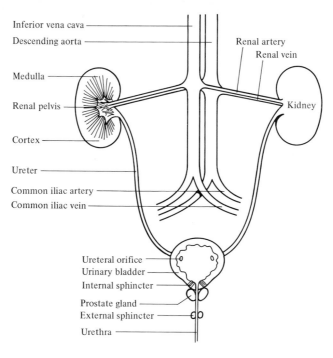

Inferior vena cava

Descending aorta

Renal artery

Renal vein

Medulla

Renal pelvis

Kidney

Cortex

Ureter

Common iliac artery

Common iliac vein

Ureteral orifice

Urinary bladder

Internal sphincter

Prostate gland

External sphincter

Urethra

FIGURE 10-8. *Kidneys.*

expelled. The same is true with food and water. There are indigestible parts of food that we expel as fecal matter, and there are forms of liquid wastes that we expel through our kidneys. The kidneys, two of them, plus two ureters, one urinary bladder, and the urethra comprise the excretory system. Without it we'd be poisoned by the ammonia our bodies create when they break down proteins. The excretory system converts this ammonia into urea, then expels it from the body. And there are other by-products created when the body converts nutrients to energy. The kidneys expel many of these along with ammonia and also maintain a chemical balance of certain materials circulating in the bloodstream.

THE KIDNEYS

The kidneys lie in the upper abdomen against the muscles of the back. They're protected by the ribs and their cartilages and a circle of fat called the adipose capsule. This capsule, a membranous tissue, surrounds each kidney.

The basic unit of the kidney is called the nephron. This is a small, coiled tube, balled on one end, containing a cluster of capillaries. This cluster, the glomerulus, is where the kidney's main business is carried on. The capillary membranes are extremely porous; and, as the blood passes by them, water and urea are filtered into the tubular space, whereas larger molecules stay in the blood.

There's a regulatory mechanism in the kidneys that keeps the chemical composition of the blood fairly constant. This composition can get thrown out of balance when other tissues exchange substances with the blood through their own capillary networks. This loss of blood balance can bring on serious physical problems. It's up to the kidneys to right the situation before any major damage is done. This can be a major task when we're sick or injured. When blood chemistry goes seriously awry, the kidneys have to work overtime. This can weaken the kidneys, of course, and makes us more susceptible to further disease or injury.

URETERS AND BLADDER

The two long, slender tubes connecting the kidney basin with the urinary bladder are called ureters. These are drains for urine leaving the kidneys. Muscles in the ureters carry out rhythmic contractions called peristalsis. These contractions force the urine to flow. The bladder, of course, eventually fills, creating a tendency for urine to back up. But at this point the ureters compress, assuring that no backflow takes place.

The bladder is a temporary container for urine and can hold about 1 pint. The bladder wall is thick when it's empty but becomes quite thin when the organ fills. It increases in length from around 2 or 3 inches to more than 5 inches.

The passageway through which urine travels from the bladder to the outside world is called the urethra. For men, it's part of the reproductive system and is much longer than the urethra in a woman. The male's urethra passes through his prostate gland, where it is joined by two ducts carrying male sex cells. It then extends through the penis to the outside. So men's urethras not only drain their bladders but also play a key role in the reproductive process. The female urethra, though, allows for drainage of the bladder only.[10]

The Digestive System

Nutritious parts of the foods we eat have to get to the cells in our bodies. This is quite a complex process, as the food has to be converted to a form that the blood can carry and that the cells can absorb through their membranes. There are two main groups of organs carrying on this work. There's the alimentary canal, the passageway beginning at the mouth and ending at the anus. And there are accessory organs—the liver, the gall bladder, and the pancreas. The alimentary canal and the accessory organs combine to form the digestive system.

Whether it's a steak sandwich, an ice cream cone, or brussels sprouts entering our bodies, the food trip starts in the mouth. Our teeth masticate the food, our taste buds let us know whether we like it, our tongues work it into the best location for swallowing. And there are glands in our mouths that provide saliva. This helps dissolve the food and helps us to chew and swallow.

Once the food leaves the mouth, peristalsis, like that in the ureter, takes over. This wavelike motion starts in the throat, or the pharynx, and continues through the entire length of the canal. After our tongues have pushed the food past the soft palate, the pharynx muscles contract, and the swallowing process begins.

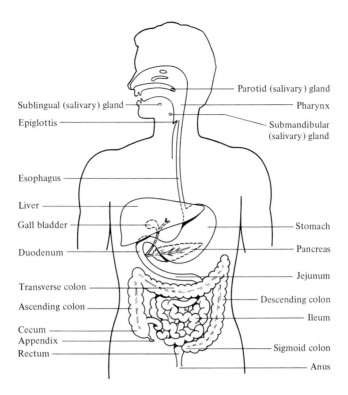

FIGURE 10-9. *The digestive system.*

The food in the pharynx passes into the esophagus, which extends through the neck and chest for approximately 9 inches. Then comes the spherical container called the stomach. The stomach produces a general churning instead of the wavelike motion that pushes food onward. When it's filled, the sphincter valve closes, letting the stomach keep the contents until the food gets thoroughly mixed with digestive enzymes called gastric juice. This breaks up and liquefies the food into what is called chyme. Chyme stays in our stomachs for between 2 and 6 hours before passing on to our small intestines.

Food entering the small intestine is almost completely digested. Saliva and gastric juice have reduced it to a state where it's nearly ready to enter the bloodstream and be carried to the body's cells. Enzymes from the intestinal wall break food down a bit further, and the pancreas provides digestive juices to complete the chemical change. The juice the liver provides is called bile, which breaks fats and oils into small drops. Bile is stored in the gall bladder until it's needed for this digestive function.

Raw food materials are now ready to enter our bloodstreams through villi, fine projections on the small intestine's mucous membrane. This process is called absorption and is the small intestine's main function. Once this absorption has taken place, the rest of the food becomes waste. We expel it through our large intestines. We have layers of muscles lining our large intestinal walls that contract to force waste (fecal matter) through our rectums prior to elimination.[11]

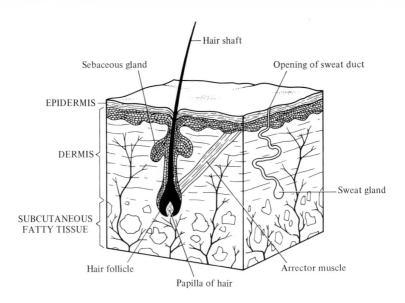

FIGURE 10-10. *The integumentary system.*

The Integumentary System

The integumentary system is the skin, the largest membrane in the body. This is the tissue that stands between us and the outside world. It protects us from mechanical injury, keeps microorganisms from getting to our cells, helps maintain the water balance in our systems, no matter what the humidity of the world around us happens to be, and helps maintain a constant body temperature, despite a very cold or very hot environment. It's a dynamic structure, this skin. It renews and changes itself constantly, and it has all kinds of thicknesses, textures, and functions. The skin over our knees, elbows, and knuckles can stretch, and the skin on the palms and soles of our feet can withstand a lot of twisting and pulling. The skin on our faces, although thin and smooth in spots, has some thick, coarse, hairy places, such as the eyebrows.

Skin regenerates itself quickly. This is important, as we average one minor skin wound per week, about 4,000 skin wounds in a lifetime. Without this fast healing process, our integumentary systems would force us to spend most of our lives in hospitals.

There are three main layers to our skin, each of which has a different function and structure. There's the epidermis, the outermost layer; the dermis, the secondary layer; and the subcutaneous tissue. The epidermis, dry and tough, covers the entire external surface of the body. Actually, there are four layers to the epidermis. It's the outermost layer that gives it a dry and tough quality. This is called the horny layer. It consists of flat, dead cells that have been pushed to the surface from the lower layer of the epidermis. The cells reach the surface and are gradually arranged into flexible patterns of horny material.

Dermis, sometimes called the true skin, is a lot thicker than the epidermis. It consists of what are known as collagenous and elastic fibers, which make the dermis tough, strong, and resilient. There's an ascending protrusion from the dermis that locks with descending ridges from the epi-

242

dermis, binding the two skin layers together. There are thousands of blood vessels and nerves in this true skin and a far greater blood flow than is necessary for the skin's metabolism. This blood acts as a temperature regulator, carrying the heat of internal organs to the body's surface. Also, the dermis houses the skin's appendages, consisting of nails, hair, and sweat and oil glands.

Subcutaneous tissue is really a way of connecting the dermis to the surface muscles. There's a lot of fat in this tissue, which provides insulation and a storage place for energy.

There are a multitude of pigment cells at the point where the dermis and epidermis meet. These produce a dark-colored pigment called melanin, which has the primary function of protecting our bodies against ultraviolet rays of the sun. We also have melanin in our hair, the iris of our eyes, and the middle coats of our eyeballs. All people have a certain amount of melanin in their skin, and darker races have a greater quantity of it than lighter people do. When we're exposed to sunlight, our melanin gets darker, and the quantity in our skin increases. That's how we become tan. Sometimes this pigmentation increases abnormally in certain localized areas of our bodies. This can indicate a glandular problem or some other type of physical disorder.

The amount of blood circulating in the surface vessels affects the skin coloring, too. So do the amount of oxygen in the blood and any chemicals, such as sulfur compounds, that may have gotten in the bloodstream.[12]

SKIN APPENDAGES

Hair belongs exclusively to mammals. It's not to be found on fish or insects or birds. It's a dead tissue, coming from our skin and growing from follicles embedded in the dermis. These follicles are in minute pits containing the hair roots. The part of our hair that people see is called the shaft.

Hair doesn't grow continuously, having several rest periods between its growth spurts. Each hair goes through what is called a cycle. It starts when the hair is formed and begins to grow, and ends when a new hair emerges from the same follicle.

All of us have thin, horny plates on our hands and feet that we call fingernails and toenails. These are made up of translucent cells that come from the outer part of the epidermis and are hard and firm enough to help protect the ends of our toes and fingers. Without them, walking and lifting would be painful, and scratching would be out of the question.

We have sebaceous glands all over our bodies, except in our palms and soles. These glands secrete a fatty substance called sebum that emulsifies and keeps water in the skin. This helps to make it soft and pliable. These glands lie in the dermis, are most numerous in the face, scalp, and the midlines of our chests and backs.

A man can always sweat, sometimes more profusely than he wants to. There are about 3 million sweat glands in our skin, originating in the epidermis, extending into the dermis. They consist of the apocrine glands, usually connected with hair follicles, and the eccrine glands, which aren't. We have apocrine glands in our armpits, genital and pubic areas, and breasts. These glands produce an odor in response to stress or sexual stimulation. That's why we use underarm sprays and deodorant creams and the like. The eccrine glands serve almost all parts of the body. They are the ones that produce the sweat because of heat. The sweat evaporates and makes us cooler, and the sweat moistens the skin, preventing the horny layer of the epidermis from becoming scaly.[13]

Metabolism and the Endocrine System

Metabolism consists of the chemical reactions going on inside our individual cells. This process is a must to have the necessary energy to carry on bodily activities and build any new structures we might need. Without metabolism, our cells wouldn't grow larger and multiply and we'd quickly wither.

Although this metabolism is an integral function of each of our cells, we have endocrine glands to increase and decrease the cells' metabolic rate. The glands do this by secreting chemical messengers called hormones directly into the bloodstream.

Each of us has a thyroid gland in his neck. It secretes the hormone thyroxin, which affects the metabolic rate in all of our tissues. If we have too little thyroxin, we get to feeling lazy and dull. If we have too much thyroxin, it's hard to slow us down. Sometimes people's thyroids become diseased and have to be removed. So, in order to overcome that lethargic feeling, they take injections of thyroid extract, which corrects the problem in an artificial way.

Two other hormones that generally influence the metabolic rate are epinephrine and norepinephrine. These are secreted by the adrenal glands just above the kidneys. These hormones regulate our circulation, speed up our heartbeat, and accelerate breathing. Also, they slow down the actions of our digestive organs and dilate the pupils in our eyes. So a large spurt of epinephrine (sometimes called adrenalin) into our systems prepares us for some threat from the world around us. This is sometimes called the "fight or flight" response.

Our sex organs have a special metabolism controlled by estrogens and progesterone in women and testosterone in men. The female hormones come from the ovaries, whereas the male variety come from the testes. The female hormones make ovulation possible, regulate the menstrual cycle, and have a strong influence on the female's emotions. The male's hormones influence emotions as well. But it's not the noticeable effect that the female experiences. Also, testosterone affects the sex characteristics in the rest of the body and stimulates sexual interest and excitement.

There are four small glands in our necks that produce the parathyroid hormone, which controls the amount of calcium in our blood. This hormone removes calcium from our bones when the blood needs it and takes calcium from the blood for the bones when it's needed there.

The pancreas gland underneath the stomach secretes insulin. This hormone decreases fat utilization and increases our utilization of carbohydrates. When the pancreas produces too much insulin, we have low blood sugar symptoms and have to eat almost continuously to keep from being dizzy or fainting. When our bodies get too little insulin, we have a condition called

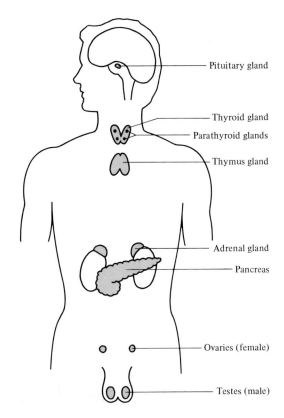

FIGURE 10-11. *The endocrine system.*

diabetes mellitus. This interferes with sugar metabolism, creating an excess accumulation of sugar in the blood. This can bring on cardiovascular or nervous system disorders. It can even cause death.[14]

The Nervous System

The nervous system is a network of billions of nerve cells under the control of our brains and spinal cords. These nerve cells, or neurons, have fibers that connect with each other at junctions called synapses, producing communication. What we think of as nerves are bundles of these long fibers that link parts of the nervous system to bodily organs and tissues. They're something like telephone cables, with a lot of small wires in them carrying impulses from one part of the body to another.

Most of our nerve cells are in our brains and spinal cords, which together comprise the central nervous system. We also have a peripheral nervous system, consisting of the major nerves coming from the central system and clusters of neurons spread throughout our bodies. Peripheral nerves are sometimes classified as cranial and spinal. Cranial nerves carry impulses to and from the brain, whereas spinal nerves perform this same function for the spinal cord.

There's a sensory branch of the nervous system that gets information from the world around us and from parts of our bodies and carries it to the brain or spinal cord. Nerves in this branch are called afferent nerves. There

245

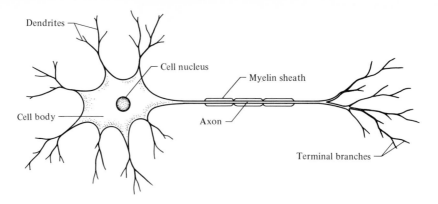

Nerves. Neurons don't enter or leave the central nervous system as individual units. Thousands of neurons, enclosed in connective tissue, combine to make up a single nerve. Some of the nerves consist solely of motor neurons whereas others contain only sensory ones. Most contain both types.

FIGURE 10-12. *A generalized neuron.*

are also efferent nerves that carry the impulses from our brains and spinal cords to muscles and glands. These comprise the motor branch of the nervous system. And this motor branch breaks down into two major subsystems. One is called the autonomic nervous system, which carries impulses to our glands, hearts, and involuntary muscles. In other words, it directs activities that our bodies carry on automatically. The subsystem that directs activities we can consciously control is called the voluntary nervous system.

THE CENTRAL NERVOUS SYSTEM

The mass in our heads that regulates our thoughts, our movements, and our reactions is extremely complex. No one has a detailed understanding of how the brain works; no one has ever come up with a satisfactory explanation of how the brain makes thinking and emotions possible. But the brain has been subdivided into various centers that generally control key parts of our behavior. And though this in no way explains our sense of awareness, consciousness, or our ability to think in abstract patterns, it does provide a crude outline of the functioning process of the most intricate, complex, efficient control system known.

The largest part of the brain is the cerebrum. Here is the area where our higher thought processes take place, where we compose poems, solve mathematical problems, make decisions. And our memories are stored in the cerebrum, the bad ones as well as the good. The cerebrum has two hemispheres, a right and a left. The right controls the left-hand side of the body, and vice versa. The deeper part of the brain, most of which can't be seen unless the brain is sectioned, is the brain stem. Here is where our breathing, blood pressure, and heart rate are regulated. The upper part of the brain stem is called the midbrain, and there's a section immediately below the midbrain called the pons. Behind the pons, under the cerebrum, is the area that controls our coordination and balance, called the cerebellum. This connects to other parts of the brain through the pons only.

246

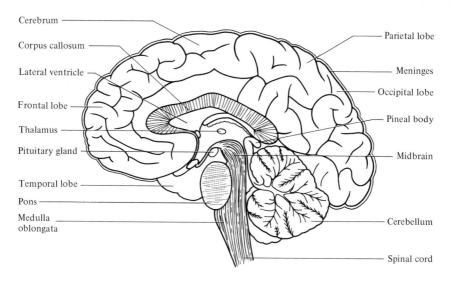

FIGURE 10-13. *The human brain.*

Gray matter called the cerebral cortex comprises the outer nerve tissue of the cerebrum. This is where our sensations like sight, hearing, and smell get registered and where we initiate voluntary actions. Involuntary actions, such as hunger, sleep, regulation of body temperature, thirst, and sexual behavior are directed by the thalamus, located just above the tip of the brain stem. The pituitary gland, just beneath the thalamus, links the nervous system to the body's endocrine system. Because the pituitary has

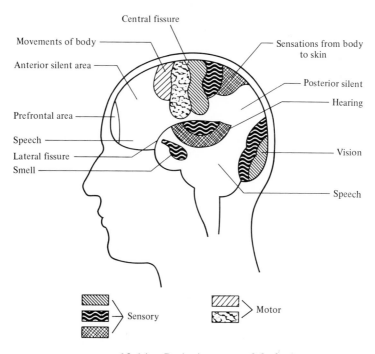

FIGURE 10-14. *Projection areas of the brain.*

such a key effect on all parts of the body, it is often referred to as the "master gland."[15]

SPINAL CORD

The spinal cord provides a kind of messenger service carrying impulses to and from the brain. If the cord is severed or seriously damaged, these impulses won't get to the desired bodily areas. Spinal cord injuries can bring on loss of control of limbs, loss of various physical functions, and loss of sensation from environmental stimuli. If we touch something too hot, the message travels through our spinal cords to our brains, where it's interpreted as pain. If we touch something soft and warm, the brain intreprets this as pleasant. But victims of spinal injury can't receive and interpret messages of this type. Sometimes they have no sensation whatever below their waists or even below their necks.[16]

The Reproductive System

Most living matter can reproduce itself. If it couldn't, life would quickly disappear. There are one-celled organisms that don't need partners to reproduce, dividing themselves through asexual reproduction only. But for higher animals sexual reproduction is a must before there can be offspring. This calls for a male and a female. The male brings a specialized sex cell, the spermatozoon, to the union, and the female brings a cell called the ovum.

Despite the differences between men and women, their reproductive apparatuses have several characteristics in common. Both have gonads to produce sex cells and manufacture hormones; both have passageways and tubes for their sex cells; and both have several accessory organs.

THE FEMALE

Female gonads, or ovaries, are on either side of the backbone in the abdominal cavity and are connected to funnel-shaped openings called fallopian tubes. During ovarian cycles, about 28 days each, eggs are produced in follicles. When the follicle gets close to the surface of the ovary, it ruptures, discharging the egg, or ovum, into a fallopian tube. Currents carry the egg through the tube to the uterus, where it develops when pregnancy occurs.

There's a glandular passageway called the vagina in which the penis is inserted during intercourse. Also, babies are delivered through this passageway at birth. So the fertilized egg, upon properly maturing, passes through the vagina to become another member of the human race.

The biological, not the aesthetic, purpose of intercourse is to get the egg and the sperm together. The male reproductive system provides lots of sperm and controls the means of getting this sperm close to the egg. The female system provides a modest number of eggs, usually one per month, and the mechanism to nurture the egg once it gets fertilized.

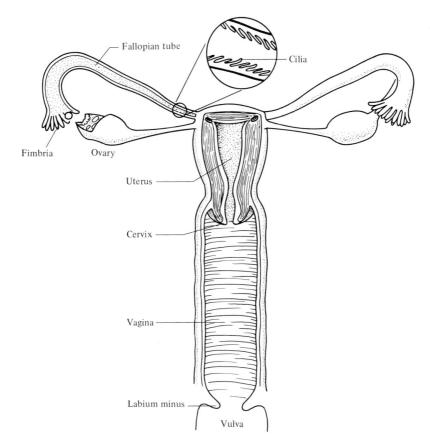

FIGURE 10-15. *The female reproductive system.*

THE MALE

Male gonads, the testes, are suspended below the penis in a sac of skin called the scrotum. There are many winding tubules in the testes with loose tissue between them. It's in this tissue that the male sex hormone is produced.

Sperm is produced in the tubules, and as spermatozoa mature they move into the epididymis and then the vas deferens. These are collecting ducts that meet the urethra just below the bladder. Accessory glands—seminal vesicles, the prostate glands, and bulbourethral glands—provide secretions that mix with the sperm to form semen. This is the fluid that eventually discharges into the female's vagina.

The urethra, in the center of the penis, can carry either urine or semen. Urine flows through a flaccid penis, but semen is discharged only when the penis is erect. The erection takes place, of course, when the male becomes sexually aroused. Extra blood fills the blood vessels and spongy tissue along the penis's shaft.

SEX-LINKED TRAITS

There's more to being a male than producing sperm that unite with female eggs. There are characteristics like beards, deep voices, firm mus-

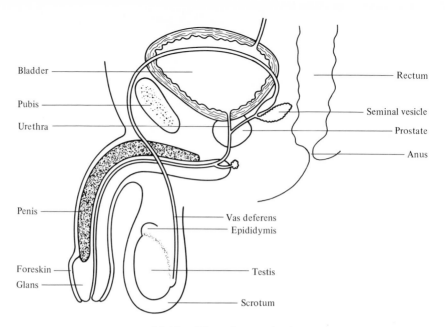

FIGURE 10-16. *The male reproductive system.*

cular development, and masculine ways of walking and gesturing that constitute the male animal. The same is true for the female. Breasts, soft bodies, high voices, heads that seldom get bald are part of the feminine image. These are sex-linked traits, conferred on all parts of our bodies by the gonads, be they testes or ovaries, which produce male and female sex hormones that constantly circulate through our systems.[17]

Processing Sensory Information

The human body can't exist by itself. Whether by domination, withdrawal, or interaction, our bodies have to adjust to the world we find ourselves in. But there's no way of adjusting until we perceive what this world is about. This perception takes place through our sensory organs—our eyes, which see; our ears, which hear; our tongues, which taste; skins, which touch; noses, which smell.

There's a difference between this world around us and what our sensory organs and brains tell the world is like, though. Physical differences, emotions, personality, and social backgrounds influence how we witness events. No two of us perceive exactly the same way. And we don't have the right kinds of receptors for certain kinds of energy forms. We can't perceive radiation or radio waves unless they're converted into some kind of energy form our senses can adjust to. And there are illusions we think of as the real world that aren't the real world at all. We can prove this when we check certain impressions against physical measurements.[18] But, distorted as our sensory impressions might be, they're essential to human life as we know it. Without them, we would exist in a state of solitary confinement, our only release being thoughts. And these would soon disappear, as we'd run out of things to think about.

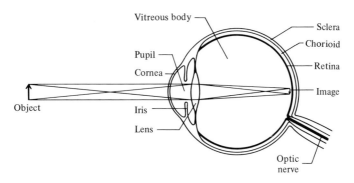

FIGURE 10-17. *The human eye.*

The Eye

The eye is a sphere, about 1 inch wide, that gives our brains visual cues. The brain organizes these cues into various patterns and shapes and constructs a picture of the outer world. The outer layer of this sphere is a glassy kind of material called the sclera. This is what we usually call the whites of our eyes. There's a transparent window in the sclera called the cornea, and there's a pigmented layer, the choroid, containing most of the blood vessels that nourish the eye. Part of the choroid is opaque, round, and richly colored. This is what makes us blue-eyed, green-eyed, or brown-eyed. It's called the iris. There's a hole in the center of the iris, the pupil, which is where light makes its entrance. The iris contracts in bright light, decreasing the pupil's diameter and reducing the amount of light entering the eye. It relaxes when the light is dim, letting the diameter of the pupil expand. More light then enters the eye, bringing on better vision in poorly lit surroundings.

The lens is a transparent, elastic structure just behind the pupil. It's through the lens that the eye adjusts for distance. Because it's elastic, it flattens when focusing on distant objects and assumes more of a spherical shape when the objects are closer. The shape of the lens and the shape of the cornea determine the point where light rays will converge on the retina—a thin layer of neural tissue lining the backs of our eyeballs. This is where light-sensitive receptor cells are located and where the image of the object we're looking at gets focused.

Light waves from any source of light come in any direction, of course. In order to get focused back onto the retina, the rays have to be straightened. This is a job for the curvilinear cornea. Also, the lens makes adjustments for distance. So the cornea and lens, along with the shape of the eyeball, determine the clarity of what we see. If the eyeball is too long for the size of the lens, images from distant objects get focused in front of the retina. Someone with this problem is nearsighted, or myopic. He can't see far-off objects clearly. If the eyeball is too short in relation to the lens, near objects focus behind the retina. Here the person is farsighted, or hyperopic.

There are two main fluid-filled compartments inside the eyeball divided by the lens. The anterior chamber is between the front of the lens and the back of the cornea. And there's a posterior chamber between the lens and the iris. Both are filled with a transparent fluid called aqueous humor. Pressure on the anterior chamber must remain constant if the eye isn't to be damaged. So there is what is known as the canal of Schlemm between the sclera and choroid. The canal allows fluid to leak when pressure in the anterior chamber builds up. Sometimes this canal gets plugged, which brings on a condition known as glaucoma. This can seriously impair vision, even cause blindness. Doctors can prevent serious damage, though, if they identify the condition when it begins. Tests for glaucoma can be given in a doctor's office by measuring intraocular pressure with an instrument called a tonometer. People should have these tests yearly. The part of the eye in the back of the lens is called the vitreous body and is filled with a gelatinous fluid called vitreous humor.

The eye is a sensitive organ. It can be injured quite easily. To protect it, you have eyelids with eyelashes; conjunctiva, a transparent membrane covering the exposed parts of the eye; and the bony frame of the orbit, which encases the eye. There are tear glands in the upper part of this orbit that secrete fluid to keep the cornea moist. And there are six ocular muscles that move the eye in its orbit up, down, sideways, and obliquely.[19]

The Ear

Ears are for hearing, of course. We do this in a highly intricate way, distinguishing about 1,600 different frequencies and 350 intensities. Frequencies range between 20 and 20,000 cycles per second, and intensities vary from very soft to very loud. Our ears also control equilibrium, or balance. They keep us from falling down when we stand up, stumbling when we go down stairs, losing our orientation between up and down, right and left.

There are three main parts to the ear. There are the external and middle parts, with the sole function of hearing, and there's the inner ear, which provides balance as well as contributing to the hearing function.

EXTERNAL EAR

The flaps growing out of both sides of our heads have the physiological designation of "conchus." These funnel the sound waves through an external auditory canal to the tympanic membrane, or the eardrum. When the waves strike the drum, it vibrates, and the first step in the hearing process begins.

The cells lining the auditory canal are coated with wax, which keeps the skin from drying and scaling. Sometimes an excessive amount of this wax accumulates, interfering with passage of sound waves.

MIDDLE EAR

The malleus, incus, and stapes are three small bones in the middle ear cavity. The cavity is separated from the external ear by the tympanic membrane. When sound waves make the eardrum vibrate, a chain reaction takes place in the small bones, which start vibrating, too. The last bone to receive the auditory signal is the stapes, which taps its message through the oval window separating the middle ear from the inner ear.

A eustachian tube links the middle ear to the throat. This lets secretions drain from the middle ear and allows the pressure on the inner part of the

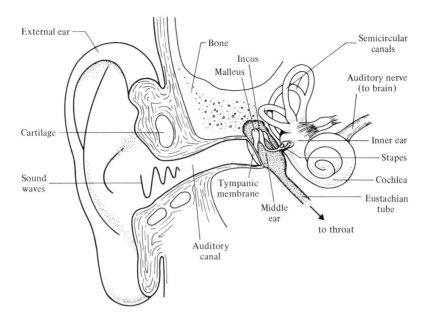

FIGURE 10-18. *The human ear.*

eardrum to equal that outside the eardrum. The outer pressure is equal to the atmospheric pressure, of course. The inner pressure becomes approximately the same when we swallow or yawn. This is when the eustachian tube opens and pressure on both sides of the drum balances. Sometimes this tube gets blocked when we have a cold or an allergy. This keeps the pressure from stabilizing, and there's a lot of pain from a stretched eardrum. Also, infection can build up in the middle ear because of the blocked drainage canal. This condition is called otitis media. Sometimes it becomes so serious that the eardrum ruptures.

INNER EAR

There is a vestibular apparatus in our inner ears that maintains our balance, and there's a cochlea to receive sound waves. Fluid surrounds both of them. Delicate nerve fibers in the vestibular apparatus get stimulated by movement of endolymph, a fluid inside the vestibular canal. These nerve fibers are connected to the brain and tell us whether we're moving right, left, up, down, or in a circle. If this apparatus doesn't function properly, we can become dizzy and nauseated, sometimes lose our ability to stand and walk.

There are three parts to the cochlea, which are sectioned by two membranes, the Reissner membrane and the basilar membrane. Parts that run the entire length of the cochlea are called the scala vestibuli, scala media, and the scala tympani. The scala media, like the vestibular apparatus, is filled with endolymph. The other two parts contain what is called perilymph.

Sound waves strike the tympanic membrane, setting up a chain reaction that causes the stapes to vibrate against the oval window, bringing on fluid waves in the perilymph of the scala vestibuli. These transfer into the perilymph of the scala tympani and set the basilar membrane into motion.

There's a specialized sound wave receptor anchored to the basilar membrane called the organ of Corti. The thousands of delicate hairs in this organ become activated when the basilar membrane moves. The hairs trigger impulses in the auditory nerve, which carries them to the brain. So sound waves in the ear get converted to fluid waves, which, in turn, become electrical impulses to the brain.[20]

Taste

There are lots of things we can't taste. It's only chemicals soluble in liquids that we can. Specialized receptor organs called taste buds sense these chemicals—about 10,000 taste buds on the upper surface and edge of the tongue, the sides of the cheeks, the insides of the lips, and the back of the pharynx. The buds are barrel-shaped structures, composed of special nerve cells surrounding small pores. The chemicals we taste apparently come in contact with sensory hairs of these nerve cells.

Taste buds become fewer and fewer as we get older, but you can't really assume sensitivity on the basis of the number of buds. Chickens have only about 12 of these receptors, but can distinguish chemicals in solutions so dilute that humans can't distinguish them.

Some have divided taste into four basic sensations: sweet, sour, bitter, and salt. But no one has found specific taste buds to support this breakdown. There seem to be specific sensations for a lot of isolated compounds chemically quite similar. Probably there are overlapping fields of taste, with different combinations giving different sensations.

There's been a lot of argument as to exactly how taste buds respond. No one has ever satisfactorily explained it. Why we like ice cream better than spinach, fried chicken better than okra, and can't stand cauliflower is still mystifying—despite centuries of research into the human body.[21]

Smell

The nerve cells sensitive to different smells lie in the mucous membranes of the upper parts of our nasal cavities. These are called the olfactory mucous membranes. These cells vary in size and shape, which could account for varying sensitivity to different smells. Because they're above the main path of air currents entering our noses, the sensations they pick up have to come from diffusion.

Possibly we distinguish groups of odors like sweet, putrid, and pungent by the way molecules are structured. But there's a big difference in our perceptions of similar chemicals. For instance, amyl alcohol stimulates olfactory cells much more effectively than methyl alcohol does.

Smelling has a lot to do with our sense of taste. Volatile food elements going through our mouths to the backs of our pharynxes penetrate our olfactory mucosa. But a bad cold plugs up our noses and sinuses and prevents this, of course. This is when we seem to lose our sense of taste. Try tasting food when you hold your nose, and notice how flat it seems.

The sensitivity of our ability to smell varies with the state our olfactory receptors are in at the moment. If you have a head cold, you can't smell as well as when you're free of congestion. When you're hungry, you can smell food odors better than after you've had a good meal. And sex affects the olfactory process. Women can smell better than men can. Also, smoking affects this sense. Nonsmokers have sharper noses than nicotine users do.

Humans seem to accommodate to odors rapidly. There's the lady who's doused herself with perfume and can't sense it a few minutes after she's had it on. People sitting in a smoke-filled room often don't realize how pungent the odor is. And there's the fellow who needs a bath. If his best friends don't tell him, he'll never know why he can't get a date.[22]

Notes

1. Sigmund Grollman, *The Human Body,* 3rd ed. (New York: Macmillian, 1974), pp. 1–39.
2. Eugene Bell, *Molecular and Cellular Aspects of Development* (New York: Harper and Row, 1965), pp. 142–160.
3. Arnost Katyk, *Cell Membrane Transport* (New York: Plenum Press, 1970).
4. Wilfred Clark and Edward Le Gros, *The Tissues of the Body* (Oxford: Clarendon Press, 1971).
5. Grollman, *Human Body,* pp. 39–56.
6. Ibrahim Adelbert Kapandji, *The Physiology of the Joints* (London: Livingstone, 1970).
7. Tuji Tonomura, *Muscle Proteins, Muscle Contraction and Transport* (Baltimore: University Park Press, 1973), pp. 6–22.
8. Robert F. Rushmer, *Structure and Function of the Cardiovascular System* (Philadephia: Saunders, 1972), pp. 1–32.
9. Charles F. Geschickter, *The Lung in Health and Disease* (Philadelphia: Lippincott, 1973), pp. 1–29.
10. Charles Roviller and Alex M. Muller, *The Kidney* (New York: Academic Press, 1971), pp. 61–157.
11. Horace W. Davenport, *Physiology of the Digestive Tract* (Chicago: Year Book Medical Publishers, 1971).
12. William Montagno, *The Structure and Function of Skin* (New York: Academic Press, 1962), pp. 14–167.
13. A. G. Lyne, *Biology of the Skin and Hair Growth* (New York: American Elsevier, 1965), pp. 267–292.
14. Ingrith Olsen, *Metabolism* (Indianapolis: Pegasus, 1973).
15. Grigorii I. Poliakov, *Neuron Structure of the Brain* (Cambridge, Mass.: Harvard University Press, 1972).
16. Neville G. Sutton, *Anatomy of the Brain and Spinal Medula* (London: Butterworths, 1971).
17. William D. Odell, *Physiology of Reproduction* (St. Louis: Mosby, 1971), pp. 20–64.
18. Carlos Eyzaguirre, *Physiology of the Nervous System* (Chicago: Year Book Medical Publishers, 1969), pp. 75–138.
19. Michael J. Hogan, *Histology of the Human Eye* (Philadelphia: Saunders, 1971).
20. Anthony A. Pearson, *The Development of the Ear,* Vol. I (Rochester, Minn.: American Academy of Ophthalmology and Otolaryngology Press, 1971).
21. Joan Steen Wilentz, *The Senses of Man* (New York: Crowell, 1968), pp. 130–154.
22. Ibid.

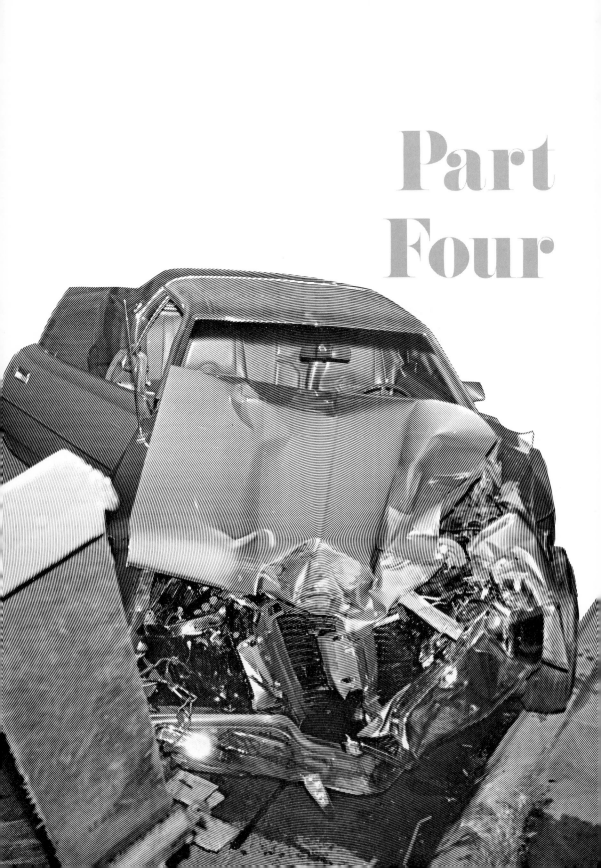

Part
Four

Health
Impairments

11 Communicable Diseases

He was a mild-mannered fellow, timid almost to the point of being afraid. And even his well-trimmed beard and spectacles didn't give him the air of distinction. But the French government was desperate. The Orleans wine was turning to vinegar, a situation striking terror into the hearts of good Frenchmen. Wars, riots, floods, and famine could be accepted with courage and stoicism—but this? This was a problem for a genius only, even if the genius didn't look and act like a genius. So in 1865, the French government sought the services of a nondescript chemist named Louis Pasteur. And they had called on the right man. By 1879, Louis had found that heating wine to 55° Centigrade would kill off the microbes and keep it from spoiling. The French nation was saved, and Louis was toasted with champagne, cognac, port, and sherry. He heated milk, too, and killed off most of the disease-producing microbes. And he studied silkworms in Alais to figure out why they were dying of a disease called pebrine. There were two microorganisms causing their problems, and Louis isolated both, advancing the theory that different kinds of microscopic bugs cause different kinds of diseases. The germ theory was born, and people literally got a new lease on life.[1]

Infectious disease had been the companion of statesmen, soldiers, scholars, peasants, and kings. Families were wiped out by it, towns and countries decimated. A life span of 25 or 30 years was accepted as normal; a face unpitted and unscarred by smallpox was extremely rare. The leper was feared

259

far more than the invading warrior, plague far more than fire and famine—and with good cause. The invading soldier was a man-made tragedy. a phenomenon man could face, could understand. Famine was the same. Grow more food, and the problem would disappear. Water would deal with fire, but the plague—this was a mystical invader that responded to nothing. What caused it? Was it some kind of divine fury taking vengeance for man's sinful ways? Possibly it was a miasma that came with the cold and darkness. No, there was a group of planets over the Indian ocean that brought on this horror. The planets would pass, and so would the plague, the leper, the quiet mutterings of the priest, and the tolling of the bells.

Historical Background

Plague reached a peak in the latter half of the fourteenth century. Black Death, as the plague was called, joined the ranks of the Tartar Army in 1346 at the Black Sea. The Army catapulted dead bodies into the city it was beseiging to make sure the enemy faced Black Death, too. Then supply ships carried it throughout Mediterranean ports. Sicily, Sardinia, and Corsica came under its spell in 1347. And Black Death ravaged Constantinople in the same year. Italy, France, and Spain succumbed to it in 1348. By 1350 all of Europe was devastated. England's population fell by nearly 50 per cent. Europe lost a third of its citizens, and it took more than 200 years to rebuild the population to pre-plague levels.

Rome, during its golden years of A.D. 96 to 180, faced the Black Death, too. This was when Rome had 700,000 citizens. A proud, vigorous, noble populace, they built magnificent temples, wrote just laws, and dug lasting roads. The Black Death claimed 10,000 of these Roman lives daily and almost wiped out the Roman Army.[2]

Louis Pasteur had given mankind an overwhelming gift. It wasn't just the plague man could now deal with. There were smallpox, cholera, diphtheria, malaria, syphilis, and thousands of other killers and cripplers. Pasteur's discoveries popularized a new way of thinking, a new and organized approach to dealing with man's health care problems. Pasteur, of course, wasn't the only leader in this area. There were giants who preceded him, men with thoughts and discoveries way before their time, men who were often laughed at, jeered, and sometimes considered insane.

Girolamo Fracastoro had a poem published in 1530 titled, "Syphilis, Sive, Morbus, Gallicus." This gave syphilis its name and identified it as a disease separate from leprosy and smallpox. Incidentally, the word originally meant "hog lover," and the poem referred to a West Indies shepherd boy who brought the malady on the human race. Fracastoro also outlined what he called the theory of "seeds" of contagion. He felt that seeds of different kinds carried illnesses from one person to another. Well people came in contact with sick people or their garments; and, lo and behold, populations began to die off. This really wasn't all that far from the truth. Fracastoro today is recognized as the father of epidemiology.

There was Lady Mary Wortley Montagu, who introduced inoculation against smallpox in 1718. When her husband was ambassador to Turkey, she learned from the Turks how to infect subjects with a mild strain of the organism. In 1722 she even inoculated the Prince and Princess of Wales. But this was a dangerous practice for the community, though it did produce immunity for the individual. The inoculated person could spread the disease while he was building up his bodily defenses.

It was up to Edward Jenner, a British country physician, to refine the process. He noticed that dairymaids never had pox-marked faces, a highly unusual characteristic in the eighteenth century. Was it possible they were immune to smallpox because they had overcome a milder disease, cowpox, at an earlier time? Jenner ran an experiment in 1796 on an 8-year-old boy, inoculating him with matter taken from a dairymaid's sore hand. He later tried inoculating him with smallpox, but the inoculation wouldn't take. Several repetitions of this experiment proved that Jenner had found an effective vaccine.

There was the episode of Dr. John Snow, a London cholera epidemic, and the Broad Street pump. Snow decided that the pump and the cholera epidemic went together and suggested to the vestrymen of St. James' Parish that the epidemic would vanish when the pump handle vanished. The incredulous vestrymen had nowhere else to turn, so in 1854 they decided to give Dr. Snow's idea a try. Sure enough, the cholera epidemic vanished. What also vanished, of course, was the drinking water from the pump, which was contaminated by seepage from an underground source. Snow had proven that cholera had something to do with the water and got people to thinking about the contents of what we drink.

Ignaz Semmelweis was put in an asylum because of his "mad" proposal that doctors wash their hands. There were Dr. Richard Mead, Lemuel Shattuck, Oliver Wendell Holmes, and hundreds of others with faith, imagination, and a sense of destiny. But none of them, including Pasteur, could have done much about the world's ills if it hadn't been for the discoveries of a humble Dutch shopkeeper named Anton van Leeuwenhoek. Anton came out with a book titled *Micrographia* in 1665, describing a newfangled gadget he had made called the microscope. He went into minute descriptions of some of the weird things he saw in water, blood, semen, and human hair and beer, and the era of bacteriology was born. People didn't get really enthused about the instrument for the next 200 years. But then Pasteur came out with his findings, and there was a mad scramble to figure out which organism caused which disease.

Robert Koch, a great German physician, isolated the bacillus of anthrax in 1876. He isolated the tubercle bacillus, the cause of tuberculosis, in 1882. There was Iwanowski, a Russian, who isolated organisms so small they could pass through the pores of an unglazed porcelain filter. These he called filtrable viruses, which were later shown to be causes for diseases like the common cold, rabies, yellow fever, chicken pox, smallpox, poliomyelitis, mumps, and measles.[3]

Microbiology

But by the turn of the century, the excitement over new bacteriological discoveries began to die down. The etiological agents bringing on many of man's woes were identified quickly. But identification alone didn't always bring the disease under control, and there were several diseases that didn't seem to have causative microorganisms. Mental illness is a good example. Another is heart disease. And there's human cancer, which may be caused by a microorganism, but no one has ever been able to identify it.

But though the excitement and wonder of bacteriology have died down, the discipline has taken on maturity, depth, and scientific sophistication in the extreme. It's even taken on a new name to describe its scope. Microbiology encompasses bacteriology and also virology. It even enters the area of antibiotics, as you can't completely separate disease prevention from treatment. Curing a disease in one individual prevents it from being transmitted to another and breaks the chain reaction of an epidemic. But the primary role of microbiology is dealing with all kinds of microorganisms, the kind that bring on disease (pathogenic), and those that don't. These organisms, harmful or harmless as they might be, don't have to live in the human world only, but can infest plants, animals, or even other microorganisms.

It's hard to envision how small microorganisms really are. They are measured in microns, or millimicrons, and these are minute indeed. A micron is 1/25,000 of an inch, or 1/1,000 of a millimeter. A millimicron is 1/1,000 of a micron. Take the polio virus. This is 10 millimicrons long, so about 6,000 of them could line up on a pinpoint. Microorganisms vary in size and shape, though, even if they're from the same strain. Like people, they're not completely uniform.

These infinitesimal specks of life can multiply rapidly. If the conditions are right, sometimes they are less than half-an-hour old when they reproduce. Usually their reproduction method is simple cell division, called fission. One cell becomes two, two become four, and so on. Some form spores as part of the reproductive cycle, and spores are harder to destroy than cells.

Like all forms of life, microorganisms have certain basic needs. These usually include nourishment; a given range of temperature; oxygen, or the absence of it; the absence of antagonists, be they biological or chemical; and sometimes moisture. So if they're pathogenic and you want to kill them you have to cut off one or more of their life requirements.

Antibiotics interfere with their nourishment and metabolism. There's heat sterilization, which destroys their life-sustaining temperature; and chemicals such as chlorine and sulfa drugs that stop their reproductive cycle or kill them outright. They're tough little bodies, though, and they don't die easily. It often takes elaborate techniques to kill them off, even though basic disease control principles are quite simple.[4]

Germs

Most microorganisms aren't of the pathogenic type, but those that are are what bring on our communicable diseases. We call them "germs," and there are about 100 different varieties of them, classified in different, complex ways. These classifications can get confusing, even for the specialist. Latin is used freely, and most of us don't know that language. So we memorize the names of the germs by rote and don't relate the names to each other. Here's

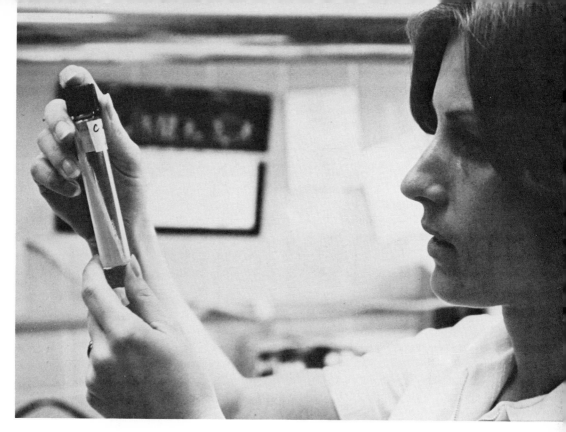

FIGURE 11-1. *Discovering a new world.*

a very loosely organized classification of germs that deals with this problem. It organizes them according to size.

VIRUS

The virus is the smallest of all the disease-producing microorganisms. It brings on sicknesses like the common cold, yellow fever, poliomyelitis, and smallpox. Viruses can have a very regular crystalline shape, or they can look like rods.

RICKETTSIA

The rickettsia organisms were named after Howard Taylor Ricketts (1871–1910), who died investigating them. They bring on diseases like typhus fever and Q fever. You can barely see them under the highest-powered optical microscope.

BACTERIA

There are three basic forms of bacteria:

1. The twisted variety, which can be spiral shaped, such as the spirochete;

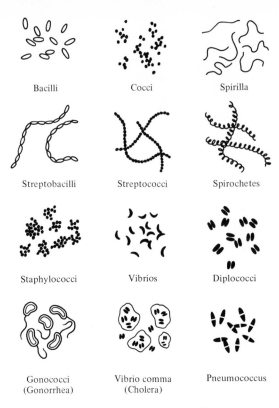

| Bacilli | Cocci | Spirilla |

| Streptobacilli | Streptococci | Spirochetes |

| Staphylococci | Vibrios | Diplococci |

| Gonococci (Gonorrhea) | Vibrio comma (Cholera) | Pneumococcus |

FIGURE 11-2. *Common types of bacteria.*

syphilis, which looks something like a corkscrew; and the vibrio of cholera, which is shaped like a comma.

2. The rod-shaped variety, associated with diseases like leprosy, tuberculosis, and typhoid fever.

3. The spherical type, which sometimes appear in clusters, like bunches of grapes. The staphylococcus organisms in infections and boils take this form. They can also be arranged in pairs or in double file. Gonococcus, associated with gonorrhea, appears this way. They can appear in chains, like the streptococcus variety associated with "strep" infections.

FUNGI

Bigger than bacteria, the fungi are plantlike organisms, present in infections like athlete's foot.

PROTOZOA

Protozoa are single-celled animals that can be as large as several centimeters. Malarial parasites are an important form of protozoa.

METAZOA

A more common name for the metazoan parasites is "worms." They're not strictly microorganisms, as you can see the adults with the naked eye.

However, the eggs or cysts may be quite small. Common varieties of them include tapeworms and roundworms such as the hookworm and the trichina worm. The last causes trichinosis in hogs and people.[5]

The Causes of Disease

Microbes multiply quickly. It takes just a few hours for one organism to become billions of organisms, and these organisms often produce toxins that interfere with the functioning of the normal cell. There's endotoxin, a poison a microbe produces when it's destroyed. And there's exotoxin, a poison released by the microorganism while it lives. These toxins can affect all cells in our bodies or just particular cells, such as the blood, nervous tissue, or connective tissue. Their effect makes them unique and allows them to be classified.

Pathogens also get classified according to their ease of invading the body. Fortunately, the most poisonous don't always have an easy time of invading. The tetanus germ is deadly but has a tough time getting in the human bloodstream. The tuberculosis bacillus can enter the human body without too much difficulty; but, in most cases, it's not too toxic.

Pathogens invade us in several ways. Their most common place of attack is the respiratory tract, entering our systems when we breathe. They settle in our throats, noses, and bronchial tissue and multiply themselves into colds and influenza. Sometimes they weaken tissues so that other less invasive microorganisms can bring on pneumonia in the lungs.

Pathogens that enter through the mouth usually concentrate in the gastrointestinal area and bring on problems like diarrhea, intestinal flu, and cholera. And there are organisms that get into our bodies through the skin and mucus membranes. Venereal disease pathogens invade this way. So do the spreaders of plague, malaria, and yellow fever. These diseases get passed around by physically contacting infected people, animals, or insects.[6]

Protection Against Disease

But man's battle against the parasites is in his favor. Even if he didn't know a thing about medicine, chemistry, or even cleanliness, he would still survive. The human race was developing a population problem long before the days of Pasteur and van Leeuwenhoek. People may not have lived as long or had the potential for happiness we do now, but survive they did. We humans are tough and flexible entities, who usually win out over fire, flood, and cold, let alone a few little bugs.

General Protection

Consider the barriers the microbe has to overcome for invasion. There's the skin. Most parasites won't get through it unless it's broken. And, if it is broken, there are usually secretions that don't lend themselves to microbial development. And our body orifices have protective barriers of their own.

There's epithelial tissue, which secretes mucus in the nose and mouth. This mucus traps most of the microorganisms trying to gain entry. And when we swallow the secretions, there is gastric juice in the stomach to take care of the few pathogens that survive the mucus. We have fine hairs called cilia in our trachea and bronchi, which carry parasites from our respiratory passages to our throats, where they can be swallowed. We've got antibiotic tears that bathe our eyes and antibiotic saliva in our mouths. There's wax in our ears to keep most of the bugs out, and urine either kills or washes away a lot of pathogens. Also, the bowel and the vagina have the kind of bacterial content that inhibits the growth of most pathogenic organisms.[7]

Cellular Protection

But, assuming the microbe does get inside the human body, it's got quite a fight on its hands. There are all kinds of barriers to its existence and growth. There are connective tissue cells that try to destroy most foreign agents they come across. And these cells are located in all parts of the body. Some are stationary and defend a specific bodily zone only. Others move about in our blood or lymph systems.

The stationary kind are called endothelial, fibroblastic, and macrophagic. The endothelial kind are flat and lie in the interior of all blood vessels and body cavities. When blood vessels get damaged by infection, the endothelial cells repair them. The fibroblastic cells surround microorganisms, forming capsules that build up scar tissue. And the macrophagic cells ingest the foreign material. They're big cells, these macrophages, and they're present in most organs that have passageways. They can be found in alveoli of the lungs, sinuses of bones, lymph glands, and the liver and the spleen.

Moving cells, those that travel through the circulatory and lymph systems, are called leukocytes. These are our white blood cells, bodies that either wall off foreign material or devour pathogens that have gotten too weak to fight for themselves. The walling-off role is carried on by granulocytes, a type of leukocyte with more than one nucleus. Monocytes, leukocytes with just one nucleus, carry out the ingestion function.

Our cells can also produce a protein called interferon. This prevents viruses that have just entered the cells from multiplying.[8]

Elevated Body Temperature

Our systems as a whole fight disease by elevating body temperature. This fever, which can make us feel pretty rough when it gets out of hand, increases cellular defense activities and antibody formation. Even the chills and shaking that sometimes go along with the fever have their good side. They're an involuntary bodily reaction to the loss of too much heat to the environment. But this helps to maintain the fever, which helps to hold down the multiplication of invading pathogens.

Antibody Formation

Another bodily defense mechanism is antigenic response. This involves the production of antibodies in response to the introduction of antigens. Antibodies fight antigens by destroying them or making them clump together so that white blood cells can destroy them. They're a kind of globulin, which all of our tissues produce; but the most active antibody producers are the spleen, the lungs, and the lymph nodes.

The very young and the very old can't produce antibodies as readily as the in-between age groups can, so the very young and very old have a tough time with infections. The same applies to people who are undernourished. They don't produce antibodies as easily as those who are well fed, and so they're more sickly. There's a host of variables affecting antibody production and the ability of these antibodies to fight off the effects of the antigens. There are even people who can produce no antibodies whatever. This condition is called "agammaglobulinemia."[9]

ACTIVE IMMUNITY

When someone makes sufficient antibodies to overcome antigenic stimulation, he's said to have "active immunity." This can take anywhere from a day or two to several months to develop, and the immunity can last for a lifetime. It can last for just a day or two, also. It depends on which specific antigen is involved and to what degree the body is exposed.

Acute infections can cause antibody formation, of course. So can what are known as "mist infections," those in which the symptoms of the disease are never apparent. And injections and oral doses in controlled amounts of the pathogen can bring on the antibodies. Sometimes the infection is so great that the immunity created lasts for a lifetime. Mumps, measles, and chicken pox are good examples. Most people contract these diseases in childhood, but it's almost never that you hear of a second infection. Immunizing by artificial techniques doesn't bring on the immunity that a case of the actual disease does, and most vaccinations have to be repeated from time to time or "boosted."[10] But this is better than coming down with something that can kill you or produce crippling aftereffects.

PASSIVE IMMUNITY

But what about the person who's never had the disease, who's never been given the vaccination for it, and then gets exposed? It certainly wouldn't do any good to give him an injection of a small amount of the pathogen at this point. It might take weeks to build antibodies, so the vaccination would just make him sicker. This is when "passive immunity" is tried. Instead of forcing the system to create its own antibodies, antibodies are isolated in other humans and animals and injected directly into the person's bloodstream. This doesn't always bring on the ideal result. Some people are allergic to foreign serum and become quite sick or even die from it. And passive immunity lasts only for a few weeks. So it's better if a person can build his own bodily defenses against microorganisms, but sometimes he doesn't have a choice.

Most babies have protection against chicken pox, measles, mumps, and whooping cough during their first few months of life. This is because their mothers have built up immunity, and maternal antibodies filter through the

TABLE 11-1
Recommended Schedule for Active Immunization of Normal Infants and Children

	Disease	Immunizing Agent	Preferred Age for Initial Dose	Number of Doses	Interval Between Doses	Booster	Remarks
Combined Antigens (Primary, Basic, or Initial Series)	Diphtheria, pertussis (whooping cough), tetanus (DPT)	A.P. Diphtheria and Tetanus Toxoids, Pertussis Vaccine	2–3 months	3	4–6 weeks	1 year after primary and 4–5 years later (see Remarks)	When primary immunization or boosters are given at 6 years or over, use Tetanus-Diphtheria Adult. Use Tetanus-Diphtheria Adult for subsequent boosters at 8–10 year intervals. After age 40, routine use of diphtheria toxoid is not recommended; use single antigen for tetanus. See below.
	Tetanus and diphtheria (Adult use)	A.P. Tetanus and Diphtheria Toxoids Combined, Adult	Age 6 and over	2	4–6 weeks	1 year after primary (see Remarks)	
Single Antigens (Primary, Basic, or Initial Series)	Poliomyelitis	Trivalent Oral Live Polio Vaccine (Sabin)	2–3 months	2	6–8 weeks	1 dose 1 year after primary and 1 dose on school entry	For primary immunization of children 2 through 5 years, give 2 doses Trivalent Oral Polio Vaccine at 6–8 week intervals, then same booster schedule as for infants. For primary immunization of children 6–18 years, give 2 doses Trivalent Oral Vaccine at 8-week intervals; no booster recommended at present.

Disease	Age	Vaccine	Doses	Interval	Booster	Remarks
Measles	12 months	Live Measles Vaccine	1	—	No booster recommended at present	It is desirable that tuberculin skin testing precede measles immunization. There is no age limit for the administration of live measles vaccine.
Rubella	12 months	Live Rubella Virus Vaccine	1	—	No booster recommended at present	At present, live rubella vaccine is not recommended for pregnant or potentially pregnant women.
Smallpox	12–24 months	Calf Lymph Virus or Dried Smallpox Vaccine	1 application	—	Every 8 years	If Immune Globulin is given, as with measles immunization, defer smallpox vaccination until 6 weeks have elapsed from the time Immune Globulin is administered. Read revaccinations at 24–48 hours and at 7–9 days. Repeat vaccination with fresh material if no reaction is observed.
Tetanus	Over 40 years	A.P. Tetanus Toxoid	2	4 weeks	1 dose 2 years after primary, every 8–10 years thereafter	Give booster dose following puncture or lacerating wounds.
Typhoid	See Remarks	Typhoid Vaccine	2	4 or more weeks	1 dose every 4 years if re-exposure is expected	If exposure is expected, whether locally or through foreign travel, consult local physician or health department. The effectiveness of paratyphoid A vaccine has never been established, and recent field trials have shown that available paratyphoid B vaccines are ineffective. In view of these data, and recognizing that the paratyphoid A and B antigens when combined with Typhoid Vaccine may increase the occurrence of vaccine reactions, use of paratyphoid A and B vaccines is not recommended.

placenta into the fetus. Probably mothers who have never had these diseases, but have built up antibodies through inoculation, don't pass on the same degree of protection that mothers who have been sick do.[11] So the girl suffering with itching and temperature and a sore throat can console herself that something good comes out of all human trial.

Warding off Communicable Diseases

If you want to destroy pathogens, the best way to do it is with moist heat. Very few germs can live in boiling water for 15 or 20 minutes. And steam under pressure will penetrate clothes and bed linen and tablecloths. Even putting items in hot water and then drying them in the sun will take care of most of the infectious agents. But sometimes these procedures aren't practical. Boiling or steaming clothes can shrink them. And sometimes you have expendable items you'd rather burn or throw away than bother to disinfect.

So some people prefer to use chemical disinfectants. There are two basic kinds of these—bactericidal and bacteriostatic. Neither one of these is "safe" to use on everything, and neither destroys all pathogens. But they can be effective when properly used. And they can be dangerous. Swallow them, and they can be poison. Put them on the skin, and they can burn. Put certain kinds of them on exposed areas of the body, and the skin absorbs them in lethal amounts. They are an essential part in the communicable disease prevention process, though. Without them we could be mighty sick and mighty dirty.

The most common chemical disinfectant, and probably the safest, is soap. It provides more of a mechanical action to get rid of germs than a bactericidal effect. Some soaps contain a phenol derivative that helps cut the number of microbes on the skin. But this is a mild disinfectant, which can't bring on much physical harm.[12]

Chemotherapy

Chemotherapy involves the treatment of a disease with chemicals. Chemicals have to destroy the parasite without destroying the host too, of course. Arsenic or strychnine might take care of a disease you had contracted, but it would take care of your stomach, heart, and bowels, too. There are two major kinds of antibacterials that have a high toxicity for certain kinds of parasites and a low toxicity for the rest of our cells. These are the sulfonamides and the antibiotics. Antibiotics usually come from living organisms, whereas sulfonamides are prepared synthetically.

Physicians use sulfa drugs to fight meningococcus, which brings on meningitis; streptococcus and staphylococcus, which cause infections of the skin and urinary and respiratory systems. Antibiotics, such as penicillin, are used in the treatment of an unlimited number of infections such as peritonitis and the various types of venereal disease. These drugs have to be used with caution, though. They can't control all infectious agents, and some microorganisms develop resistance to them. They can't cure the common cold or influenza. Nothing can. They have no effect on certain strains of staphylococci and some cases of tuberculosis and gonorrhea. And people can develop an allergy to antibiotics and become extremely sick or even die from them.[13] The cure can be worse than the disease.

Communicable Diseases

There are an almost infinite number of microorganisms that can bring on infection in man. But before they can do it they have to work their way into his body from one of three entry points: the respiratory system, the intestinal tract, or openings in the skin. All pathogens attack along one of these three routes, and the diseases they bring on can be grouped by the way the cause of the disease got in the body.

Respiratory Diseases

Respiratory diseases are hard to control because people have to breathe. And there's plenty of space in the atmosphere for microscopic organisms to survive. So the most common of illnesses to plague us are the respiratory kind. Some lead to prolonged disability, some to death, and some are pretty minor. Viruses bring on most of these diseases, but bacteria and fungi play their parts, too.[14] Some of the more common of these respiratory ailments are the following:

THE COLD

It happens once or twice a year to most of us. Our eyes water, we're chilled or feverish, our stomachs hurt, our throats hurt, our noses drip, and we cough and sneeze. We have the medical malady that plagues even the hardiest of the Miami Dolphins, the most sophisticated of *Vogue* models, the sharpest of the astronauts. Everybody suffers with colds, and there's not much anybody can do to prevent them or cure them. Antibiotics don't affect cold-producing viruses. Neither do hot baths, exercise, bed rest, or bourbon. Aspirin can relieve the discomfort a little. Caffeine can reduce depression. Decongestants can reduce nasal secretions and shrink mucus membranes. These can make the cold more tolerable, but they won't make it go away.

Colds, of course, usually won't kill you, so you might as well bear them stoically and wait for better days. But they can bring on complications that call for medical treatment. There are bacterial pneumonia, tracheobronchitis, sinusitus, ear infections, and laryngitis. There are also temperatures of 102° or 103°F or higher. At this point, the doctor should be given a chance to demonstrate scientific medicine.

There have been claims that taking massive doses of vitamin C or other kinds of vitamins prevents colds, cures colds, makes the colds you get less severe, reduces the number of colds you get each year or each decade. There's no accepted scientific evidence to back these claims, and there's no scientific evidence that a light diet and a lot of fluids help a cold, either. Keeping out of drafts and in a warm temperature won't help the cold disappear. And increasing humidity with a vaporizer or a pan of water on a

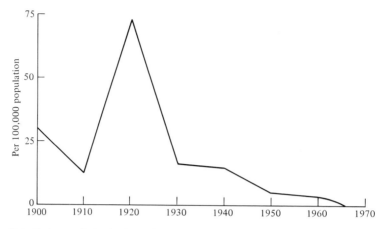

Note the increase in deaths that took place during the influenza epidemic shortly after World War I. Since that time the influenza death rate has undergone a steady decline.

SOURCE: Randolph Clark and Russell W. Cumley (eds.), *The Book of Health* (New York: Van Nostrand Reinhold, 1973), p. 155.

FIGURE 11-3. *Deaths as a result of influenza.*

hotplate won't give more relief than an amulet made of ground lizards' ears or doing a handstand on a crocodile's grave during a full moon. But sometimes you think certain actions make you feel better. And if you think you're feeling better, maybe you do feel better.

Actually, there's not just one kind of cold. There are more than 40 viruses that bring them on, and they consist of different kinds of maladies. There are head colds, or rhinitis, chest colds, or tracheobronchitis, and colds that center around the throat, pharyngitis. How these miseries get spread, no one is quite sure. It would seem logical that pathogens come out of infected people when they cough, talk, sneeze, or blow on their coffee; and the pathogens invade another poor human when he breathes in things from an unwashed cup or rubs his nose after touching a contaminated article. But no one is sure. Cold viruses are extremely elusive and don't seem to have regular patterns of behavior and growth. Probably there are several things we do that make us more susceptible to colds. We can get ourselves overly fatigued or chilled, or follow poor nutrition habits. But no one is quite sure.[15]

INFLUENZA

A lot of people think of influenza as a cold, but it is different. It can make you sicker than a cold, and there are vaccines that tend to prevent it. It's caused by one of four viruses—A, B, C, or D—and it's spread through the air or through contaminated towels or dishes or through intimate contact with someone who's suffering from the malady. Air passages of people who are infected get inflamed. They have chills, headaches, muscular aches, and malaise. Temperatures rise sharply; their throats get red; their noses run; and they usually have a dry cough. Two or three days of these symptoms leaves the sufferer pretty exhausted, and it takes 2 or 3 weeks before he feels himself again. Sometimes there are secondary infections, and the recovery period is longer yet.

There's a "flu season" that hits sections of the country every 2 or 3 years. This is when proponents of flu vaccines have a chance to show how they can control an epidemic. And they have been moderately successful. Around 50 per cent of the people who get vaccinated are protected. So, despite the skeptics, it does pay to get that shot, especially if you're in a high-risk group. Pregnant women, people with chronic and debilitating diseases, old people, and people who have just gotten over a long siege of illness should get a flu vaccination; and it doesn't hurt healthy young college people to get one, either.

Treatment for the sickness is like treatment for the common cold. You can't cure it, but you can make yourself feel a little better while you have it. There are aspirin to reduce fever, decongestants and nose drops to keep air passages open, bed rest, and patience. If fever gets out of control, or if you have rapid pulse or extended trouble with breathing, it's best to see a doctor.[16]

BRONCHITIS

Bronchitis is a form of cold or influenza that settles in the trachea and bronchi. There's usually coughing, which produces a thick sputum. There's sometimes a mild fever, and sometimes there are laryngitis and sinusitis. For short periods of time, this isn't a serious condition. It usually doesn't keep you in bed or away from work. But bronchitis doesn't last a short time for some. The expectoration and coughing can go on for several months and recur on a yearly basis. This continual irritation of the bronchi forces the membranous linings to thicken. There are changes in the epithelium, which bring on more inflammation and more mucus, which plugs the small bronchioles. The sickness lasts longer and longer, gets worse and worse, until streaks of blood begin to appear in the sputum. Then comes shortness of breath and a lung condition called emphysema, which slowly brings on death.

The causes of bronchitis are airborne. There are viruses that bring on the cold and influenza, and there are smoke and pollution. Man probably irritates his own bronchioles more than any germ does. It's almost never that a case of emphysema occurs in a nonsmoker. True, factory smoke, automobile exhaust, and dust wreak their havoc; and the Asian flu virus doesn't soothe the trachea. But the major cause of this malady, particularly the crippling form of it, is Lady Nicotine.[17]

PNEUMONIA

Pneumonia was almost always fatal prior to the days of antibiotics, and it can still be fatal. But more than 95 per cent of pneumonia victims recover when they've gotten proper treatment. It's a lung inflammation, a filling of the air sacs with pus or some other kind of fluid. Aspiration of chemicals or other irritants can cause it, but usually it's brought on by bacteria. Viruses can cause pneumonia in the very young and the elderly.

273

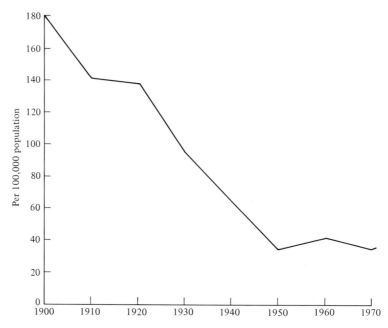

SOURCE: Randolph Clark and Russell W. Cumley (eds.), *The Book of Health* (New York: Van Nostrand Reinhold, 1973), p. 159.

FIGURE 11-4.   *Deaths as a result of pneumonia.*

Most pneumonia victims have severe chest pain or a "stabbing" feeling, and they have a high temperature and a shaking chill. Often there's a cough that brings up bloody sputum. Usually antibiotics reverse the symptoms about 24 hours after they've been administered.[18]

TUBERCULOSIS

Tuberculosis was once a serious respiratory infection in the United States, and it still is. About 15 per cent of the American people are infected with the tubercle bacillus, and about one in 20 of this group will develop active tuberculosis. Of course, the statistics are much better than they were in the 1870s or the 1770s, but tuberculosis is still an American health problem to be reckoned with. Also, more than 75 per cent of newly discovered cases are in the advanced stage, when it's most contagious. Only one case in five is found in the early stage, a time when treatment is most effective and recovery is most likely.

A tubercle bacillus creates this disease, but there are several factors that help it enter the human body and grow. There are sex, age, body build, and race; and, apparently, we can inherit a tendency toward picking up tuberculosis. Gender is the most important influence. Males are twice as likely to develop the disease as females are, and they're twice as likely to die from it. As to age, nearly half of all male tuberculosis victims are over 45 years old. And though Whites seem less likely to develop the disease than Blacks, it's hard to separate race from living conditions as a cause. Poverty and poor nutrition go together, and poor personal hygiene and crowded conditions are part of poverty, too. So race may not be the cause of a high incidence of tuberculosis among Blacks—maybe society is.

Since the days of Pasteur, milk hasn't had a lot to do with spreading the disease. Pasteurization keeps it quite safe, and dairy herds are inspected constantly for bovine tuberculosis. The bacillus makes its rounds through the air like other respiratory disease organisms. People who are infected cough or sneeze in a victim's direction or contaminate a towel or tablecloth with droplets, and suddenly he's picked up their germs. Within a few weeks all of his body cells are allergic to the bacillus or its protein, and he reacts positively to a skin test. A few months later, there are changes in the alveoli of his lungs and their surrounding lymph nodes.

The body starts a healing process at this time that is often successful. White blood cells surround the bacilli and form "tubercles." Lime forms around the lesions, and they eventually become calcified, with the bacilli walled inside. Although most of the bacilli don't die, they exist in a dormant state only. This isn't always the perfect process, however. Sometimes the germs multiply so fast that the body defenses can't handle them. They move to new locations to set up new infection sites. The calcified lesions that have been formed break down along with the general breakdown in health of the victim, and the dormant bacilli become active and spread. There is modern chemotherapy, though, which can pretty well arrest the pathogens or

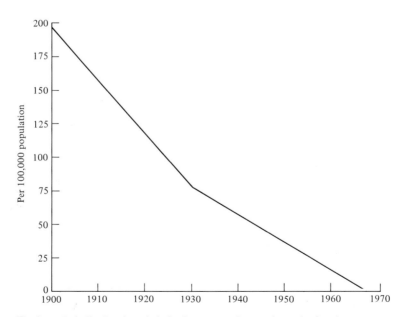

The dramatic decline in tuberculosis death rate came about as the result of modern detection and treatment methods.

SOURCE: Randolph Clark and Russell W. Cumley (eds.), *The Book of Health* (New York: Van Nostrand Reinhold, 1973), p. 162.

FIGURE 11-5. *Deaths as a result of tuberculosis.*

destroy them. The trick lies in discovering the disease before it's widespread. Then the patient has a better than 20-to-1 chance of staying alive and living a productive and nonsickly type of life.

The Mantoux skin test is used to screen people who might be infected with the tubercle bacillus. There are other skin tests used for the same purpose, but the Mantoux is the one most widely accepted. It consists of injecting a little tuberculin between the layers of the skin and waiting to see if the skin develops a red wheal. If so, a series of X-rays and laboratory exams are initiated to look further for live tubercle bacilli. Sometimes they're found; sometimes the red wheal is just a false warning. But it's better to waste time checking than save time by not identifying who has the disease.

There is a vaccine against tuberculosis called BCG (Bacillus Calmette-Guerin). This is about 85 per cent effective in preventing tuberculosis for a 6- to 7-year period. But there's a lot of disagreement on how or whether it should be used, so it's usually not used with most elements of the population. Nurses and physicians exposed to tuberculosis patients get the vaccine, and often children and members of households where the disease has been identified get it, too. There are some health departments that make it available in areas where the tuberculosis incidence is high. But most people in this country have never been immunized and never will be.

Many authorities oppose the widespread use of BCG, because this would eliminate an effective TB screening program. People who receive the vaccine have positive skin tests, so using it on a widespread basis would make the skin test worthless. It would be impossible to tell whether someone was infected or had been immunized.[19]

Gastrointestinal Diseases

By and large, the more sanitary the community and the higher the standards of personal cleanliness of its populace, the lower is the gastrointestinal disease incidence. These are diseases of filth and ignorance, of inadequate facilities. Not that everyone who gets a case of diarrhea or a bad stomach ache has been careless about bathing or washing his hands or cleaning his food and utensils. Possibly he lives or associates with others who have bad habits of this type. Or, possibly, he's just plain unlucky. But protozoa, tapeworms, and roundworms don't survive well in soap and hot water. These little one-celled organisms and multicelled animals are the etiological agents of gastrointestinal disease. Viruses can bring on problems of this type, too, and so can bacteria.

VIRAL INFECTIONS

Viral Enteritis. Viral enteritis is a disease that spreads almost as easily as respiratory infection does, and most of us get it from time to time. It gets passed around by fecal contamination of the hands, and young children are usually the carriers. It brings on diarrhea, fever, vomiting, and nausea. But it makes you sick for just a few days and usually disappears without any type of significant treatment. It can be controlled, of course, by washing hands after defecation.

Hepatitis. There are two types of hepatitis. There's infectious hepatitis, spread by food and water contaminated with feces; and there's serum hepatitis, spread by unsterilized needles entering the skin. Both varieties make their victims extremely sick, and both can cause death. The infectious variety brings on heavy diarrhea, fever, and headache. It usually makes the victim turn a yellowish color, or become jaundiced, and causes nausea, vomiting, loss of appetite, and a lot of tenderness around the liver area. Rest is the only specific treatment for the ailment, and it takes about 3 months of it to get the victim back on his feet.

Serum hepatitis creates similar symptoms and calls for similar treatment. It can be controlled by sterilizing hypodermic needles, syringes, and surgical instruments the way they should be, and by making sure that blood donors don't have a history of jaundice. This isn't too hard to accomplish in a hospital or a clinic. But with drug addicts it's a big problem. They're usually anxious to get the heroin or speed into their veins as quickly as possible, so they don't take the time to sterilize their needles or even clean them. This has increased the incidence of serum hepatitis markedly in some sections of the country. The age bracket most commonly affected is 15 to 24 years old. Another group particularly vulnerable to serum hepatitis are laboratory workers. They work with equipment that is often contaminated with infected blood or sera, and it's possible for this contamination to work its way into a cut or some other break in the skin. But this is an occupational hazard that most laboratory workers are aware of and don't seem to mind facing.

There's a serum globulin used for immunization against both forms of the disease, but it's more effective with the infectious than with the serum type. In fact, the overall outlook for infectious hepatitis is much more favorable than for the serum variety. Infectious hepatitis is easier to prevent, it is much less likely to produce permanent damage, and immunity lasts longer. A dirty needle produces more misery than a dirty drinking glass.[20]

BACTERIAL INFECTIONS

Salmonella bacteria are the organisms that bring on most of the intestinal tract sickness in the United States. There are other organisms in other parts of the world that play leading roles in creating man's inner maladies, but salmonella is number one bacterium in this country. A couple of the sicknesses caused by salmonella organisms are the following:

Typhoid Fever. Salmonella typhosa is the agent that causes typhoid fever. It is excreted in the feces and can live in the soil for several months. Flies can then be the vectors that carry it. Or it might get transmitted through fecally contaminated water. Good sanitation can control this type of transmission, of course, but there are people who are already infected who transmit it directly. If they work in a food-handling occupation, many other people can come down with the disease very quickly.

There are a few who get over the effects of the disease but become chronic carriers of it for years. Typhoid bacilli locate themselves in their gall bladders and breed and multiply and enter the feces. Usually the only way to

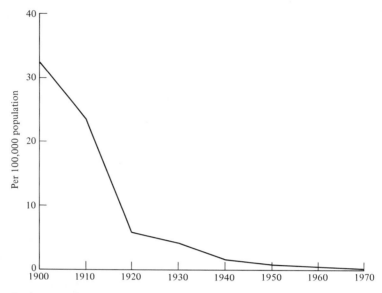

Sanitation and immunizations have practically eliminated typhoid fever as a cause of death in the United States.

SOURCE: Randolph Clark and Russell W. Cumley (eds.), *The Book of Health* (New York: Van Nostrand Reinhold, 1973), p. 469.

FIGURE 11-6. *Deaths as a result of typhoid fever.*

remedy the situation is through surgery. Remove the carrier's gall bladder, and he spreads the disease no longer.

Not many die from typhoid in this modern day of chemotherapy. People get mighty sick from it, though. There are an enlarged spleen, rose spots on the trunk of the body, fever, bronchitis, and both constipation and diarrhea.

Paratyphoid. Paratyphoid comes from other salmonella organisms, which usually breed in animals or their products. Poultry products carry a lot of these organisms, particularly eggs. Also, beef carries its share. Some surveys have indicated that as high as 58 per cent of meat sold in the marketplace contains salmonella pathogens. And home cooking temperatures usually won't kill them. Many live ones can be found in freshly boiled or fried eggs.

Luckily, man isn't too susceptible to paratyphoid. He's got to swallow a lot of salmonella before symptoms develop. And if he's got good general health his bodily defenses destroy the bacteria.[21]

Integumentary Diseases

There are three ways microorganisms can get through our outermost organ, the skin. They can enter through a break, such as a cut, burn, scratch, or skin infection. They can enter through an insect bite or sting. And sometimes they penetrate healthy skin through the pores.

Some of these pathogens are just nuisances, and some are barely contagious or not contagious at all. There's hookworm, which makes you itch and scratch a lot, but that's about all. And there are microorganisms attacking through the skin that can bring on serious handicaps. Syphilis is a good example. And there's one, rabies, that always brings death. The following are some of the more common skin-acquired sicknesses:

TETANUS

Sometimes called "lockjaw," tetanus is a disease that can, and often does, kill. About a third of those diagnosed as having it die, and those who don't die sometimes wish they would. They have muscle spasms of the neck, abdomen, and face, particularly around the jaws. There are difficulty in breathing, difficulty in swallowing, and restlessness combined with an overwhelming sense of exhaustion. It's an extremely painful and shocking disease, which can leave the patient in a depressed and exhausted state months after the main symptoms have passed.

Most people associate tetanus with a deep puncture wound from a rusty nail. This isn't necessarily so. Tetanus comes from *Clostridium tetani,* which can get in the body through any break in the skin. The break doesn't have to be caused by a nail, and rust has nothing to do with the problem. Twigs, burns, sewing needles, insects, thorns, and hypodermic needles can create openings for the tetanus pathogens to enter.

Humans carry *Clostridium tetani* in their intestinal tracts in spore form. So do cows, horses, and other mammals. And it exists in the soil, in house dust, and in the dust in hospitals and in operating rooms. So the disease could become widespread if it weren't for the effectiveness of the immunization. It gives almost 100 per cent protection and lasts from 3 to 10 years. Physicians usually administer booster shots at the time of an injury if it's been more than a year since the last injection. This almost guarantees immunity.

What doesn't guarantee immunity is antiseptics. Putting iodine in the wound, or Merthiolate or Listerine, will in no way destroy the pathogens. They're hardy germs and sometimes even survive antitoxins. Cleansing the wound of dirt and removing damaged tissue helps to reduce infection. But the only way of being sure, or almost sure, of not being stricken by tetanus is keeping vaccinations current.[22]

RABIES

A person showing symptoms of rabies will almost surely die. This doesn't mean that someone exposed to the disease will die. Antiserum and vaccine can be very effective in keeping the disease from taking hold. But if it does take hold the victim suffers unbearable pain, goes into convulsions, often becomes maniacal, sometimes becomes paralyzed. There are few maladies that produce more dramatic symptoms.

Children seem more susceptible to the disease than older people. This is probably because children are more likely to get bitten by dogs or cats or other warm-blooded animals. It's the saliva of these creatures that carries the rabies virus.

279

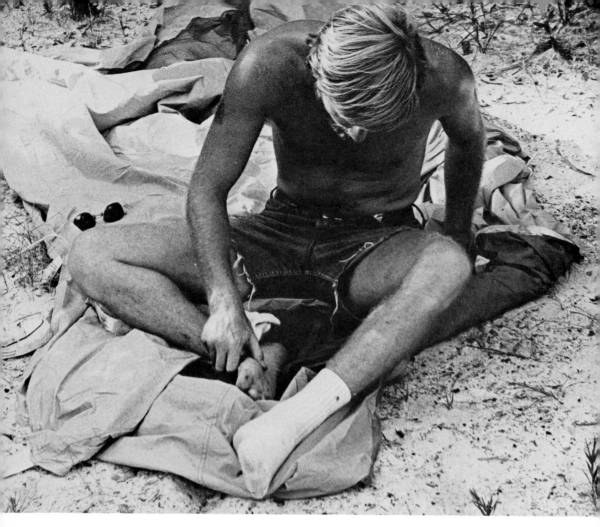

FIGURE 11-7. *If he hasn't had his teta-nus immunization, he might have a problem.*

There are two kinds of the disease: the "sylviatic" type that bats, raccoons, foxes, coyotes, and skunks carry; and the "domestic" type, carried by dogs and cats and sometimes cows. Either type is deadly.

The severity of the wound and where it's located have a lot to do with whether the disease develops. Bites on the face and the neck are the most serious. Also, the amount of virus in the saliva plays a key role in the overall danger. And these factors affect the incubation period as well. Incubation can be as short as 10 days or last for several months, even a year. It depends on just how serious the bite is.

Dogs are usually the carriers of rabies in rural areas, but you can't always be sure whether a dog is infected or not. Sometimes it's erratic and aggressive, but that can be a natural part of some dogs' personalities. The animal may growl a lot, bite anything that comes near it, or it may just seem listless. But if a dog or any other animal bites someone it should be suspected. Contact a doctor—immediately.

280

Although you can't do much about wild animals until after they've bitten you, you can see that your dogs and cats get rabies vaccine. This keeps them from getting infected and indirectly protects people as well. All states have laws regarding this practice, and most have laws involving the control of stray dogs.[23]

VENEREAL DISEASE

It was 2 years after Columbus discovered America that France's Charles VIII laid siege to Naples. The amorous Spanish were defending the city—an army that traveled with harlots as well as cannons and rifles. Apparently the Spanish general got the idea that his women could do more damage than his gunpowder. He sent the ladies to meet the French army, and it wasn't long before Charles' campaign was in complete disarray. The French were too diseased to fight, too demoralized to remain an army, so they disbanded and spread the sickness of the harlots throughout Europe. The disease got tabbed the "French disease." The French, of course, didn't call it that. To them, it was the "Spanish sickness" or the "Neapolitan disease." Germans called it the "Polish pox"; the Poles called it the "German pox"; the Turks called it the "disease of the Christians."

People used to think that syphilis *was* venereal disease, that there was no other form of the malady. An eighteenth-century Scottish surgeon, John

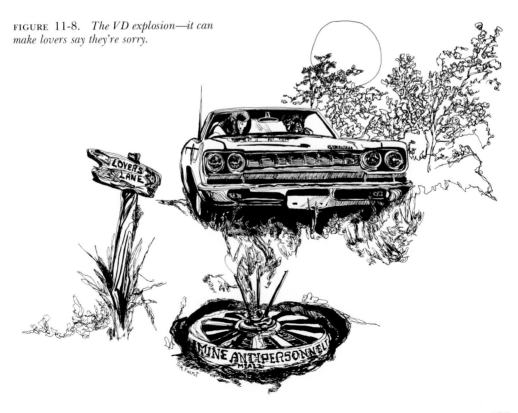

FIGURE 11-8. *The VD explosion—it can make lovers say they're sorry.*

Hunter, set out to prove this by infecting himself with both syphilis and gonorrhea. The brave soul wrongly concluded that he had just one disease, and many people believed him. Benjamin Bell, another Scotsman, didn't believe him, though. And this physician was a little less noble in his studies than Hunter had been. He inoculated his students with the two scourges and came to the conclusion that the diseases were clinically different. There was a lot of argument and superstition surrounding the matter, however, until 1879, when the gonococcus was isolated.

Syphilis and gonorrhea are the two most common venereal diseases in the United States, but there are three others: chancroid, lymphogranuloma venereum, and granuloma inguinale. These create their own brand of misery, but they don't create it as often as the two popular varieties do.

Syphilis. The spirochete *Treponema pallidum* enters through the skin to cause syphilis, and it's almost always the skin that covers the genital organs. The disease gets transmitted from person to person by direct physical contact. And, of course, the physical contact usually involves sexual relations. There's an incubation period from 10 to 90 days after exposure, with an average of 21 days. Then the disease process begins.

The first sign is usually a chancre in the place where the germs entered the body, the genital area. The chancre is usually painless, just a small sore or lesion. Sometimes it doesn't appear at all, and sometimes it's so small it's not noticed, particularly by women. But, whether noticed or not, it disappears in about 2 weeks. So quite often infected people don't worry about it. They don't realize that primary syphilis has become part of their lives.

A few weeks to 6 months later, secondary syphilis signs appear, and these are pretty hard to ignore. Although different people have different symptoms, the most common are lesions, which can appear all over the body

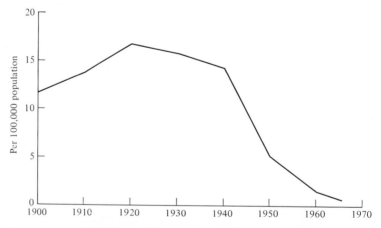

The big decline in syphilis deaths since 1940 was probably caused by the introduction of antibiotics.

SOURCE: Randolph Clark and Russell W. Cumley (eds.), *The Book of Health* (New York: Van Nostrand Reinhold, 1973), p. 522.

FIGURE 11-9. *Adult deaths as a result of syphilis.*

or on various parts of it. Along with the lesions, there is usually a rash from head to toe and white patches in the mouth or the throat. There can also be patches of falling hair, swelling of the lymph glands, a low fever, and pain in the bones and joints. By the time these signs appear, the entire body is infected.

While these primary and secondary signs are being manifested, the disease becomes highly contagious. Lesions around the moist body areas, such as the mouth and the anus and the genital areas, teem with spirochetes that are usually ready to invade a new body. But the secondary symptoms, like the primary ones, don't last long. In less than a month, the rash, the lesions, the spots in the mouth, and the fever are gone. And the ease of contagion goes, too. Not that syphilis can't be transmitted by someone not suffering from the primary or secondary stages. As the disease enters the early latent period, secondary lesions occur from time to time. And through these the spirochetes can find new victims. So syphilis is communicable for about 2 years after the initial infection.

The noncommunicable, latent phase of the disease may not harm anyone other than the victim, but the suffering it creates is tragic. Insanity, blindness, paralysis, heart disease, or death can be the outcome. And the germs bring the suffering to a climax very slowly. It's often 10 to 30 years before the end results of untreated syphilis finally take place.

Gonorrhea. Unlike syphilis, gonorrhea stays in the locality of the infected parts. It doesn't spread itself throughout the body, or attack the central nervous system or any system away from the locality of where the germs entered the body. The germs are called *Neisseria gonorrheae.* They're vigorous bacteria, which take around 5 days to incubate in males, and often a shorter time in females. The mode of transmission, of course, is sexual intercourse. People claim to have gotten it from toilet seats, towels, and dirty bathtubs, but the claims are highly questionable.

It's a quite painful disease for the male. He gets an excruciating burning sensation and discharges pus when he urinates. If he doesn't seek medical attention, the infection can spread to other parts of his urinary or genital system. He might even become sterile. For the infected woman, the pain isn't nearly as great. She might notice a little discomfort when she urinates, but she often doesn't become aware of the seriousness of the problem until the disease has entered her fallopian tubes or ovaries. Then the pain does get severe, and sterility becomes likely.

Gonorrhea can involve the rectal areas in both sexes, but victims often don't know that they're infected. The only symptoms may be an occasional wetness or itching around the anus.

The Other Venereal Diseases. Chancroid—In the military, where young men associate with people in other parts of the world, chancroid is sometimes more common than syphilis. It's characterized by lesions in the genital area, painful inflammation, swelling, and ulceration of the lymph nodes. The tongue, lip, breast, chin, and umbilicus may develop lesions, too. *Hemophilius ducreyi,* a bacillus, is the causative agent, and sexual intercourse and lack of cleanliness let the agent travel from one person to another. The incubation period for chancroid can be only 24 hours and is seldom longer than 5 days. It's communicable as long as the infected person has draining lymph nodes or lesions.

Lymphogranuloma venereum—A venereal disease quite common in the tropics, and not unknown in some of our southern states, is called lymphogranuloma venereum. As the name implies, it's a venereal infection of the lymph channels and lymph nodes. The agent is a virus that causes elephantiasis of the genitals and swelling of the lymphatic gland in the groin. The groin becomes inflamed and ulcerates, and the victim usually suffers from fever, headache, pains in the joints, and abdominal aches. Eventually the swelling around the groin disappears, but this doesn't mean that the disease has disappeared. Even though it's not fatal, lymphogranuloma venereum stays with the victim for many years and creates limitless suffering.

Like all venereal disease, it's usually spread by sexual intercourse. And, like syphilis, it can be diagnosed by a blood test. Its incubation period is from 5 to 21 days and it is contagious as long as the victim has lesions. This can be just a few weeks or several years.

Granuloma inguinale—A relatively rare disease that occurs only in temperate and tropical areas is known as granuloma inguinale. Males seem to contract it more often than females do, but neither sex dies from it. If the disease isn't treated by antibiotics, however, it can bring serious harm to the genital organs and spread to other organs in the body. Granuloma inguinale manifests itself by skin lesions around the external genitals. The lesions often ulcerate, but they're usually painless. As long as these lesions exist, the disease is contagious.

Venereal Disease in the Newborn. If a girl giving birth has gonorrhea, she can transmit it to her baby as it passes through the cervix and vagina. Usually, it is the baby's eyes that are infected. So, in most states, silver nitrate or penicillin ointment must be applied to a newborn's eyes. As for syphilis, a mother can infect her unborn child after the seventeenth week of pregnancy. The spirochetes pass through the placenta and attack the fetus. But if a mother receives proper treatment, even after pregnancy has occurred, the unborn child won't become infected.

Venereal Disease in the Female. The male usually knows when he has VD. If it's syphilis, although the chancre may not hurt him, he can certainly see it. If it's gonorrhea, he can usually see a discharge, and he'll almost always notice the pain when he urinates. But the female usually doesn't get such obvious signs. Quite often the syphilitic chancre is located on her cervix, which has no nerves. So the lesion is completely painless and not visible. Gonorrheal infection is usually located in the cervix, too, usually within the opening of the womb. Because her urinary system isn't involved, she feels no pain in this area. So she can be a reservoir of infection for years without knowing it. Eventually, though, one or both of her fallopian tubes can become inflamed, and she can become sterile.

Finding People Who Need Help. It's just about impossible to get venereal disease without having intimate contact with someone else. And he or she who has VD often passes it on to others. One recorded case initiated 42 cases of syphilis within less than a year. Another passed on 78 cases of gonorrhea. The sick aren't just endangering their own well-being and the well-being of their offspring. The public's well-being is involved, too, so public health personnel have the responsibility for tracking down carriers.

Health departments provide VD clinics, also. They examine people free of charge for the presence of VD; and, if they have it, treat them for free as well. In some states, minors can get examination and treatment without parental consent.

But, despite the preventive and treatment measures available, many consider that America is in the midst of a VD epidemic. Gonorrhea and syphilis together account for more cases of reported communicable disease than all of the other communicable diseases combined. During the 1960s, the incidence of gonorrhea increased over 50 per cent. The incidence of syphilis has decreased slightly, but not nearly enough to offset the increase in gonorrhea.

Of course, statistics of this type are highly questionable. People suffering from these problems often don't see physicians. They treat themselves or get treatment from illegal sources. And a lot of physicians (some estimate as high as 90 per cent) don't report VD cases to their health departments. Why? Maybe they feel these reports violate patients' confidence. Maybe they don't like the fuss and bother of the paperwork. Or maybe they identify with people who contracted the disease through extramarital or homosexual relations. Reports of this type can ruin reputations, can ruin lives, can ruin families. But, whatever the reasons, the physician who doesn't report this information is gambling with his community's health, and the odds are poor.

It's not the girl with the red light over her door or the one standing under a street light who spreads most VD. She passes on her share, of course. But most of it comes from promiscuous sexual relations—some heterosexual, some homosexual—between people who go to school, hold jobs, and raise families. Infection sources of this type are hard to track down. People who get the disease from them often won't name them because of some perverse kind of loyalty. And, if they do name them, the contacts have often moved away before public health officials can find them.

Obviously, venereal diseases must be controlled. They're not just something that would be nice to control, a meddlesome harassment we can learn to live with, particularly if we're not personally infected. This is foolishness. These diseases bring suffering, humiliation, and decadence to communities as well as to individuals. They're costly, they're tragic, and they are spreading. And though human nature might keep them from being eradicated, it certainly doesn't keep them from being controlled. People who are infected have to be located, treated, and counseled—quickly. Physicians have to assume a deeper sense of responsibility in this area, reporting all VD cases they run across to their public health departments. And parents have to assume a greater sense of responsibility, too. Do their children know the dangers of VD, how it's contracted, what to do if they get it? Do the parents themselves know how to deal with the problem? And then there are the schools. Teachers are blamed for all ills the world faces. Why should VD be an exception? Have they passed on the key facts to children in the fourth, fifth, sixth, seventh, and eighth grades? Or is it an embarrassing subject, something that's best to ignore? The children in the fourth and fifth grades are the ones who really need the education in this regard. When they get to high school or college, they've usually been informed, correctly or incorrectly, one way or another. VD can be controlled. It's a terrifying animal, but one that can be tamed. All we need are a little determination, a little responsibility, and a little concern for somebody else.

VD in Today's World. Penicillin would eliminate VD. No doubt about it. One massive dose of the "miracle drug" would cure the worst case of syphilis or gonorrhea, and it wouldn't be long before all sufferers received their shots and the disease disappeared. This was the thinking in 1943. Thirty-some years later, with VD coming on stronger than ever, this type of thinking seems ludicrous. But there's nothing really funny about it.

What to do? Obviously, penicillin by itself will not totally eradicate or effectively control the problem. There are a lot of aspects to it—educational, social, moral, personal, and legal, as well as medical. But with a little common sense, a little knowledge, and a little restraint, anyone can assure, or almost assure, that he doesn't get VD or suffer the consequences. There's no other class of disease so amenable to prudence. If everyone used the following precautions, venereal disease wouldn't exist within a generation.

1. Obviously, don't knowingly expose yourself to VD. There are types of people more likely to have it than others. And though you may want to associate with them, avoid circumstances that bring on exposure.
2. If you're a male, and you're having intercourse with a girl who is suspect (just about all girls you're not engaged or married to are suspect), use a condom and wash the genital area well after the act is completed. This won't assure the prevention of VD. But, if the condom doesn't break, it makes catching it unlikely.
3. A girl having intercourse with a suspect male should insist that her partner wear a condom, which can prevent VD as well as pregnancy.
4. If you get exposed, take prophylactic measures as soon as possible. If prophylactic measures such as ointments and cleansing devices aren't available, or you don't know what to do, see a physician.
5. Look out for the danger signals—the chancre, pain during urination, pus. If they appear, get medical help, and quickly. And have a blood test taken yearly as part of the physical examination. This won't show whether you have gonorrhea, but it will reveal syphilis.
6. If you do have VD, report all sexual contacts to public health authorities. You're doing them a favor, a very big favor.[24]

Diseases of Childhood

There are some diseases that affect the younger generation much more readily than they do older folks. And when people over 20 contract them, they usually have severe symptoms. Viruses bring these diseases on, and chemotherapy does little to make them go away. These childhood diseases make you feel miserable, even if you're a child; can produce residual damage, even if you're not a child; and can kill you when your childhood is far in the past. Here are some of the more common ones.

RUBELLA

Also known as German measles, rubella usually occurs during late childhood or early adolescence. The infection lasts just a few days and causes a mild fever, red itchy spots, and a general feeling of malaise. It's really not a serious disease at any age, except when it's contracted by pregnant women. Then the seriousness involves the unborn child, not the mother. The fetus can develop without limbs, be blind, deaf, or mentally retarded. Even gamma globulin or immune serum globulin doesn't protect the unborn child once the mother has been exposed. The mother receives protection. But, of course, she's not the one who's really threatened. There are vaccines that provide better than 95 per cent protection against rubella, but these should be administered to children between the ages of 1 and 12, never to pregnant women. The vaccine can do as much harm to unborn children as the disease itself can.[25]

MUMPS

Mumps is a disease that can make you very sick but by itself causes little permanent damage. Most people have heard the story of the fellow who got

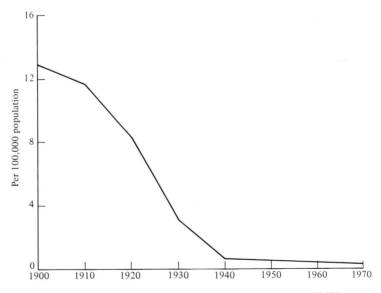

The death rate in 1900 from measles was greater than one person in every 10,000. Today it's less than one person in every 100,000.

SOURCE: Randolph Clark and Russell W. Cumley (eds.), *The Book of Health* (New York: Van Nostrand Reinhold, 1973), p. 73.

FIGURE 11-10. *Deaths as a result of measles.*

287

mumps and became sterile, and the story is true. But this happens in less than one case in a hundred, and it's almost always a case that was untreated. There are some serious complications that can grow out of mumps, though, such as pancreatitis, orchitis (swelling of the testes), vision impairment, nerve deafness, myocarditis, meningoencephalitis, and mastitis. There's a vaccine available that is 95 per cent effective in preventing this disease. And, if you've never had mumps, it's a good idea to discuss the vaccination with your doctor. It's one of the most common communicable diseases in this country.[26]

RUBEOLA

Rubeola is the red, or regular, measles. The disease is very contagious and attacks all who are susceptible, regardless of age. And though the disease itself is almost never fatal, it can lead to complications. There is pneumococcus, which brings on pneumonia, and streptococcus, which brings on infection of the middle ear. A number of children die from these secondary bacterial infections each year, and a small percentage develop encephalomyelitis, which can cause permanent brain damage.[27]

HEMOLYTIC STREPTOCOCCUS

There are streptococci in all of our bodies, but they usually don't bring on disease. There's a specific type of them, however, group A, that can cause a multitude of illnesses. There are scarlet fever, erysipelas, puerperal fever, cellulitis, and a plain sore throat. Sometimes these pathogens cause a rash, sometimes not. A lot depends on the overall health and age of the victim.

The pathogens almost always get spread by direct contact with a sick person. Sometimes contaminated food carries the germs, sometimes it's dirty towels or eating utensils. The onset of the sickness is usually quite sudden. A person doesn't have a headache, and then he does. He also has chills, a high fever, and probably nausea and vomiting. This may mean nothing more than the common cold, but it can mean scarlet fever or "strep throat."

Strep throat encompasses several types of throat infections. There are acute tonsillitis, pharyngitis, and several others. People with a variation of this infection who get a rash have scarlet fever.

Children from 5 to 15 years old are the most common victims of scarlet fever and strep throat. Either of these diseases can lead to a complication called rheumatic fever. Rheumatic fever can lead to serious cardiac damage if it isn't treated immediately with chemotherapy. Actually, the disease doesn't have to take place at all. If strep throat is identified in its early stages, by means of a culture, chemotherapy can keep complications from developing.[28]

INFECTIOUS MONONUCLEOSIS

In the strictest sense of the term, infectious mononucleosis isn't a childhood disease—unless you consider a teenager a child. Most people who come down with this ailment are in their late teens or early 20s. Some call it the "kissing disease," which says something for this age bracket. But no one is exactly sure what causes it or how it's spread. Probably a virus is at the root of the problem, and probably close contact with someone who is infected is what brings it on. It seems to reach its peak with the college group around examination time. So fatigue and emotional stress probably play a part in giving the infection a chance to take hold.

Like all diseases, it can make you feel miserable. But, unlike many, it won't kill you or do any permanent damage. There is usually a fever of somewhere between 100° and 103°F. There are headache, sore throat, a feeling of complete listlessness; sometimes there is enlargement of the liver. Occasionally the victim has a mild case of jaundice, or yellowing of his skin. It takes 4 or 5 days for these symptoms to develop, and they usually last from 2 to 8 weeks. Complications almost never develop, and recovery is usually complete.

Rest is the only treatment for the disease. Medications can ease the discomfort a little, but there's nothing known that can cure the headache or the sore throat or the fever other than bodily defenses. And these need time to overcome the unwelcome invader. But they almost always triumph eventually.[29] After all, it would be a tragedy if the kissing disease were fatal. The human race could become extinct.

Notes

1. Louis A. Baron, *Man Against Germs* (New York: Dutton, 1967), pp. 13–24.
2. William Bulloch, *The History of Bacteriology* (London: Oxford University Press, 1960), pp. 67–129.
3. Ibid.
4. R. N. Doetsch and T. M. Cook, *Introduction to Bacteria and Their Ecobiology* (Baltimore: University Park Press, 1973), pp. 1–15.
5. André Siegfried, *Germs and Ideas* (Edinburgh: Oliver and Boyd, 1965), pp. 21–23.
6. William A. Nolte, *Oral Microbiology* (St. Louis: Mosby, 1973), pp. 67–124.
7. Franklin H. Top, *Communicable and Infectious Diseases* (St. Louis: Mosby, 1968), pp. 20–27.
8. J. P. Revillard, ed., *Cell Mediated Immunity: In Vitro Correlates* (New York: Karger, 1971).
9. J. F. P. Hers and K. C. Winkler, eds., *Airborne Transmission and Airborne Infection* (New York: Wiley, 1973), pp. 282–285, 290–294.
10. G. Sermont, *Genetics of Antibiotic Producing Microorganisms* (New York: Wiley, 1969), pp. 1–23.
11. R. H. Regamey, ed., "Symposia Series in Immunobiological Standardization," *International Symposium on Biological Assay Methods* (New York: Karger, 1969), pp. 2–43.
12. G. Sykes, *Disinfection and Sterilization* (Philadelphia: Lippincott, 1965), pp. 9–38.
13. William B. Pratt, *Fundamentals of Chemotherapy* (London: Oxford University Press, 1973), pp. 5–19.
14. D. Court, "Fact and Fancy in Acute Respiratory Disease," *Australian Pediatrician Journal*, Vol. 7 (June 1971), 64–72.
15. Abbas M. Behbehani, *Human Viral, Bedsonial and Rickettsial Diseases* (Springfield, Ill.: Thomas, 1972), pp. 135–138.

16. Ibid., pp. 206–211.
17. Carl C. Dauer, Robert I. Korns, and Leonard M. Schuman, *Infectious Diseases* (Cambridge, Mass.: Harvard University Press, 1968), pp. 181–188.
18. Hobart A. Reimann, *The Pneumonias* (St. Louis: Green, 1971), pp. 3–13.
19. R. Finn et al. "Immune Supression Gliomas and Tuberculosis," *British Medical Journal*, Vol. 1 (January 8, 1972), 111.
20. Rudolph Schindler, *Gastroenterology* (New York: Grune and Stratton, 1957), pp. 12–16.
21. Dauer, Korns, and Schuman, *Infectious Diseases*, pp. 16–21.
22. Ibid., pp. 60–63.
23. Top, *Communicable and Infectious Diseases*, pp. 453–462.
24. Stewart M. Brooks, *The V.D. Story* (South Brunswick, N.Y.: Barnes, 1971).
25. Top, *Communicable and Infectious Diseases*, pp. 506–513.
26. Behbehani, *Human Viral, Bedsonial and Rickettsial Diseases*, pp. 231–235.
27. J. A. O'Connor et al., "Measles, Morbilli, Rubeola, Rubella," *Pediatrics* Vol. 49 (January 1972), 150–151.
28. Top, *Communicable and Infectious Diseases*, pp. 579–604.
29. Richard L. Carter, *Infectious Mononucleosis* (Oxford: Blackwell, 1969).

12 Chronic Diseases

Uncle Harry died from a heart attack. At least, the doctor said so. Now isn't that strange? People hardly ever die from something that far out.

If the year were 1900 or earlier, this would be true. Only one in seven died from heart disease or stroke. There weren't too many who passed on from cancer or emphysema, either. But these were the "good old days" when all you had to worry about were pneumonia, influenza, and tuberculosis. These were the major killers of the time. These provided excellent immunity from heart disease and stroke.

Forty-two years was the average life span in 1850. Then along came Louis Pasteur and his heating of milk; engineers who built septic tanks and sewage disposal systems; and Procter and Gamble, who made the daily bath a way of life. There were vaccinations that all but eliminated smallpox and diphtheria, penicillin and sulfa, which got VD pretty well under control—or should have gotten it under control.

The good old days of communicable diseases are largely gone. Now we have 20 more years of life and the chronic and degenerative diseases to face. This is the day of coronary thrombosis, pulmonary embolism, myocardial infarction, lung cancer, emphysema, and senility. There's no holding progress back.

You might live to be 90 or even 100 in this modern day of medical miracles. And though at 18 this may not sound like the greatest of prospects, liv-

TABLE 12-1
Leading Causes of Death Among Americans

Rank	Cause of Death	Number of Deaths	Death Rate per 100,000 Population
	All Causes	1,921,920	951.9
1.	Heart diseases	739,265	366.1
2.	Cancer	323,092	160.0
3.	Stroke	207,179	102.6
4.	Accidents	116,385	57.6
	Motor vehicular	55,791	27.6
	All other	60,594	30.0
5.	Influenza and pneumonia	68,365	33.9
6.	Diseases of early infancy	43,171	21.4
7.	Diabetes mellitus	38,541	19.1
8.	Arteriosclerosis	33,063	16.4
9.	Bronchitis, emphysema, and asthma	31,144	15.4
10.	Cirrhosis of liver	29,866	14.8

Source: U.S. Public Health Service.

ing under any conditions beats the devil out of the alternative. There are degenerative diseases, granted, that take old men's eyes and make them dim; take happy, self-confident personalities and make them cantankerous and forgetful; take hearing and replace it with silence; take beauty and replace it with varicose veins, twisted fingers and swollen knuckles, bald heads and sagging chins. But there's a price for living that all must pay. The only fellow who can cancel the debt is the man in the black cape with the scythe.

Dimensions of Debilitating Disease

Some pay the price of debilitating disease much earlier than others, and some pay much more than others. There are about 2 million cases of chronic epilepsy in the United States, 600,000 of cerebral palsy. The mentally retarded comprise $5\frac{1}{2}$ million, and there are another million with multiple sclerosis, parkinsonism, and muscular dystrophy. People with mental and emotional disorders, the chronic type, comprise over 20 million. Many of these have never known a happy day, had a friend, enjoyed a moment of self-satisfaction. There are 14 million with heart and circulatory and cerebrovascular diseases. Some of these can hardly sleep because of the pain, hardly know their own names or those of their loved ones. There are 16 million with asthma or hay fever, 17 million with chronic sinusitis. These aren't dramatic debilitators, of course, but they make life less pleasant than it could be and enjoyment and relaxation periodic visitors.

Then there's cancer, a chronic and awesome debilitator. Probably the million people who have it suffer as much from fear and doubt as they do from pain. There's emphysema, which afflicts $\frac{3}{4}$ million people, who can barely breathe enough air to walk across a room, to cough, to ask for a cigarette.

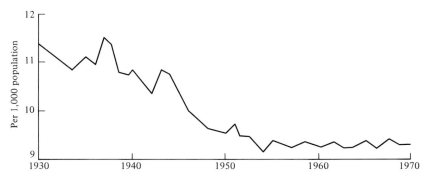

SOURCE: *Monthly Vital Statistics Report,* Department of Health, Education, and Welfare (Nov. 1973).

FIGURE 12-1. *Crude death rates: 1930–1970.*

A million and a quarter still suffer with tuberculosis. Nearly 4 million have chronic visual problems. Nearly 7 million are hard of hearing.[1] It's a tough world for many, a less than happy place, sometimes a less than tolerable place.

Cardiovascular Disease

If you die between the ages of 45 and 64, the odds are almost 50-50 that a cardiovascular problem did you in. "Cardiovascular" refers to the heart and

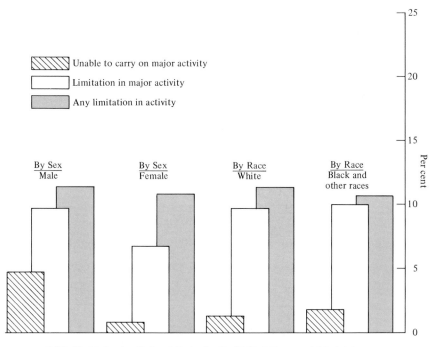

SOURCE: Public Health Service, National Center for Health Statistics, unpublished data.

FIGURE 12-2. *Persons limited in activity as a result of chronic conditions (by sex, race, and degree of limitation), 1971.*

TABLE 12-2
Death Rates for Major Cardiovascular Diseases in the United States
(Based on a 10 per cent sample of deaths. Rates per 100,000 population in specified group.)

Year	All Ages*	1–14 Years	15–24 Years	25–34 Years	35–44 Years	45–54 Years	55–64 Years	65–74 Years	75 Years and Over
1968	511.0	1.6	4.5	17.3	90.4	304.5	856.6	2,236.1	6,897.6
1969	499.7	1.2	4.4	16.8	86.3	293.5	816.9	2,155.5	6,752.7
1970	494.0	1.4	4.4	16.8	86.3	293.5	816.9	2,155.5	6,752.7
1971	490.4	1.7	3.9	17.3	85.7	294.2	801.3	2,114.5	6,597.3
1972	493.9	1.7	4.5	14.7	80.0	282.8	767.9	1,990.8	5,190.4
1973	494.4	1.6	4.0	14.3	73.3	268.1	762.6	1,914.5	5,229.4

* Includes deaths at under 1 year of age.

Source: Monthly Vital Statistics Report, Department of Health Education, and Welfare. Collected from January issues of years 1969, 1970, 1971, 1972, 1973, 1974.

the blood vessel system. This system consists of arteries, veins, capillaries, venules, and arterioles. If something goes seriously wrong in any of these areas, it can place a strain on the heart that can cause it to fail. Or maybe a defect will develop in the heart itself. The cardiovascular system is extremely complex, and there's a lot that can go wrong with it. Take the arteries supplying the brain. If they don't function properly, part of the gray matter in our heads can get starved for blood. Suddenly there's a stroke, bringing on paralysis, blindness, loss of speech or even the ability to think. Sometimes a condition of this type brings on slow, progressive senility, the reversion of a healthy and vigorous personality to childishness, irritability, and forgetfulness.

Arteries supplying the kidneys will cause them to fail if they don't function properly. Over three-fourths of all cardiovascular-renal deaths are brought on by the heart itself. Then there's coronary artery disease, a malfunction of the arteries of the heart.[2] It's such a complex network, with so many parts dependent on so many others, no wonder it fails so many people eventually. The miracle seems to be that the cardiovascular system serves so many so well for so long.

Atherosclerosis

Probably most college students have the beginnings of atherosclerosis. It's a condition brought on by the buildup of fatty deposits in the arterial blood vessels. This constricts them, of course, impairing their ability to carry blood. The fatty deposits consist of cholesterol plaques, which are sometimes so rough that they injure blood platelets when they flow by. This causes a clot to form, which often attaches itself to the roughened spot and becomes a "thrombus." Sometimes the clot breaks away and becomes an "embolus." In this case, it circulates through the bloodstream and sometimes will be swept into a small artery where it can cause a blockage. A thrombus can cause a blockage, too, if it becomes large enough.

Arteriosclerosis

Arteriosclerosis means "hardening of the arteries." They harden from calcium deposits that build up as the person ages, making his arteries less and less elastic and impeding circulation. Quite often, the first symptom of arteriosclerosis is high blood pressure. This comes from calcium deposits in the arterioles, which lie between the arteries and the capillaries.[3]

Coronary Artery Disease

He had had a great meal. There were two helpings of potatoes with thick gravy, chicken roasted dark and moist and buttery, cherry cobbler, and after dinner brandy. What a meal! He was reveling in that pleasantly stuffed and satisfied feeling when the pressure in his chest started. For a moment it was mild, a sensation he had had before, a sensation that had gone away. But this time the pressure became greater and greater until it felt as though his chest wall was being crushed by a tightening band. And there was

295

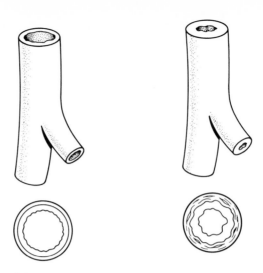

The lining of the vessels on the left is comparatively thin. This permits normal blood flow. The arteries on the right are thickened by fat-like deposits that tend to block the flow of blood. This is atherosclerosis.

FIGURE 12-3. *Atherosclerosis.*

pain—sickening, paralyzing, frightening throbs of it extending into his neck and down his left arm into his fingers. This was angina pectoris, that unwelcome visitor to many a man in his 50s, his 40s, even his 30s and 20s. The cause of angina is coronary insufficiency—a major reduction in the supply of blood to the heart. Women face angina pectoris just as men do, but the rate for men is about twice as great. The rate for smokers is about twice as great as that for nonsmokers. The rate for the sedentary is about twice as great as for the active.

Sometimes an artery gets suddenly closed off by a clot because of atherosclerotic plaque. If the clot is a thrombus and plugs an artery supplying the heart, you have coronary thrombosis. Sometimes this clot comes from an embolus, but in either case you have a condition known as coronary occlusion. The part of the heart that suffers this sudden lack of blood dies, but quite often the victim survives. This being the case, an alternate blood supply route develops around the dead heart tissue. This dead tissue is called a myocardial infarct.

The myocardial infarction rate is five times as great for men as it is for women. A third of the people experiencing them don't live beyond 48 hours. Fortunately, for the two-thirds who do survive these first few days, the chances of returning to a nearly normal life are excellent. Sometimes they can return to activities like golf, swimming, tennis, and bowling. They can't return to overeating and overdrinking, though. Myocardial infarctions are twice as likely to occur among people who are 15 per cent above average in weight. And they shouldn't return to smoking, either. Cigarette users have twice the number of myocardial infarcts that nonsmokers do.[4]

Congestive Heart Failure

Congestive heart failure really isn't a disease. It's a condition that disease of the heart brings on. "Congestive" refers to the presence of an unusually large blood supply in some part of the body, so in congestive heart failure the heart gets so much blood that it fails.

The beginnings of this condition sometimes take place in childhood, when the victim comes down with rheumatic fever. This can bring on thickening and scarring of heart valves, which keeps them from completely opening or closing. Hypertension can bring the condition on, too. A person who suffers from it for an extended period demands an excessive work load from his heart, which can seriously weaken the muscle. Sometimes a heart that has been damaged by myocardial infarction or coronary thrombosis finally goes into failure. This is extremely serious, of course. But people can survive this condition, often live with it to a ripe old age.

The congestion can take place in either of the heart's two pumps. If it's the left pump (the left ventricle) that fails, fluid backs up into the lungs. The patient's chest "rattles," he's short of breath, and he usually has a deep cough. This is called cardiac asthma. If it's the right ventricle that fails, fluid backs up into the legs and abdomem, bringing on a swelling called edema. Sometimes both pumps fail, and the edema becomes generalized over the entire body. You can press your finger into the skin of somebody who has this condition and the indentation remains after you take your finger away.

Treatment for this condition includes diuretics to remove water from the body and sodium along with it. Also, the victim usually goes on a salt-free diet. Since the weakened heart muscle can't pump enough blood to the kidneys for them to excrete salt in the urine, excess salt accumulates. This holds water, which contributes to the edema. Digitalis is usually another part of the treatment. This improves the heart's ability to pump and deals with hypertension.[5]

Congenital Heart Disease

There are 40,000 American babies born each year with defective hearts. Many of these hearts don't pump enough blood to the lungs for oxygenation, so the babies' skin and mucous membranes have a bluish tint. This condition is known as cyanosis, and the children are "blue babies." Inborn defects aren't always this severe, though. Sometimes cyanosis occurs only during exertion. Sometimes it doesn't happen at all. And quite often the cyanotic effect shows only on the lips and fingertips.

Why these inborn heart defects occur nobody really knows. Some are due to German measles and other viral infections of the pregnant mother, but most of them just seem to happen with no good explanation. A lot of them can be corrected by surgery. The heart-lung machine has been a big boon in this area. It takes over the pumping function of the heart on a temporary basis and certain functions of the lungs as well. This allows certain delicate procedures to be performed while the heart is given a rest from its life-sustaining mission.[6]

Cerebrovascular Accidents

Sometimes called apoplexy, stroke, or CVA, a cerebrovascular accident is some kind of interference with the blood supply to the brain. This can cause death, but usually it doesn't. It often causes speech disorders, paralysis on one side of the body, and loss of memory. But even these impairments often improve after a few weeks. A lot depends on how serious the damage to the brain tissue was and the exact location where this damage took place.

The signs of CVA usually develop suddenly. There are severe headache, nausea, and then unexpected convulsions and a coma. Sometimes stroke victims get preliminary warnings like dizziness, weakness that comes and goes, and a temporary loss of sensation on one side of the body. Over 75 per cent have had some kind of cardiovascular disorder.

One in every hundred people suffers a stroke. Most of them are over 60 years old and suffer from a clot called cerebral thrombosis. Another group, usually over 50, suffer from hemorrhage.

Sometimes surgery is called for to remove cranial pressure or repair damaged arteries. And usually the victim gets anticoagulants to bring down his blood pressure and dissolve clots. Then comes the rehabilitative part of this treatment. There's speech therapy, if this function has been lost or hampered. There are massage and exercise to improve the functioning of affected muscles.

About half of all stroke victims have severe permanent handicaps. But many return to work, and 70 to 80 per cent who survive for 1 month can learn to care for themselves.[7]

High Blood Pressure

About 22 million people have high blood pressure in one form or another. The medical term is "hypertension," a condition in which someone's blood pressure is always higher than it should be. Actually, there are two measures of blood pressure: systolic pressure, produced when the heart contracts, and diastolic pressure, produced when the heart relaxes. A doctor or nurse who puts a blood pressure cuff around your arm measures both. Young people normally have a systolic pressure of somewhere between 100 and 120, whereas that of the older generation ranges between 120 and 140. For healthy people at any age, the diastolic pressure should be 90 or below. Of course, blood pressure readings vary from time to time. Usually they increase with excitement and exercise and decrease when you relax. But the average reading is what counts, and for a healthy college student it should be about 120/80. Someone with an average blood pressure of 150/100 is suffering from hypertension.

Age may not cause this condition, but the aging process contributes to it. About half of all people over 50 years old have this disease to some extent. It brings on episodes of nervousness, weakness, dizziness, and headaches. It can lead to myocardial and cerebral occlusions, congestive heart disease, kidney disorders, and retinal damage to the eyes. But, with proper treatment, hypertension usually isn't fatal. After onset, the victim can live 20 years or more.

About 90 per cent of all people suffering from hypertension have a form of it known as essential hypertension. It happens when the small arteries throughout the body become constricted. This decreases the amount of blood that can be carried and raises the pressure of this blood. But no one is sure what causes the small arteries to constrict. Also, there's no treatment that completely cures this malady. Tranquilizers have helped some patients. Changing living patterns to reduce emotional stress has helped others. Losing weight can help, and eliminating tobacco can help, too. Sometimes an operation called a sympathectomy can bring dramatic relief. Here the nerves that bring on the arteriole constriction are removed. But the disease can be alleviated only, not cured.[8]

There is a condition of abnormally low blood pressure called hypotension, but there's no disease of hypotension. It can create problems only if the victim is in shock or is hemorrhaging. But under normal conditions low blood pressure brings on no ills.

Heart Transplants

Doctor Frankenstein used to do it, and sometimes Doctors Barnard, DeBakey, Cooley, and a host of others do it, too. They take hearts from some people and put them in other people. It seems like a ghoulish type of procedure, but it has been a blessing to some who had no other hope of survival.

The heart donor has to be dead, of course—at least, dead in a legal sense. In some countries this means that he can't produce brain waves on an electroencephalogram. Other countries require that the donor has also stopped breathing and that his heart has stopped pumping blood. And once the death is announced the heart has to be removed almost immediately. Within 30 minutes after it ceases function, the heart begins to degenerate, and there's irreparable cell damage. Sometimes this damage can be slowed a little by cooling the body. But, still, speed in this procedure is of essence.

Also, not just any donor heart will do. The recipient and donor should have similar blood-tissue types in order to reduce the chance of the body's rejecting the new heart tissue. Lymphocytes, a type of white blood cell, protect us from disease pathogens and other foreign materials that enter our bodies. But the lymphocytes can't tell the difference between the kind of foreign materials we want and those we don't. Strange hearts get attacked just as germs and viruses do.

There's a drug called antilymphocyte globulin (ALG) that suppresses the action of lymphocytes. But although this keeps them from destroying a foreign heart, it keeps them from warding off diseases, too. So recipients sometimes have to be kept in sterile environments. The idea is to give patients just enough ALG to keep their lymphocytes from attacking their new organ, but not enough to stop them from warding off disease. It's a difficult balance to strike, but doctors are striking it more often as experience with this new procedure accumulates.[9]

Preventing Cardiovascular Disease

You're going to die. This is an absolute certainty from the day you are born. And if you don't die from an accident, cancer, some kind of infectious disease, or a riot, the chances are that cardiovascular disease in one form or another will eventually get you. The key word here is "eventually." There's no such thing as completely eliminating diseases of this type, but they can be forestalled and controlled. Most physicians recommend the following measures to stave off problems of this type:

1. Maintain a normal weight or a weight that's slightly below normal. Typical heart-attack victims have jowls and large waistlines.
2. Participate in some kind of vigorous physical activity each day—preferably running, swimming, or bicycle riding. This keeps circulation up and blood pressure down.
3. Don't smoke, particularly cigarettes. This is preaching, true, but it's a sermon with a highly meaningful message. The typical heart victim inhales around two packs a day.
4. Go easy on animal fats or other foods that have high cholesterol levels. All the evidence isn't in yet, but a lot of the data gathered so far indicate that cholesterol brings on constriction of the arteries. This, in turn, brings on coronary occlusions, myocardial infarctions, hypertension, and cerebrovascular accidents.
5. If you're feeling fine, have your heart and blood pressure, as well as other parts of you, checked once each year. If you're not feeling fine—particularly if you have dizzy spells, if your heart seems to be skipping beats, if you have a lot of recurring pains in your chest—have your heart and blood pressure checked immediately.[10]

Cancer

Cancer isn't a disease that strikes only grandmothers and World War II veterans. A lot of people think that it is, that cancer affects only people who have been through their best years, who long ago played their last game of football or put on a bikini. Not so. Half the people who die from cancer are under 65. For women between the ages of 30 and 54, it's the leading killer. And though it's a frightening disease, often a painful and long-lasting one, it's not necessarily fatal. One-third of those diagnosed as having cancer survive. And it could be two-thirds who survive, if the disease were diagnosed in its early stages and if the victim received proper treatment.

What Is Cancer?

Cancer really isn't one disease. It's a class of diseases that affect different parts of the body with different symptoms at different stages of life. But these diseases have one characteristic in common—irregular cell growth. Cancer is more a disease of the cells than it is of whole bodily tissues or systems. Not just humans are subject to it. All members of the animal kingdom can become the prey of this unwelcome predator. And plants can become its victims as well.

Life starts as a single cell, be it plant life or animal life. And this cell divides and multiplies, and identity begins to take shape. A new tree is being formed, a new tadpole, a new human being. With humans, some of the cells

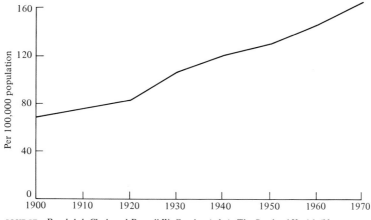

SOURCE: Randolph Clark and Russell W. Cumley (eds.), *The Book of Health* (New York: Van Nostrand Reinhold, 1973), p. 642.

FIGURE 12-4. *Deaths as a result of cancer.*

multiply into skin, some into nervous tissue, some into bone. And then there's birth and more cell division, which brings on childhood, adolescence, and maturity. Cell division slows down a bit by the time you enter college, but there's enough of it to replace worn-out cells or those that have been injured. From the time we're born until the time we die we're constantly

FIGURE 12-5. *A typical cancer cell.*

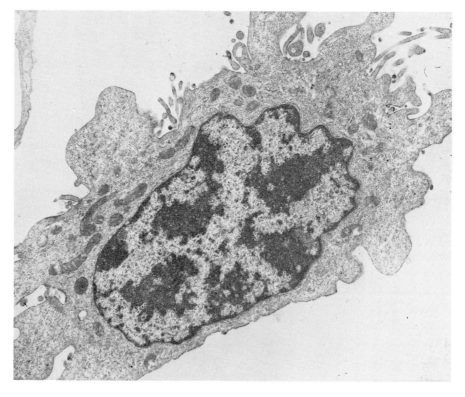

TABLE 12-3
Cancer: The Casualty Figures, Warning Signals, and Safeguards

	Estimated New Cases 1970	Estimated Deaths 1970	Warning Signal (When Lasting Longer Than 2 Weeks See Your Doctor)	Safeguards	Comment
Breast	67,000	29,000	Lump or thickening in the breast	Annual checkup; monthly breast self-examination	The leading cause of cancer death in women.
Colon and rectum	73,000	46,000	Change in bowel habits; bleeding	Annual checkup, including proctoscopy	Considered a highly curable disease when found early during routine physical examinations.
Lung	68,000	62,000	Persistent cough, or lingering respiratory ailment	Prevention: heed facts about smoking; annual checkup; chest X-ray	The leading cause of cancer death among men, this form of cancer is largely preventable.
Oral (including pharynx)	14,000	7,000	Sore that does not heal; difficulty in swallowing	Annual checkup	Many more lives should be saved because the mouth is easily accessible to visual examination by physicians and dentists.
Skin	112,000	5,000	Sore that does not heal, or change in wart or mole	Annual checkup; avoidance of overexposure to sun	Readily detected by observation, and diagnosed by simple biopsy.
Uterus	42,000	13,000	Unusual bleeding or discharge	Annual checkup, including pelvic examination and Papanicolaou smear	Mortality has declined 50% during the last 25 years. With wider use of the "Pap" smear, many thousands more lives can be saved.

Kidney and bladder	32,000	15,000	Urinary difficulty; bleeding, in which case consult your doctor at once	Annual checkup with urinalysis	Protective measures for workers in high-risk industries are helping to eliminate one of the important causes of these cancers.
Larynx	7,000	3,000	Hoarseness; difficulty in swallowing	Annual checkup, including mirror laryngoscopy	Readily curable if caught early.
Prostate	35,000	17,000	Urinary difficulty	Annual checkup, including palpation	Occurring mainly in men over 60, the disease can be detected by palpation and urinalysis at annual checkup.
Stomach	17,000	16,000	Indigestion	Annual checkup	A 40% decline in mortality in 20 years, for reasons yet unknown.
Leukemia	19,000	15,000	Leukemia is a cancer of blood-forming tissues and is characterized by the abnormal production of immature white blood cells. Acute leukemia strikes mainly children and is treated by drugs that have extended life from a few months to as much as 3 years. Chronic leukemia strikes usually after age 25 and progresses less rapidly. Cancer experts believe that if drugs or vaccines are found that can cure or prevent any cancers they will be successful first for leukemia and the lymphomas.		
Lymphomas	23,000	18,000	These diseases arise in the lymph system and include Hodgkin's disease. Some patients with lymphatic cancers can lead normal lives for many years.		

Source: 1970 Cancer Facts and Figures, American Cancer Society.

changing. If this process proceeds in an orderly fashion, the person affected is looked on as healthy, a normal part of nature's life cycle. But sometimes the replacement of worn-out cells gets out of hand. Suddenly, for reasons unknown, cells begin to break nature's rules. They grow wildly, like weeds. And, like weeds, they steal the food supply from normal cells and choke off areas they occupy. If nothing can be done to stop this wild cell growth, bodily tissues cease to function, and the victim dies.

Cancer cells can grow in any part of the body, but they're wanderers and often don't stay where they originate. Clusters of them break off and enter the bloodstream to travel to the lungs, the breasts, the armpits, the stomach. The term for this spread is "metastasis." Not all growths do this. There are benign ones that grow in place, producing tumors that doctors can easily remove and patients can forget about. But the cancerous growths, the malignant ones, spread wildly and destroy tissues throughout the entire body.

No one knows what causes cancer. It can't be "caught" from someone who has the disease. It doesn't come from a germ, from a certain kind of food or drink, from a blow, from animals, from petting or kissing. Prolonged physical or chemical irritation, such as smoking, can contribute to it, but this doesn't cause it. The same is true for X-rays, solar rays, and extended exposure to the sun and wind. Cell nutrition, the chemical composition of cells, hormones, viruses and their behavior, enzymes, and environmental stress are somehow at the root of the problem. But which ones acting in which ways on which tissues is yet to be worked out.[11] A lot of research has gone into the cause of cancer, and there will probably be much more before man gets any real insight into this complex tragedy.

Cancer Protection

There's no way of keeping cancer cells from growing in your body. In truth, there's no sure way of keeping them from killing you. If they're discovered early, the doctor might be able to destroy them. Then again, he might not. There's no sure protection from this invader, but there is protection that isn't sure. It's known as "See your physician once a year to have an overall physical checkup." You've heard this before, of course, and possibly you've already established the routine. If you haven't, start now. The only one who can tell if you have cancer is a physician. And if it's caught in its early stages the odds of getting rid of it are usually pretty good.

Sometimes, though, it's better not to wait for that routine checkup. There's a sore you've got that's been giving you a lot of trouble or a deep cough that just won't go away. Everyone should be suspicious of cancer, highly suspicious. There's a condition known as "cancerophobia," which applies to a neurotic who's in constant fear of the disease. This, of course, has to be dealt with in its own right. But most don't have this problem and should be on the alert for the following danger signals:

1. A sudden loss of weight without any apparent explanation.
2. A lump in the breast or elsewhere that suddenly begins to thicken.
3. An expansion or a change in color of a wart or a mole.

4. Bleeding or discharge that seems unusual.
5. Constant problems with indigestion or problems with swallowing.
6. Hoarseness or a cough that won't go away.
7. A major change in bowel habits.
8. Frequent headaches that are quite severe.

Also, women should examine their breasts monthly. If they change in shape, if one breast is higher than the other, or if a nipple is discharging or retracted, it's time to see a doctor. The same applies if glands under armpits are swollen.[12]

Cancer Treatment

The real key to treatment, of course, is diagnosing the cancer when it's in an early stage and totally removing all malignant cells from the body. These cells, in almost all cases, have to be removed by one of two means—X-ray or surgery, which unfortunately destroys healthy tissue along with the cancerous growth. The ideal is to come up with some kind of agent that selectively destroys malignant cells only and leaves the healthy ones be. But this ideal hasn't been achieved and possibly won't be achieved for many years. Chemotherapeutic cancer agents cause regression in certain kinds of cancer cells for varying periods of time, but they don't cure cancer. Nitrogen mustard prolongs life for people suffering from cancer of the blood, such as Hodgkin's disease or chronic leukemia. And there are chemicals used to treat lung cancer and cancer of the ovaries. Sometimes sex hormones are used to alter endocrine balance, which can bring on remission of cancer of the reproductive system. But if it's a cure the physician is seeking, not just temporary relief, he has to resort to the knife or the X-ray tube, drastic as these measures might be.

There has been some research on using viruses to cure cancer, and this has had some measure of success. Viruses localize in many types of cells and destroy them, and cancerous cells are no exception. If this technique could be perfected, the ideal cure for certain types of cancer would be available. Researchers have also tried to use immunological techniques on the disease. They inject tumor material from one patient into another with a similar type of tumor. The second patient builds up antibodies to fight this foreign substance in his body, and these antibodies are then extracted and injected back into the first patient. This has brought a certain measure of success, but the technique is more of an experiment than an accepted form of treatment.[13]

Emphysema

Emphysema has been around for a long time, but no one paid much attention to it until the last 20 or 30 years. Suddenly physicians became aware that it was one of the greatest killers and cripplers of all the debilitating conditions. One out of four deaths in the over-65 age group is caused by emphysema, or diseases related to it. The rate is one in 20 for men under 55. Those, who don't die from the ailment often have poor attendance records at work, often have trouble meeting the work demands of their jobs when they do show up. Some finally have to abandon their occupations. Many emphysema victims reach the stage where they can't take care of their personal lives. Moving from room to room, brushing their teeth, or taking a bath is completely exhausting and sometimes impossible. There's no known cure for this sickness, and once you have it you have to learn to live with it. Quite often it just gets worse.

What Is Emphysema?

Emphysema is a disease where the lung sacs, or alveoli, lose their elasticity. The lungs fill with air, which can't be completely exhaled, and the victim's blood starts getting more and more carbon dioxide and less and less oxygen. This puts quite a strain on his heart. It works harder and harder to pump more oxygen through his system so that more oxygen can get to his tissues, but often it reaches the limit of its endurance and fails. This is a kind of heart disease called cor pulmonale.

It starts subtly. No one thinks he is getting emphysema, assuming that he knows what emphysema is. He thinks that he has a cigarette cough, is having a little bronchial trouble, can't quite get over a chest cold or the flu. Sometimes he coughs up sputum for months, but he's done this before; a couple of weeks' vacation and a warmer climate should fix him up fine. It doesn't fix him up fine, of course. He begins experiencing shortness of breath out of proportion to activity. His coughing attacks get more frequent and more violent, and veins in his neck and head become distended. At this point, he might see his doctor, be told what his problem is, and start treatment. If not, his chest will become barrel-shaped, his shoulders rounded, his lips a bluish color. Eventually, his fingers will become club-shaped at their ends.

Ninety per cent of all emphysema victims admit to being heavy smokers. Another 10 per cent are light smokers, or people who claim they've never smoked, or liars. All victims seem to have had several bouts with influenza, pneumonia, and other respiratory diseases. Victims often work at jobs like paint spraying, welding, mining, and foundry work, where they're exposed to a lot of foreign particles in the air. Also, air pollution seems to contribute to this condition.

A lot can be done to help someone with emphysema, particularly if his case is diagnosed in the early stages. The most important part of the treatment is to convince him to quit smoking. The physician can give him medications that liquefy his mucus and let him cough it up more easily and medication to relax his bronchi and bronchioles. Also, there are breathing exercises and warnings to stay away from dust and smoke-filled rooms and gasoline fumes. Once lung tissue is destroyed it can't be regenerated. But the patient can learn to use more efficiently the respiratory potential he has left.[14]

Diabetes

Diabetes was recognized as a disease before Hippocrates wrote his oath. Since humans emerged from the caves, many have complained of constant

TABLE 12-4
Death Rates for Bronchitis, Emphysema, and Asthma in the United States
(Based on a 10 per cent sample of deaths. Rates per 100,000 population in specified group.)

Year	All Ages*	1–14 Years	15–24 Years	25–34 Years	35–44 Years	45–54 Years	55–64 Years	65–74 Years	75 Years and Over
1968	16.6	0.4	0.4	0.8	2.7	9.8	41.6	101.1	138.4
1969	15.6	0.3	0.5	0.6	2.6	9.9	38.0	89.4	138.4
1970	14.9	0.3	2.7	4.1	9.4	18.2	40.5	106.9	429.6
1971	14.5	0.3	2.1	3.5	8.1	16.7	36.8	91.2	374.2
1972	13.8	0.3	0.2	0.7	1.8	8.0	31.1	117.7	106.8
1973	14.4	0.1	0.2	0.5	1.9	8.3	32.2	79.8	134.2

* Includes deaths at under 1 year of age.

Source: Monthly Vital Statistics Report, Department of Health, Education and Welfare. Collected from January issues of years 1969–1974.

TABLE 12-5
Death Rates for Diabetes Mellitus in the United States
(Based on a 10 per cent sample of deaths. Rates per 100,000 population in specified group.)

Year	All Ages*	1–14 Years	15–24 Years	25–34 Years	35–44 Years	45–54 Years	55–64 Years	65–74 Years	75 Years and Over
1968	19.2	0.2	0.6	2.4	5.4	12.7	38.3	100.7	200.2
1969	18.5	0.1	0.7	2.1	5.4	12.2	38.7	93.1	190.8
1970	18.5	0.3	0.7	2.1	5.4	12.2	38.7	93.1	190.8
1971	18.2	0.1	0.7	2.0	5.2	12.2	35.1	92.7	195.6
1972	18.8	0.2	0.5	2.6	4.3	13.2	34.6	95.5	176.2
1973	17.4	0.1	0.4	1.7	4.4	11.4	33.1	82.0	171.1

* Includes deaths at under 1 year of age.

Source: Monthly Vital Statistics Report, Department of Health, Education, and Welfare. Collected from January issues of years 1969–1974.

hunger, thirst, a feeling of weakness, and the need to urinate more often than they should. Diabetes shortened the life span of many, made the lives of many others dull, insignificant, emotionally unstable, exhausting. Then, in 1922, Frederick G. Banting and Charles H. Best announced that they had isolated animal insulin. This could be used to replace the insulin human diabetics lacked, providing a normal life and a normal life span for millions.

Despite Banting and Best's discovery, diabetes (its complete name is "diabetes mellitus") is among the ten top causes of death in this country. One in every 50 persons has it, and many cases aren't detected until there has been vascular damage to the kidneys. Sometimes there's vascular damage to the eyes as well. These problems grow out of a malfunction of pancreatic cells in the islets of Langerhans. These pancreatic cells usually produce insulin and place it directly into the bloodstream. When they don't, the victim suffers from insulin deficiency, and insulin plays a key role in sugar metabolism. So the diabetic accumulates an excess amount of sugar in his blood and excretes an excess amount in his urine. Insulin also plays a key role in the utilization of fats, so untreated diabetics have a weight problem.

There are really two kinds of diabetes, the juvenile type and the type that primarily affects adults. The juvenile type is more serious and usually strikes the victim when he's 10 to 12 years old. The adult variety centers in the over-40 population who are overweight. Both types are caused by a deficit in the amount of insulin the pancreas synthesizes. But with the younger group the deficit is much more severe. Apparently, inheritance plays a role in this sickness, as two-thirds of juvenile diabetics have relatives with the same problem.

Not all diabetes patients have to take insulin. People who develop a mild form of it in later life can usually control the sickness by diet and exercise alone. And there are hypoglycemic compounds that patients can take orally to lower their blood sugar levels. Some patients with more severe cases do have to take insulin, of course. This can be a bother, as they have to learn to inject themselves with needles. But it's the kind of bother worth enduring. It saves lives.[15]

Arthritis

There are two types of arthritis. Rheumatoid arthritis involves inflammation of the joints and osteoarthritis comes from deterioration of the cartilage between bones.

Rheumatoid arthritis is by far the more crippling variety and the more painful. Nobody knows what really causes it. It's certainly not an infection. You can't catch it from someone who has it. But once you've got it there are an unlimited number of things that seem to make it worse. Cold, emotional problems, a light blow, the flu can make a victim truly miserable. Women get it more often than men do, and infants are afflicted as well as the old. But the most common time for rheumatoid arthritis to strike is between the ages of 20 and 50. It can make hands twist to claws, knees swell like massive bubbles, feet become twisted clubs. But complete crippling by this disease is rarer than it once was. Rest seems to help. Light exercise, physical therapy, and occasionally splints seem to prevent deformity. About 25 per cent of all sufferers from the illness recover completely. Another 50 per cent have periods of remission and a little deformity.

Osteoarthritis comes to almost all people past the age of 40. It's the most common of all joint ailments. Even animals get it, if they live long enough. After all, cartilage is in their joints as well as in human ones, and these specialized connective tissues degenerate in time. So does bone—particularly if we injure it, put a lot of weight on it by getting fat, let our muscles get weak so our skeletons have little help in keeping the body together. These and age bring on osteoarthritis, and there's nothing that can cure it. The victim can be helped, though. He can get drugs to ease his pain and an orthopedic appliance, if it's necessary. He can be given physical therapy and encouraged to stick to his diet.[16]

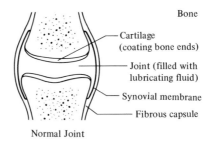

Normal Joint

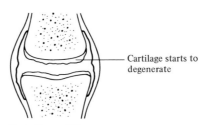

Early Stage of Disease

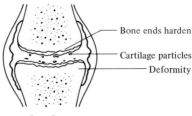

Late Stage

Note the marked physical and mechanical changes that take place in body joints affected by osteoarthritis.

FIGURE 12-6. *Osteoarthritis.*

Rheumatism

There are aches and pains people get that don't involve joints. Possibly there's a sore back, a stiff neck, or a calf or a thigh that hurts when you walk. These problems fall under the category of nonarticular rheumatism. Obviously, this is a pretty broad category covering most of the aches and pains man suffers, whether he's in grade school, in college, or drawing social security. For instance, there's lumbago. This refers to pain in the back. Fibrositis, an inflammation of the white fibrous tissue, can bring it on. Or maybe one of the discs between the bones and the spinal column has ruptured. This is a painful, possibly an incapacitating form of rheumatism. It sometimes calls for surgery, sometimes a cortisone injection, almost always aspirin, rest, and a hot bath. Emotional disorders can trigger this problem, strain can bring it on, so can fatigue and cold. Like other forms of rheumatism, man learns to live with it, ignore it when he can, see a physician when he can't.[17]

Gout

Henry VIII suffered from gout. So did William Pitt and thousands of others who enjoyed the best of food, drink, and the good life. So gout has been

FIGURE 12-7. *Suffer!*

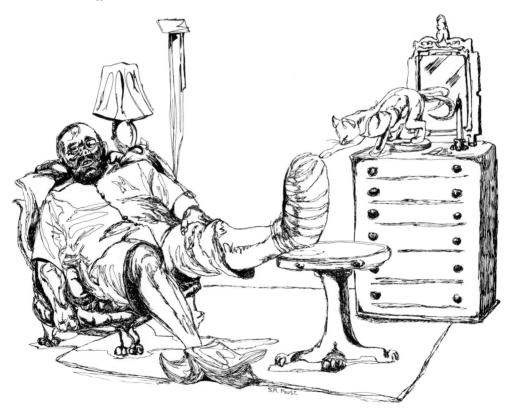

regarded for years as payment for excesses of the body, deprivation of the soul. Not so. There are teetotaling preachers who get gout, too, straight-laced bankers, retiring professors. Old-maid librarians usually don't get it, as the illness almost always occurs in men, not women. But the men's character and personal habits aren't what bring the disease on. Inheritance plays a key role, as gout runs in families. Drugs, infections, and emotional upsets contribute to the problem, too.

The gout-prone individual has a metabolic disorder that lets uric acid build up in his blood. Sodium urate crystals deposit in the linings of his joints and bring on inflammation. The metatarsal joint in the big toe is the one most commonly afflicted, but ankles and knees can become involved. Attacks last for several days, and pain is excruciating. Even a sheet brushing against the afflicted toe or a breeze passing over it can bring on throbs of anguish.

Colchicine helps to keep gout under control by reducing the sufferer's uric acid level. Also, a low-purine diet—restricting the intake of alcohol, fatty food, lentils, cereals, and meats—can help. And there are exercise, rest, and avoiding tension.

Gout will get worse if it isn't treated. It can eventually bring on permanent deformities or kidney disease. But with proper care the gout victim can usually keep his malady pretty well under control.[18]

Neurological Disorders

Neurological disorders are often the cruelest of diseases that afflict man and can interfere with his ability to think or function as a complete person. They can bring on spasms, convulsions, total helplessness. Sometimes accidents cause them, sometimes disease, sometimes metabolic defects. Sometimes no one has any idea. People with these problems often suffer the scorn, the rejection, the fear and pity of mankind. They need help, and they usually get it, in a clinical and monetary way. They need understanding and friendship, which they often don't get.

Cerebral Palsy

People with cerebral palsy can have a mild coordination problem, and they can have spasms or severe convulsions. Usually their gait is awkward and irregular. Often they grimace and drool. No two cerebral palsy victims are afflicted to the same degree, and no two of them act exactly the same. Some have extreme difficulty in speaking. Some have little control over their eyes, their movements, their arms. Some—about 60 per cent—are mentally retarded, and some have very high IQs. Over 600,000 people in this country are afflicted with this problem, and a new victim joins the group with each 170 births.

Damage to the central nervous system is what brings the disease on. This usually happens shortly before birth, during birth, or before the victim becomes 3 years old. Head injury is a cause; malnutrition is another; German measles contracted by the mother during the first trimester of pregnancy is another yet. There are also Rh incompatibility between the mother and the fetus, encephalitis, meningitis, and oxygen deficiency.

There's no medical treatment that can repair damaged brain tissue, but there is treatment that can control the number and severity of seizures and training that can teach people to live to the fullest within the limits of their handicaps. Over 20 per cent of cerebral palsy victims can be taught to be completely self-sufficient. Another 20 per cent can become partially self-sufficient. The remaining 60 per cent can gain a greater degree of self-assurance, even though they need partial or complete care.[19]

Epilepsy

The devil played a big role in ancient medical thinking. He was the fellow who brought on the plagues, the famines, and the lepers. And he was the fellow who brought on the fits, the convulsions, and the blackouts. *Epilepsy* is a Greek word for "seizure." In ancient times, it was thought that someone having an epileptic attack was being seized by the devil. The devil seized animals, too, which occasionally had uncontrolled muscular spasms. Epilepsy has never been confined to humans. It's a neurological impairment that can affect any organism with a brain.

About 1 per cent of the American population suffers from it, and this includes some very intelligent and gifted people. Van Gogh and Julius Caesar were afflicted with epilepsy. So was Alexander the Great. Yet there are still states that prevent epileptics from going to school, from marrying, from participating in community programs, from getting a driver's license. The driver's license restriction might make sense. The other restrictions reflect misunderstanding, bigotry, and just plain stupidity.

Epilepsy isn't communicable. It does no one other than the victim any harm, and it's a transitory affliction, one that usually leaves the victim without a handicap when he isn't having seizures.

No one is sure what causes epilepsy. Inheritance probably plays a role. Brain injury, minute brain tumors, or bodily chemical imbalance can affect the problem, too. Erratic discharge of brain cell impulses is what brings on the convulsions, but there's a lot of disagreement over what causes the erratic discharge. There's even disagreement over what constitutes a convulsion. There are different types of them, some of which bring on loss of consciousness, some which don't. All cause involuntary muscular spasms, but sometimes these spasms are so mild that an observer isn't aware of them. Most investigators agree, however, that any type of unexplained seizure that interferes with conscious human behavior is a form of epilepsy. Usually the disease is subdivided into the following three categories:

GRAND MAL

Grand mal is the most severe of the attacks, by far the most dramatic. Quite often the victim screams, his body stiffens, his muscles go into spasms. The attack can last for 10 seconds or for 10 minutes. It can strike once a year, once a month, or several times a day. When the attack is over, the victim is usually confused, sleepy, and sick to his stomach.

313

PETIT MAL

Petit mal isn't just a mild grand mal. The victim loses consciousness for only a matter of seconds, usually doesn't fall, and is alert as soon as the attack is over. Sometimes there are minor head and eye movements, a little staggering, a minor twitch. Petit mals usually occur in children who grow out of them when they reach their teens. And some people have them for years without knowing that they're having them. They're epileptics and don't know it.

PSYCHOMOTOR EPILEPSY

In psychomotor epilepsy, the victim exhibits unusual behavior and attitude. He may clap his hands, run aimlessly, or exhibit abnormal rage, anxiety, fear, or incoherent speech. Sometimes he hallucinates. Occasionally he's violent. Quite often he can't remember what he did during his attack once it's over.

Sometimes an operation can relieve the cause of epilepsy, but usually it has to be controlled by drugs and psychological counseling. The counseling is often directed at the patient's family as well as the patient. There's such a stigma attached to this disorder that both need bolstering.[20]

Muscular Dystrophy

Most of the victims of muscular dystrophy are between 3 and 13 years old. And most don't reach their twenty-first birthday. There's a gradual wasting away of their muscle tissue, usually starting with their legs and lower backs. The children become clumsy at first, eventually can't walk, eventually become helpless.

When this condition develops in adults, the muscles of the pelvic and shoulder girdle often become involved, sometimes the facial muscles. Sometimes the victim can't smile, frown, grimace.

There's no cure for muscular dystrophy. Physical therapy can reduce the effects of the muscular debilitation. Antibiotics can prevent and treat infection, which is important because respiratory muscles eventually are affected. And psychological counseling can help to control emotional problems. But, until research comes up with better answers concerning the nature of the illness, victims have to live with it and hope.[21]

Multiple Sclerosis

No one knows the cause of multiple sclerosis, either, and treatment for it is about the same as the treatment for muscular dystrophy—physical therapy, psychological counseling, rest, a balanced diet. This disease usually strikes people between the ages of 20 and 40, can cripple quickly or progress gradually. The myelin sheaths covering the nerve fibers in the brain and spinal cord disintegrate, and scar tissue forms. The scar tissue blocks the nerve functions, and the victim loses muscular coordination, his ability to maintain his balance, and sometimes control over his bowels and bladder. There can be paralysis, speech impairment, impairment of vision, trembling, and numbness of various bodily parts. Although the disease is progressive, there are usually several periods of remission before multiple sclerosis reaches the acute stage. Fortunately, it's seldom fatal.[22]

Parkinson's Disease

There are young people who have Parkinson's disease, but usually it afflicts the over-60 group. Around 2 per cent of our senior citizens have tremors in one of their limbs. This is how Parkinson's disease begins. The tremor is slight at first, but with time it increases in intensity and spreads to other parts of the body. Then come rigidity of the muscles, a face that looks like a mask, a shuffling gait, a loss of equilibrium.

In the strictest sense of the term, this isn't a disease, but a syndrome. The basal ganglia in the nervous system malfunction, which brings on the syndrome of tremors. There are drugs that can control these tremors and reduce the muscular rigidity. Physical therapy can help, too. But there's no sure way to deal with the basal ganglia, the cause of the problem. Sometimes neurosurgery helps. Sometimes pinpoint freezing with liquid nitrogen can help. But these treatments control symptoms only. They don't cure. They don't prolong life.

There are 500,000 people in this country who suffer from this ailment. It can bring on death or contribute to death. It can make the living years pretty unpleasant, too. The sufferer is usually accident prone because of his clumsiness and stiffness. Strangers stare at him, pity him. Sometimes loved ones feel uncomfortable around him, so they avoid him.

To make his life as bearable as possible, his environment should be designed to reduce the chance of stumbling and falling. Hand rails in his home can be helpful, and couches and chairs that are high make it easier for him to stand up and sit down. Also, he can usually do just one thing at a time. He can't cut his meat while he carries on a conversation or concentrates on television. So he has to alter his behavior pattern. His family, if he has one, has to make allowances.[23]

Huntington's Chorea

Just as in Parkinson's disease, malfunction of the basal ganglia causes Huntington's chorea. But the symptoms are much more severe. There are involuntary jerking movements throughout the entire body; there's usually severe mental impairment; and there's often an early death. People as young as 1 year old can become afflicted with it, and people in their 60s can, too. But the disease usually strikes people in the 30- to 45-year-old bracket.

The illness was named for an American physician, Dr. Huntington. And the term *chorea* is a Greek word for "dancing." Dr. Huntington's patients appeared to have dancelike movements, and often other members of their families exhibited these movements as well. Apparently, this is an inherited disease that passes from parent to child by a single dominant gene. Children of afflicted parents have about a 50 per cent chance of becoming victims themselves.[24]

315

Allergies

Almost 20 per cent of the people in the world have runny noses, hives, watery eyes, rashes, twitches and itches, headaches, coughs, and sneezing and wheezing. They don't suffer from these symptoms all the time. Only when there's a certain type of pollen in the air, when a cat enters the room, when they've eaten some nuts or strawberries, when they've come in contact with certain kinds of plastics or dyes, when they've taken a certain kind of medication do they turn from healthy, well-adjusted people into sniffling, swollen, short-of-breath examples of human misery.

Allergy isn't a specific disease. It's an overcompensation on the part of the immune system of the body. And there are as many things people are allergic to and as many varying responses to them as bits of pollen on a pussy willow.

Some people are extremely sensitive to ragweed. So, when they're exposed, their system develops antibodies. This produces no symptoms. Problems can develop, though, with a second encounter. The ragweed, or "antigen" (a foreign substance), reacts with the antibodies that it brought on in the first place. So someone's reaction to a given stimulus changes, and this changed reaction is allergy.

Most allergies are annoying, but that's the extent of the problem. No one likes to sniffle and sneeze from hay fever, to scratch hives or not be allowed to scratch them. Watery eyes ruin a girl's appearance, and a headache can keep you home from a party. There is an allergy, though, that goes beyond the annoying stage—bronchial asthma. This can bring on suffocation during acute attacks. And if it doesn't kill outright, it can cause emphysema or slowly cause heart disease. The problem starts in the bronchi, which narrow and get plugged with mucus. This creates breathing problems in the asthmatic, who makes a typical wheezing sound when he exhales. Some claim this sickness is entirely psychosomatic, that only the neurotic and insecure suffer from it. This isn't true. But emotional stress can trigger an asthmatic attack and make one that's in progress more severe.

Heredity has a lot to do with asthma. Most who suffer from it have relatives with the same kind of ailment. This is true of the other allergies, too. But allergies have one good point; unlike most diseases, age tends to mellow them. They become less severe when victims enter adolescence and sometimes disappear during adulthood.

The key treatment for an allergy is avoiding the cause of it. This might involve giving up a certain kind of pet, restricting a diet, using only a certain kind of cosmetic, avoiding wool and camel's hair in clothes. Sometimes it involves changing where you live. There can be a certain kind of pollen or dust in one section of the state or country that isn't present somewhere else.

And sometimes the sufferer can be desensitized by a physician. The physician (usually an allergist) injects small but increasing amounts of the offending agent into the patient until he builds a tolerance, in the hope that he then won't suffer from exposure to ragweed, dog hair, strawberries, and the like, unless he faces excessive amounts of them. Also, symptoms can usually be alleviated with antihistamines and steroids such as cortisone. Eighty per

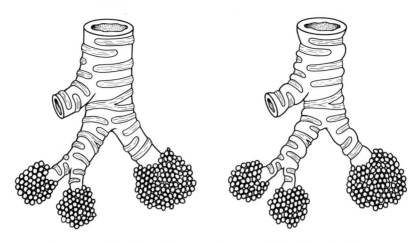

Normal bronchioles (the small air passages) appear at the left. The asthmatic's bronchioles become constricted by bands of muscles, as shown on the right. Mucus forms in the passages, and air flow to the alveoli is restricted.

FIGURE 12-8. *Asthma.*

cent of the time an allergy sufferer can get relief by a combined program of desensitization, avoidance, symptom alleviation, and just plain rest.[25]

Notes

1. P. W. Conover, "Social Class and Chronic Illness," *International Journal of Health Service,* Vol. 3 (1973), 357–368.
2. A. M. McIntyre, et al., "Unified Approach to Health, Disease," *American Journal of Nursing,* Vol. 71 (December 1971), 2369–2374.
3. H. Keen, "Glucose Tolerance, Plasma Lipids and Atherosclerosis," *Proceedings of the Nutrition Society,* Vol. 31 (December 1972), 339–345.
4. Don Carlos Peete, *The Psychosomatic Genesis of Coronary Artery Disease* (Springfield, Ill.: Thomas, 1955), pp. 106–136.
5. Wilhelm Raab, *Prevention of Ischemic Heart Disease* (Springfield, Ill.: Thomas, 1966), pp. 100–106.
6. Forrest H. Adams, H. J. C. Swan, and Victor E. Hall, eds., *Pathophysiology of Congenital Heart Disease* (Los Angeles: University of California Press, 1970).
7. T. Fyfe, et al., "Comparison of Seasonal Incidence and Mortality of Stroke and Myocardial Infarction," *Health Bulletin,* Vol. 30 (April 1972), 159–161.
8. Milton Mendelowitz, *Hypertension* (New York: Grune and Stratton, 1961).
9. Thomas Thompson, *Hearts: Of Surgeons and Transplants* (New York: McCall Publications, 1971).
10. Gösta Tibblin, Ancel Keys, and Lars Werkö, *Preventive Cardiology* (New York: Halsted Press Books, 1971).
11. Lauren V. Acherman and Juan A. del Regato, *Cancer* (St. Louis: Mosby, 1970), pp. 33–69.
12. Ronald W. Roven and Francis J. C. Roe, *The Prevention of Cancer* (New York: Appleton-Century-Crofts, 1967).
13. Acherman and del Regato, *Cancer,* pp. 69–120.
14. S. Costas, "Renal and Perirenal Emphysema," *British Journal of Urology,* Vol. 44 (June 1972), 311–319.

15. Max Ellenberg and Harold Rifkin, eds., *Diabetes Mellitus: Theory and Practice* (New York: McGraw-Hill, 1970).
16. Sydney Licht, ed., *Arthritis and Physical Medicine* (Baltimore: Waverly Press, 1969), pp. 17–61.
17. James A. Boyle and W. Watson Buchanan, *Clinical Rheumatology* (Philadelphia: Davis, 1971).
18. Ibid.
19. Lord Brain, *Clinical Neurology* (London: Oxford University Press, 1964).
20. W. R. Gauers, *Epilepsy* (New York: Dover, 1964).
21. R. J. Pennington, "Biochemical Aspects of Muscle Disease," *Advances in Clinical Chemistry,* Vol. 14 (1971), 409–451.
22. W. R. Russel, "Multiple Sclerosis: Occupation and Social Group at Onset," *Lancet,* Vol. 2 (October 16, 1971), 832–834.
23. John Gillingham, ed., *Third Symposium on Parkinson's Disease* (London: Livingstone, 1969).
24. R. W. Wells, "Huntington's Chorea: Seeing Beyond the Disease," *American Journal of Nursing,* Vol. 72 (May 1972), 954–956.
25. Howard G. Rapaport and Shirley Motter Linde, *The Complete Allergy Guide* (New York: Simon and Schuster, 1970).

13 Accidents and Safety

There are 1,800 of us getting out of bed this morning who will be killed before the week is out. Cars will smash some of their bones, rip their muscles, and spread blood. Hunting rifles will destroy a few others. Electricity and overturned boats will make a contribution to senseless tragedy. More Americans have died from accidents than from all of our wars combined. But who wants to start a protest movement against accidents?

There will be 173,000 injured this week. No one, other than their families, will worry about them. There will be 731 deaths, or about that number, caused by automobiles. Accident rates are quite constant and predictable. There will be 138 people who drown, 121 smokers who have their last cigarette as they fall asleep and set fire to their bed. Around 50 will die from leaking gas or accidental poisoning. Eleven hundred will injure or kill themselves or their companions with firearms, and there will be another 31 firearm deaths in the home, in the barroom, and on the street. A good percentage of these will be children between the ages of 5 and 14. In the senior citizen group, 385 will die of falls in bathtubs, on slick floors, or on slippery pavements. There will be 18 do-it-yourself hobbyists who get electrocuted. They'll forget to turn off the current. People are consistent. They're consistently absent-minded, careless, thoughtless, irresponsible, and often just plain stupid.

The annual accident toll is consistent, also. There are about 150,000

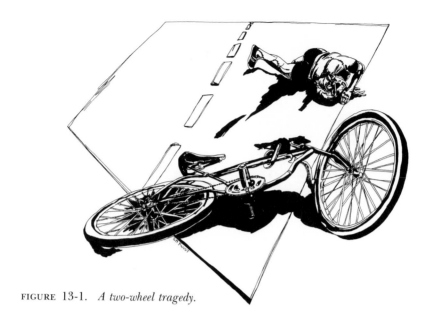

FIGURE 13-1. *A two-wheel tragedy.*

TABLE 13-1
U.S. Deaths from Accidents

Type of Accident	Deaths (1,000)			
	1950	1960	1967	1969
All Accidents	91.2	93.8	113.2	116.4
Railway accidents	2.1	1.0	1.0	0.9
Motor vehicle accidents	34.8	38.1	52.9	55.8
Other road-vehicle accidents	0.5	0.2	0.3	0.2
Water-transport accidents	1.5	1.5	1.5	1.7
Aircraft accidents	1.4	1.5	1.8	1.8
Accidental poisoning by				
Solid and liquid substances	1.6	1.7	2.5	3.0
Gases and vapors	1.8	1.3	1.6	1.5
Accidental falls	20.8	19.0	20.1	17.8
Blow from falling object	1.6	1.4	1.4	1.3
Accidents caused by				
Machinery	1.8	2.0	2.1	N.A.
Electric current	1.0	1.0	1.0	1.1
Fire and explosion	6.4	7.6	7.4	7.2
Hot substance, corrosive liquid, others	0.8	0.4	0.4	0.3
Firearms	2.2	2.3	2.9	2.3
Inhalation and ingestion, causing obstruction				
or suffocation	1.4	2.4	2.0	3.7
Accidental drowning	4.8	5.2	5.7	6.2
Excessive heat and sunstroke	0.1	0.2	0.1	0.3
Complications due to nontherapeutic proce-				
dures, thereapeutic misadventure, others	0.6	1.1	1.5	2.6
All other accidents	6.1	5.9	6.9	8.7

Source: U.S. Public Health Service.

fatalities each year; 11.1 million injuries. About 400,000 of these injuries result in amputation, blindness, or some other permanent disability. Although the totals have remained fairly constant, the accident rates, by type of accident and age of victims, have changed some. The rate for 5- to 14-year-olds has gone down significantly since the stress on health education programs in the schools. Also, bicycle accidents have decreased, probably because of the schools' efforts. But schools haven't made much of an impression on the 15- to 24-year-old group. Nearly half of all their fatalities come from automobile accidents, and another 10 per cent result from drownings, accidents with firearms, and fires. Maybe people listen when they're very young and get a little hard-headed when they enter their teens. And maybe there aren't enough young people taking driver education courses. Those who do take them commit only 20 per cent of the vehicular infractions of those who don't.[1]

Causes of Accidents

Accidents don't just happen, of course. You can pretty well generalize the causes for them. Here are some of the key ones:

The Accident-Prone Individual

Sam has been in the hospital three times this year. There had been that evening in February when his car skidded on gravel and sideswiped a tree. This had only brought on a concussion and the loss of two teeth—nothing to be too concerned about, really. Sam had gotten a cheap lesson on being a little more careful. Then had come the incident in May with his lawnmower. His right foot had gotten badly mangled; but, luckily, he didn't lose any toes. Dr. Childress did an excellent job in surgery. Then came the October incident and the broken hip. Sam had been walking downstairs in new shoes. You really can't trust leather heels.

There are still a couple of months left in the year, and Sam might give the hospital a little more business before January 1. And let's not forget the number of times he scraped himself, stubbed his toe, or got a burn that didn't call for medical attention. Sam is accident prone, and he's certainly not unique. Everyone knows somebody who has more than his share of sick leave and is always stumbling over things; cuts himself so badly shaving that it's hard to plug the leak; burns himself when he gets near a stove; falls from the ladder when he paints his house. There are certain personality traits these people usually display. They're often the kind who enjoy a rousing party or screaming thrills for entertainment. They're impulsive people who don't think much about what they're going to do before they get on with it. They resent authority more than most people do, and they're not much on establishing close interpersonal relations. Some psychiatrists feel these people are subconsciously trying to have accidents. After all, an injury can bring on a lot of personal attention and sympathy—something these people really want but don't know how to seek in a direct way. And injuries let them escape from responsibilities and worries. The boss really can't blame you for doing a poor job when you're lying in a hospital bed. Sometimes these people, psychiatrists say, have subconscious guilt feelings that demand punishment. The accidents satisfy this need. These people can sometimes be helped with psychotherapy. But those who aren't helped make a big contribution to the accident picture.[2]

Temporary Emotional Problems

It was almost 5 o'clock when he got called into the office. Mr. Porter, the boss, wanted to talk with him—or yell at him. Charlie's report on the November personnel picture was about as inept, incomplete, poorly worded, and confused a study as Porter had seen. Where had Charlie gone to school? Or had he gone to school? Was the problem laziness or just plain stupidity? Charlie had worked hard on that report and had thought it was pretty good. He muttered this to Mr. Porter, who told him he was too stupid to think. "Get out!" They would talk about this more in the morning. Charlie's stomach felt like some animal was clawing it. Rage made him shake a little. His body was weak as he headed for his car. How long would it take him to find a new job, he wondered, as he slid behind the wheel. He pressed hard on the accelerator. The wheels screeched as he cut onto the highway; and then there was the car at the crossroads that he didn't notice. His mind wasn't on his driving. Too bad. In an instant, his problems with Mr. Porter vanished.

How many accidents grow out of disagreement with a neighbor, an argument with a wife, or resentment of a boss, nobody knows. Researchers estimate that the number is considerable. Painful memories, fury, and regret get in the way of concentrating on tasks at hand. Nothing is a greater accident producer than lack of concentration.[3]

Physical Causes

Anger does have a side benefit, though. It keeps you from falling asleep. You can't drive too well or safely operate an electric saw without being awake. And fatigue and drowsiness take their toll. It's been shown that the greater the number of consecutive hours you drive, the greater your chance of having an accident. State and federal laws limit the number of daily working hours per truck driver to 12. The limit is 10 hours for people driving commercial passenger vehicles. The operators of privately owned vehicles could take some guidance from these regulations. And it wouldn't hurt them to get in the habit of taking driving breaks, too. About every 2 hours it pays to stop, stretch, and have a cup of coffee, if it's available.

Illness is a factor in accidents. Epileptic seizures bring them on, heart attacks, sometimes temporary dizziness. Dizziness contributes to more accidents among the older generation than it does the younger set, and so do poor vision and poor hearing.

Then there's drug abuse to consider. This changes physical and mental makeup in bizarre ways and brings on bizarre tragedies. Many have heard of the speed freak who decided he would fly from a tenth-story window or derail a speeding train. But you seldom hear of the head-on collision

FIGURE 13-2. *You can really lose with pills and booze.*

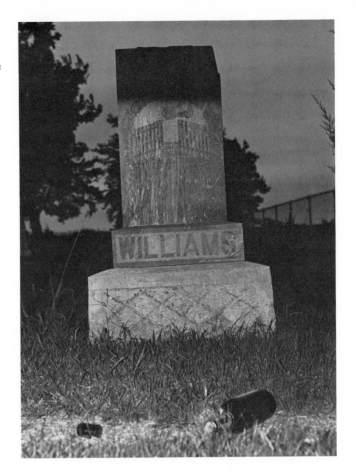

brought on by legitimate drugs prescribed by a physician. A pill purchased legally can make you every bit as drowsy or dizzy as one picked up from the slinky pusher. Legally dispensed medications have warning labels on them, though. When they do interfere with your alertness—and this applies to both the prescription and nonprescription variety—it's foolish to ignore the warnings. Someone who drives or performs a dangerous act when he's under the influence of a drug of this kind can get problems he's not asking for. And don't forget alcohol. Whether it's beer, vodka, or tequila, it's a drug that can cause every bit as big an accident as heroin, cocaine, or morphine.

And there are stimulant drugs, too. Amphetamines of one variety or another help to keep us alert for hours and days. So why not take a few when you want to drive a long distance? No sense in wasting money on a motel room. This kind of logic has brought on more tragedy than most tornadoes and plagues have. Stimulants can cause hallucinations and other perceptual problems. They can make you think a truck is in the left-hand lane when it's in the right or that a curve is really a straight road or that a two-lane highway carries one-way traffic. If you rely on amphetamines for an extended period, you have a tendency to fall asleep suddenly. This can happen when you're traveling 90 or passing a truck on a downhill grade.[4]

Environment

Weather can cause accidents. There are fog and ice and sleet, as well as people who don't make allowances for these conditions. Put the two together and an accident is a natural. Also, don't forget some of the poor environments that are man's fault—carbon monoxide in enclosed garages, machine shops that are poorly lighted, stairs with frayed rugs, and winter walks that haven't been scraped. Man may be capable of conquering the elements, but he doesn't always do it.

Equipment

If you believe Ralph Nader, a good percentage of our automobile accidents aren't the driver's fault at all. Some underpaid mechanic, ineffectively supervised by an overpaid manager, who's carrying out the plans of a yes-man engineer, who's working for a power-greedy corporation, is really responsible. If you don't believe Ralph Nader, you might suspect that a few automobile accidents result from a wheel coming off on a curve or the brakes failing or the engine exploding. Certainly equipment failure does cause accidents—just how many, no one can be quite sure. The airlines have certainly got problems in this area; so have coal companies. But a lot of accidents blamed on equipment are really brought on by human error. Sometimes equipment in fine working order when it's new isn't properly maintained and deteriorates. If you blame equipment when it causes an accident, the maintenance crew shouldn't be forgotten when blame is passed out. Also, people don't always use equipment the way they should. They don't use the right equipment for a given job; they overload equipment; they run it too fast. A lot of the problems equipment failures supposedly cause can be avoided with a little safety education and a lot of caution.[2]

Social Pressure

We're all victims of our society in one way or another. You say we're not—we're really our own men? This just isn't so. We speak English, not French. And though society is free, English is the tongue to use in this country. We could learn French, of course, but most of American society wouldn't know what we were talking about if we used it. Society also dictates to a large extent how we dress, where we work, how we treat relatives, and what our relationships with friends should be. Society can be a pretty cruel taskmaster. Take children. The world can be a tough place for them when their parents are old or poor or their mothers are pregnant with another child. It can be tough when their parents quarrel and when the family moves to a new environment. This increases their accident rate. Other factors increasing their accident rate are limited space and time to play, a lot of exposure to an immature babysitter, and easy access to harmful agents.

Peer groups apply a lot of social pressure to teenagers. Show that you're not "chicken." "Dare you!" "What a mama's boy!" It's hard not giving in to the crowd. Strong souls will stand fast. But most teenagers aren't all that strong—and neither are the older folks.

Older folks give way to social pressure in their own right. Few men would think of driving down a highway at 40 or not passing a slow-moving truck. After all, you don't want to drive like an "old woman." Seat belts are things grownups sometimes don't fasten because it makes them appear "fussy." And Dad isn't about to get a ladder to change a light bulb. The chair has always been good enough, hasn't it? Do you think he's getting old?[6]

Accident Agents

The agent is the mechanism involved in the accident. It didn't cause the accident. People, the weather, and certain elements of the environment are the causes. But the agent, passive as its role might be, is an essential part of the tragedy picture. How could you have a motorcycle accident without the agent "motorcycle"? Could you have a poisoning without the agent "poison"? The agent doesn't have the magnificent brain we humans have and doesn't have the intelligence to bring on misery—in fact, it's usually inanimate. But, without it, the accident picture isn't complete. Here are some of the more common agents that round this picture out:

Poisons

Over 2,000 people die each year from ingesting something that eats the lining of the stomach, poisons the bloodstream, or interferes with the heart and the lungs. Some people do this intentionally, of course, to commit suicide. But these cases don't come under accident statistics.

Most of the people killed or injured by poisons are children. They like to drink battery acid stored in Coke bottles and swallow bottles of candy-flavored aspirin and tasty little biscuits labeled "rat poison." You just can't train a 2-year-old to be selective about what he puts in his mouth. Kids are stubborn. And their parents and older brothers and sisters are stubborn, too. They'll store cleaning fluid and polishing fluids under the sink or on easy-to-reach kitchen shelves. And why not? Isn't this the easiest place to find them and get at them? And lighter fluids belong in the living room and bedside tables, don't they? And let's not forget the bathroom medicine cabinet. This should be well stocked and easily accessible to anybody who needs pills in a hurry.

Most accidents with these agents, as with any other agents, could be prevented by the smallest touch of common sense. Poisonous things and medications should be kept under lock and key and placed on high shelves. Obviously, poisons should never be stored near food, and they should be destroyed when they've outlived their purpose. The same applies to prescription drugs.

But we often don't use the smallest touch of common sense, and suddenly there's a nightmare. Who can help? If a physician is nearby, he can take over and probably solve the crisis. A physician is seldom nearby, though, is often hard to locate, and harder yet to get to the scene of the poisoning before it's too late. But there are 560 poison control centers in the

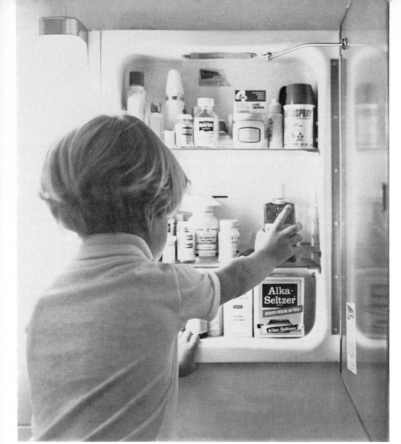

FIGURE 13-3. *"She had so many children. . . ."*

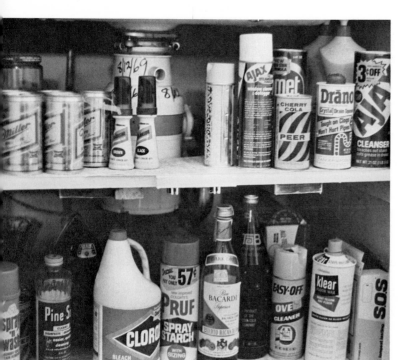

FIGURE 13-4. *Want a drink?*

TABLE 13-2
Counterdoses for the Home

DO THIS FIRST

- Send for a doctor—immediately.
- Keep the patient warm.
- Determine if the patient has taken
  (1) a poison.
  (2) an overdose.
- While waiting for physician, give appropriate counterdose below.
- But do not force any liquids on the patient if he is unconscious.

- And do not induce vomiting if patient is having convulsions.

To Find the Correct Counterdose
- In one of the lists printed below find the substance causing the trouble.
- Next to that substance is a number. This refers to counterdose bearing same number in the section below.

KEEP ALL POISONS AND MEDICINES OUT OF REACH OF CHILDREN

Poisons
Acids—18
Bichloride of mercury—1
Camphor—1
Carbon monoxide—12
Chlorine bleach—17
Detergents—1
Disinfectant
  with chlorine—17
  with carbolic acid—4
Food poisoning—7
Furniture polish—16
Household ammonia—15
Insect and rat poisons
  with arsenic—2

Poisons (Cont.)
with sodium
  fluoride—11
with phosphorus—13
with DDT—7
with strychnine—6
Iodine tincture—3
Lye—15
Mushrooms—7
Oil of wintergreen—9
Pine oil—16
Rubbing alcohol—9
Turpentine—16

Overdoses
Alcohol—9
Aspirin—9
Barbiturates—10
Belladonna—6
Bromides—7
Codeine—5
Headache and cold
  compounds—9
Iron compounds—8
Morphine, opium—5
Paregoric—5
"Pep" medicines—2
Sleeping medicines—10
Tranquilizers—10

1
Induce vomiting with
- Finger in throat, or
- 1 tablespoonful of syrup of ipecac, or
- Teaspoonful of mustard in half glass of water, or
- 3 teaspoons of salt in warm water.

2
- Give glass of milk, or
- Give 1 tablespoonful of activated charcoal, mixed with a little water.
- Finally, induce vomiting but not with syrup of ipecac (see #1).

3
- Give 2 ounces of thick starch paste. Mix cornstarch (or flour) with water.
- Then give 2 ounces of salt in a quart of warm water to induce vomiting. Drink until vomit fluid is clear.
- Finally give glass of milk.

4
- Induce vomiting (see #1).
- Then give 2 ounces of castor oil.
- Next give glass of milk or the white of 2 raw eggs.

5
- Give glass of milk, or activated charcoal in water.
- Give 2 tablespoons of epsom salts in 2 glasses of water.
- Keep patient awake.

6
- Give glass of milk, or activated charcoal in water.
- Next induce vomiting (see #1).
- Give a tablespoon of bicarbonate of soda in a quart of warm water.

7
- Induce vomiting (see #1).
- Next give 2 tablespoons of epsom salts in 2 glasses of water except in cases where diarrhea is severe.

8
- Induce vomiting (see #1).
- Give 2 teaspoons of bicarbonate of soda in a glass of warm water.
- Finally give glass of milk.

TABLE 13-2 (continued)

9
- Give a glass of milk.
- Next induce vomiting (see #1).
- Give a tablespoon of bicarbonate of soda in a quart of warm water.

10
- Induce vomiting (see #1).
- Give 2 tablespoons of epsom salts in 2 glasses of water.

11
- Give glass of milk or lime water.
- Then induce vomiting (see #1).

12
- Carry victim into fresh air.
- Make patient lie down.
- Give artificial respiration if necessary.

13
- Induce vomiting (see #1).
- Then give 4 ounces of mineral oil. Positively do NOT give vegetable or animal oil.
- Also give 1 tablespoon of bicarbonate of soda in a quart of warm water.

14
- Give glass of milk, or
- Give 1 tablespoon of activated charcoal, mixed with a little water.
- Next induce vomiting (see #1).
- Finally give 1 ounce of epsom salts in a pint of water.

15
- Give 2 tablespoons of vinegar in 2 glasses of water.
- Now give the white of 2 raw eggs or 2 ounces of vegetable oil.
- Do NOT induce vomiting!

16
- Give water or milk.
- Then give 2 ounces of vegetable oil.
- Do NOT induce vomiting!

17
- Give 1 or 2 glasses of milk.

18
- Give large quantities of water.
- Give 1 ounce of milk of magnesia.
- Do NOT induce vomiting!

United States that operate on a 24-hour basis. Most of them are located in large hospital emergency rooms and have telephone numbers listed in the front of the phone book. If the number isn't listed, the information operator will furnish it. These centers recommend treatments that should be administered immediately, depending on the medicine or type of household product swallowed. They administer a more comprehensive type of treatment when the patient is brought to the emergency room.[7] But the most effective kind of treatment, of course, is good judgment prior to the accident. This keeps it from happening.

Fires

Smoking is such a common practice that we get used to the sight of people lighting matches and lighters or ashes burning under their noses. We see people get away with it so often that danger from fire seems almost nonexistent. But more than 8,000 people die from burns each year. Thousands more are maimed and disfigured. It's a horribly painful accident, often a needless one. There's the fellow who wants a cigarette while he watches TV in bed. It could be his last gamble with lung cancer if he dozes off during a commercial. There are people who drink more than their share of bourbon and scotch who smoke, too. They're not just taking chances with their own lives. They put everyone in their vicinity in danger.

328

FIGURE 13-5. *He lit my fire.*

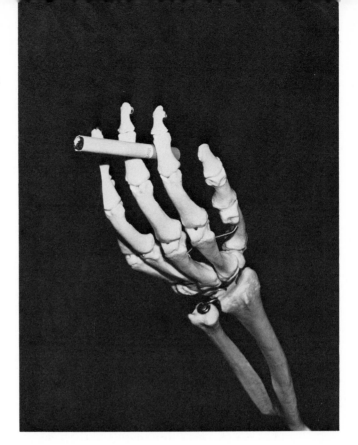

About half of all burning deaths involve people over 65 years old and those under 5.[8] A lot of these deaths are the result of someone else's gross negligence. But older people and children do tend to get forgetful and careless with matches. Older people, of course, are hard to control, but you can keep matches and lighters out of the reach of children.

Firearms

Everybody knows crime is rampant. Corner grocery stores are robbed on a daily basis, purses are snatched, homes are ransacked. And don't forget muggings, beatings, and rape. The answer? Get a gun. Wrong! At least, this is the wrong solution for over 2,500 people each year who die in firearm accidents. Rifles and pistols may seem rather harmless, because we've played with cap guns and pop guns and water pistols without having to worry about safety. And though we know we ought to be careful with the real weapons we bought, they look so much like toys it's a temptation to treat them like toys.

Nobody worries about leaving caps in a cap pistol or water in a squirt gun. Why make a big thing about whether a pistol or rifle is loaded? If it isn't loaded, how is it going to do you any good when you need it? This kind of reasoning has brought on more heartbreak than all the robberies since the fall of Rome. About half of all people who die in firearm accidents are children.[9]

Of course, storing ammunition and weapons in separate locations isn't always the answer, either. A lot of accidents come from "unloaded" guns. It's best to treat a gun as though it's loaded even when you're sure there's no ammunition in the chamber. This is particularly true when you clean the weapon. If you point a gun at someone, be sure you want to kill him. If killing isn't your thing, then don't own a gun. It can only cause misery.

Electricity

Ben Franklin took quite a risk when he flew his kite in a rainstorm. There were many people who died about that time proving that electricity and lightning are the same thing. People go on dying from electrocution in the 1970s by dropping electrical appliances in their tubs while they bathe, by repairing electrical equipment instead of letting a qualified electrician do it, by letting their children chew on electric wires or stick their fingers into electric outlets. Electricity burns, disfigures, maims, and kills. If you don't know how to handle it—and there are lots of people who don't have the slightest idea—avoid it, but respect it.

Power Lawnmowers

Power lawnmowers are wonderful gadgets for cutting off toes and fingers and sometimes even amputating a whole leg. They're a necessity for modern suburbia, of course. Your lawn has to be every bit as well trimmed as the Joneses'. Not only Jones says so, but your wife does, too. So you push those rotating blades over your front yard at least once a week. You want to get out on the golf course, though, so you don't bother to clear the yard of rock, wire, and other debris before you start. Can't you worry about that after the golf game? There's no sense in worrying about your pet dog wandering in the yard, either. He knows how to take care of himself. Besides, you're getting a little tired, and you want to go in the house for a beer. Let's forget the lawn for a while, but don't bother to turn the mower off. It's too much work to start the darn thing again. It's amazing that there aren't more accidents with lawnmowers than there are.

A couple of other practices suburban gardeners follow is mowing hill-sides from side to side rather than up and down. The up-down motion can get pretty tiring. And, after all, Columbus took a chance, didn't he? There are people who refill the tanks when the motor is hot and running. A lot get away with this, and there are some who go down in flames. And there are people who avoid the problem with gasoline engines entirely. They use an electric mower—even in the rain and when the grass is soaking wet.[10] These people go down in flames, too.

Power Tools

Why people won't read operating manuals before using power tools is beyond understanding. The things look lethal, they sound lethal, and they are lethal. A chain saw can take off a hand in an instant. A power lathe can grind a hand to mush. But some hardy souls are convinced they can learn to operate these tools by trial and error. Who wants to waste his time guessing at what some writer thinks? This theoretical bit gets in the way of common sense. And then there are those who read the manuals but won't follow them. They won't keep their tools in decent repair; they use their tools for tasks they weren't designed for; they won't wear safety goggles or safety lenses when their manuals warn that they should. Sometimes these people carry lucky charms and rabbits' feet, and sometimes Lady Luck treats them just fine. Sometimes, though, she's not the perfect lady.

Glass Doors

It happens a lot when people have had too much to drink. There is this glass door. They would have sworn it was open; the glass was so clean and all. So they really couldn't be blamed for stumbling into it. They knew exactly what they were doing right up to the accident. Injuries of this type can involve a simple bump in the nose, disfiguring and painful lacerations, death. Children often get involved with glass door accidents when they play hard and don't watch where they're running.

These doors should always be made of safety glass and be marked with some easily seen device, like a decal. And, if you're throwing a party, point out the glass door when guests arrive. Some may forget about it after the second highball, but a reasonable number will keep it in the backs of their minds.[11]

Motorcycles

Marlon Brando looked great in a leather jacket and boots, and a lot of his imitators look pretty fine, too. So the motorcycle is popular with the 16- to 24-year-old group. Seventy per cent of motorcycle operators are at this age level, and 90 per cent are males. They're a daring lot, something like the carefree musketeers in an earlier era. Each road leads to an adventure; each adventure brings victories, a deeper sense of manhood, fun. There are roads, though, with unexpected curves, and there are dead ends.

Automobiles are dangerous. For every 100 million miles they travel, there are 5.5 deaths. For motorcycles, this figure is 23. If you have an accident in a car, particularly a heavy car, there's some metal and rubber and a steering wheel between you and the point of impact. With a motorcycle, you meet the colliding vehicle, tree, or pavement head-on. And heads don't hold up too well under this kind of treatment. More than 50 per cent of people involved in motorcycle accidents get cranial injuries, many of which bring on serious incapacitation or death. And other parts of the body get hurt in these kinds of accidents. Knees and legs almost never escape unharmed. The motorcycle is an exciting toy, but it can be a cruel one.

A lot of people who drive motorcycles don't have the experience or training they should. Probably they have a license to operate the cycle, but there are people with licenses to operate automobiles who don't have enough experience or training, either. And there are protective clothing and headgear motorcycle riders should wear, which a lot of them don't. After all, it's just a short trip. They're not going to get on the highway or do much

331

TABLE 13-3
Motorcycle and Total Motor Vehicle Data, 1960–1971

| | Vehicles | | | | Deaths | | | |
| | Motorcycles | | Total Motor Vehicle | | Motorcycle Riders | | All Motor Vehicle Occupants | |
Year	Number	Yearly Per Cent Change	Number	Yearly Per Cent Change	Number	Yearly Per Cent Change	Number	Yearly Per Cent Change
1960	575,497		74,500,000		731		29,750	
1961	595,669	+3.5	76,400,000	+2.6	697	− 4.7	29,850	+0.3
1962	660,400	+10.9	79,700,000	+4.3	759	+ 8.9	32,300	+8.2
1963	786,318	+19.1	83,500,000	+4.8	882	+16.2	34,700	+7.4
1964	984,763	+25.2	87,300,000	+4.6	1,118	+26.8	37,900	+9.2
1965	1,381,956	+40.3	91,800,000	+5.2	1,515	+35.5	39,450	+4.1
1966	1,752,801	+26.8	95,900,000	+4.5	2,043	+34.9	42,800	+8.5
1967	1,953,022	+11.4	98,900,000	+3.1	1,971	− 3.5	42,700	−0.2
1968	2,100,547	+ 7.6	103,100,000	+4.2	1,900	− 3.6	44,100	+3.3
1969	2,315,916	+10.3	107,700,000	+4.5	1,960	+ 3.2	45,200	+2.5
1970	2,814,730	+21.5	111,200,000	+3.2	2,330	+18.9	43,500	−3.8
1971	3,293,400	+17.0	115,000,000	+3.4	2,410	+ 3.4	43,200	−0.7

Source: Accident Facts 1972, p. 56.

over 60. And there are people who take a few drinks before getting on the cycle so they'll be loose, or so they'll have a little more nerve. Gotta show your buddies what you're made of. People following these practices often show in gory detail what they're made of. They don't hide a thing.

The federal government entered this motorcycle accident picture in 1966 by passing the Highway Safety Act, which applies specifically to motorcyclists. The act requires that each motorcycle driver and passenger wear approved safety helmets and eye protection devices. And the act requires that motorcycle operators pass certain kinds of theoretical and practical tests before they're given their licenses. This hasn't eliminated the motorcycle accident problem, of course, but it has helped. There has been a slight decline in the motorcycle accident rate since 1966. And, because of this, several states have enacted motorcycle safety laws of their own. Most require additional equipment on motorcycles, such as crash bars, turn signals, windshields, and one or more rear-view mirrors. Some states require that cyclists and passengers wear heavy clothing, boots, and gloves. This holds down injuries to the skin when you slide along the pavement or gravel.[12] But the most effective regulations are the ones the motorcyclist sets for himself. Half-hearted compliance with laws doesn't create an effective safety program for the state or for the individual driver. Anyone operating a vehicle of this type should emphasize road courtesy and safety procedures. So should people driving automobiles, but it's not as imperative for them as it is for the two-wheel driver. Although he may not be the fellow with the most to lose, he is the one who has the greatest chance of losing what he has.

Automobiles

More than 50,000 Americans die in motor vehicle accidents each year—about the total number killed in Vietnam. In fact, all wars we fought in haven't killed as many Americans as the automobile has. It's a deadly weapon all right, one that's always loaded, and one that goes off when you least expect it.

DRIVER ERROR

The 18- to 24-year-old is the most common victim. More than 10,000 people of this college-age set lose their lives to automobiles annually. Drivers in this age group have accident rates 2 to $2\frac{1}{2}$ times higher than older drivers do. When you consider that youth is the time when reaction time, alertness, and manual dexterity are at their peak, the statistics make you wonder. Is it driving knowledge that's creating the problem? Certainly, students who have taken driver education programs have dramatically lower driving accident rates than those who haven't taken them. But knowledge and education are superficial solutions for every ill from drug addiction to pregnancy. They are important. But there doesn't seem to be that much knowledge required for driving a car on the right-hand side of the road, not exceeding the speed limit, and staying sober when you get behind the wheel. Poor driving attitudes seem to be the real cause of high accident statistics, and a lot of youths don't rate too high in the good attitude department.

TABLE 13-4
Motor Vehicle Accidents—Persons Killed or Injured: 1960-1972
(Estimates based on summaries of motor vehicle accidents prepared by various states.)

Item		Persons Killed					Persons Injured*				
		1960	1965	1970	1971	1972	1960	1965	1970	1971	1972
Number of persons	(1,000)	38	49	55	54	56	3,682	4,100	5,100	4,700	4,850
Driver action	(1,000)	30	42	45	46	(NA)	2,600	3,682	4,513	4,136	(NA)
Pedestrian action	(1,000)	8	9	10	10	10	256	275	301	319	277
Per cent distribution		100.0	100.0	100.0	100.0	100.0	100.0	100.0	100.0	100.0	100.0
Driver action:											
Exceeding speed limit		36.1	41.1	39.3	36.1	(NA)	38.5	42.2	21.9	22.7	(NA)
On wrong side of road		17.0	16.4	13.8	14.1	(NA)	6.7	6.8	9.3	5.1	(NA)
Had not right-of-way		12.8	13.0	14.0	14.6	(NA)	22.5	18.9	15.7	19.9	(NA)
Drove off roadway		16.6	10.5	14.5	15.6	(NA)	8.3	6.9	11.2	10.9	(NA)
Reckless driving		12.5	14.9	14.3	12.6	(NA)	13.5	19.2	37.0	36.2	(NA)
Other†		5.0	4.1	4.1	7.0	(NA)	10.5	6.0	4.9	5.2	(NA)
Pedestrian action:											
Crossing at intersection		29.2	20.8	22.4	21.1	20.0	32.7	26.2	31.4	31.2	29.7
Crossing between intersections		37.2	40.8	41.8	42.9	37.6	32.2	31.6	26.4	26.9	24.3
Children playing in street		5.3	3.3	3.1	2.2	3.0	6.6	6.3	5.5	5.1	5.3
At work in road		2.9	2.8	2.0	2.2	2.5	2.2	1.8	2.0	2.0	2.2
Coming from behind parked car		6.2	6.9	3.1	3.3	2.8	25.7	26.8	9.3	8.7	10.3
Walking on rural highway		20.0	25.6	24.3	24.3	18.9	2.4	7.6	23.2	8.8	10.2
Not on roadway		4.2	4.7	4.1	4.1	6.3	4.5	3.6	4.4	4.7	4.8
Other‡		5.1	5.2	9.2	9.9	8.9	3.7	6.1	8.9	12.6	13.2
Collision with											
Automobile		39.5	41.2	40.6	39.6	40.2	74.9	72.5	73.2	72.7	71.4
Pedestrian		20.0	18.6	17.8	18.2	17.8	8.3	6.7	5.9	6.8	5.7
Fixed object		10.7	10.5	10.1	9.9	11.8	4.8	5.1	5.7	5.8	7.7
Other§		4.8	4.5	3.8	4.0	4.2	2.1	2.4	1.9	2.2	2.7
Noncollision		25.0	25.2	27.7	28.3	26.0	9.9	13.3	23.3	12.5	12.5

Weather condition:										
Clear	87.4	84.8	84.1	83.3	83.3	83.9	78.6	80.7	80.1	80.5
Fog	1.2	2.0	2.0	3.7	2.3	0.7	1.5	1.4	1.6	1.4
Rain	9.0	11.0	12.1	11.1	12.4	10.6	15.4	14.2	13.3	14.3
Snow	2.4	2.2	1.8	1.9	2.0	4.8	4.5	3.7	5.0	3.8
Road condition:										
Dry	79.2	77.4	78.8	75.9	77.0	71.5	69.1	72.7	68.0	70.2
Wet	15.1	17.9	17.2	18.5	18.3	16.5	22.4	20.4	22.2	21.2
Snowy or icy	5.7	4.7	4.0	5.6	4.7	12.0	8.5	7.9	9.8	8.6
Day of accident:										
Sunday	17.7	18.7	17.6	17.2	16.3	15.2	13.6	13.7	13.9	12.6
Monday	11.6	10.9	11.4	11.5	11.7	13.5	13.2	13.2	13.0	13.4
Tuesday	11.6	10.0	10.5	10.7	10.2	12.2	11.9	13.2	12.6	12.6
Wednesday	10.5	11.2	11.2	10.9	11.0	12.1	12.9	13.4	12.8	12.9
Thursday	11.2	11.9	12.2	12.6	12.0	13.5	13.9	13.2	13.9	13.9
Friday	16.0	15.4	16.3	16.5	17.1	16.0	16.5	16.6	17.1	17.6
Saturday	21.5	21.9	20.8	20.6	21.7	17.5	18.0	17.7	17.4	17.0
Hour of accident:										
Midnight–6 A.M.	22.3	22.2	21.6	21.5	21.4	10.9	10.7	11.8	11.1	10.5
6 A.M.–noon	15.6	14.8	15.6	15.7	15.1	22.0	21.8	20.7	20.8	21.6
Noon–6 P.M.	27.8	28.7	28.4	28.5	28.1	40.5	39.7	40.0	40.7	41.1
6 P.M.–midnight	34.3	34.3	34.4	34.3	35.4	26.6	27.8	27.5	27.4	26.8
Age of victims:										
Under 10 years	(NA)	7.6	(NA)	6.9	7.2	(NA)	8.9	(NA)	8.3	7.8
10–19 years	(NA)	15.9	(NA)	18.9	19.9	(NA)	21.4	(NA)	22.3	23.8
20–34 years	(NA)	28.4	(NA)	29.6	31.9	(NA)	31.6	(NA)	35.0	36.4
35–54 years	(NA)	24.3	(NA)	21.7	29.6	(NA)	25.7	(NA)	22.5	20.9
55 years and over	(NA)	23.8	(NA)	22.9	21.4	(NA)	12.4	(NA)	11.9	11.1

NA, Not available.

* Includes persons injured attributable to action of both parties and those for whom action could not be determined.

† Cutting in; improper passing; no or improper signaling; movement of driverless car; miscellaneous.

‡ Standing on safety isle; getting on or off other vehicle; riding or hitching on vehicle; miscellaneous.

§ Railroad train; bicycle; other vehicle; miscellaneous.

Source: The Travelers Book of Street and Highway Accident Data (Hartford, Conn.: The Travelers Insurance Companies, annual).

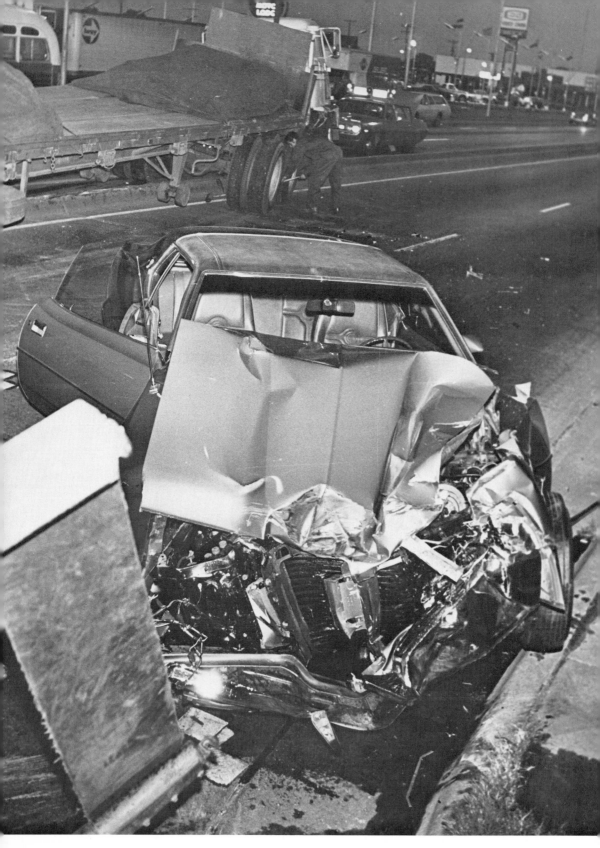

FIGURE 13-6. *A four-lane dieway.*

This is natural. Young years are the time to rebel, the time to question tradition, regulation, and the time to break out of the nebulous prison known as society. Why should other drivers be treated with more courtesy, respect, and consideration than anyone else? This might sound selfish and irresponsible, because it is. But it's the kind of attitude a lot of young people get, regardless of the generation. Youth in the 1920s had their raccoon coats and bobbed hair and flasks of bootleg whiskey. Youth in the 1930s and 1940s had their hot rods, bobby socks, and jazz festivals. There were the panty raids of the 1950s, the love-ins of the 1960s. But, no matter what the year, this attitude is a tough one to change. And it does influence highway performance.

Of course, age can be a problem at the other end of the scale. No one likes to admit that he's too old to drive a car or too old to focus his attention on the road or keep his mind on vehicles, pedestrians, and traffic lights; too old to respond quickly to unexpected crises or possibly even see or hear crises that do develop. Some people are more alert at 80 than others are at 40. And there are people in their 30s who already have started to "slow down." But, no matter the age, there are people too old to drive.

And then there are people in their 20s, 30s, and 40s who shouldn't be operating cars, either. People of any age with serious heart conditions, epilepsy, diabetes, or any condition that can bring on sudden unconsciousness have no business behind a wheel. But laws often don't keep these people from driving, and these people often won't disqualify themselves. How many accidents have been caused by an unexpected coronary, a sudden convulsion or fainting spell? Who knows? Dead men tell no tales, and those who live aren't about to admit that they can't control their own faculties. And there are people who are seriously nearsighted who won't wear glasses, people with night blindness who shouldn't touch an accelerator after sundown, those with tunnel vision, those with sight in just one eye. There are excitable people, the kind who become unnerved when a horn honks or a truck gets too close. There is the absent-minded type who uses his time behind the wheel to solve his business or home problems. There is the fellow with a quick temper who would like to ram his grillwork right into that road-hog's tail pipe. Regardless of age, these people have no business driving. But there's no way of keeping them from doing it. All you can do is make allowances for them when you get behind the wheel yourself.[13]

MECHANICAL ERROR

It's not always the driver who causes the accident. Usually it is. Human error is a lot more common than mechanical error. But, according to Ralph Nader, mechanical faults in the automobile have brought on their share of misery. In *Unsafe at Any Speed,* Nader advances the theme that with the knowledge and technology we have today we could make the automobile a lot more crashworthy. We need more research in this area, Nader says. But, more important, we should apply the know-how we have. Manufacturers have shown almost no concern, Nader feels, for automotive-design safety since Walter Chrysler incorporated his mechanic shop and Henry Ford started his assembly line. So it's up to the federal government to set the same

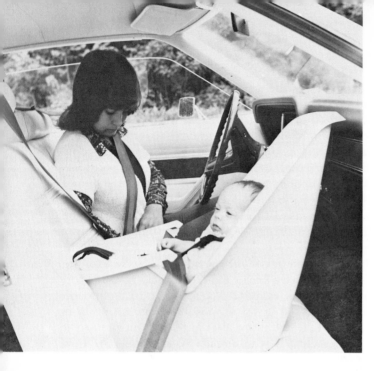

FIGURE 13-7. *Harnessing safety.*

type of safety standards that have been established for the aviation industry, the railroads, and other kinds of public transportation.

Some aren't too impressed with Nader's arguments. They feel he's a publicity seeker, that he's making headlines by attacking an unpopular dragon. After all, what better enemy could you want than a capitalistic giant?[14]

SEAT BELTS

But even his critics admit that Nader has created a lot of consumer interest in automotive safety. And when the consumer gets interested, Congress does, too. So there have been House and Senate investigations on the subject, and legislation has been passed forcing manufacturers to put seat belts and antipollution devices on their cars. Antipollution devices are controversial, and they have little to do with automotive safety. But there's nothing controversial about the roles seat belts can play in reducing automotive injuries and fatalities. Cornell University conducted a study called "The Automotive Crash Injury Research Project" and came up with the following facts:

1. There would be a 25 per cent reduction in fatalities if motor vehicle accident victims couldn't be ejected from their cars. Fifty-five hundred American lives would be saved each year.
2. The chance of injury in any kind of motor vehicle accident is $2\frac{1}{2}$ times greater for the person without a seat belt than for the person with one.
3. Some claim that if you're going to die in an accident, you'll die. Seat belts can't materially change the odds. Not so. The mortality rate of people not belted in their cars at the time of vehicular impact is 8 times greater than for those with seat belts fastened.

Then why would anyone be foolish enough to drive without fastening his seat belt? It doesn't seem to be all that much bother. But apparently it is that much bother to some. The belts make them feel tied down and uncomfortable, restricted. Not surprisingly, people with this attitude get high scores on tests measuring impulsiveness and risk-taking. They've usually had more than one traffic citation, enjoy the excitement of fast driving, and even rate themselves as drivers who aren't too cautious.

But even people who rate themselves as cautious aren't always as cautious as they think. Less than half of those who carefully buckle their seat belts before entering the highway bother with this safety measure around town. After all, they feel, they're just going to the store or the office. What can happen in a mile or two, or even in a few hundred yards? And they're not really going all that fast. If you're not going 70 miles an hour, you're not going fast. Unfortunately, this reasoning is completely false. Two-thirds of all automobile deaths take place within 25 miles of the home. More than half of the accidents causing serious injury and death involve speeds of 40 mph or less.

Of course, a lot of automobiles don't have seat belts. This is particularly true of cars owned by young people. They're old cars, which didn't have seat belts as part of their standard equipment. And the present owners won't go to the trouble or expense to have them installed. They'll buy new cars one of these days; they'll get their seat belts then. Obviously, this is foolish. The older the car, the greater the need for seat belts becomes. Cars made in the 1940s, 1950s, and 1960s have much higher accident rates per mile than the newer ones do.[15]

A lot of cars have seat belts for those in the front seat but none for those in the back. Since the rear-seat passengers take about the same risk as the front-seat passengers do, this makes about the same sense as waiting to buy seat belts until you get a new car. They're really not all that expensive or tough to install. A few dollars and a few minutes' effort can prevent a few tragedies.

LAW ENFORCEMENT

Something that Ralph Nader hasn't recommended, but has reduced traffic fatalities and injuries, is tougher law enforcement. This is a state problem, of course, one that the federal government has little control over, and one that doesn't always make for good headlines and popular politicians. But some of the following measures have been effective in reducing the death rate:

1. Tougher driver's license exams, and exams that have to be retaken on a periodic basis. The person who has the knowledge and physical ability to qualify for a license when he's 18 doesn't always have the same abilities when he's 68.
2. Mandatory automobile inspection programs. This is again done on a periodic basis.
3. Increasing the number of policemen patrolling the highway. This isn't always popular with taxpayers, as it is an expensive measure. But it's one

of the better ways known to keep people within the speed limit and on the right side of the highway.

4. Hiring special forces to reinforce the police during heavy traffic periods, such as quitting times and holiday weekends.
5. More use of radar devices to trap speeders. This seems like a sneaky way of catching a speeder. He doesn't really get fair warning that he's being checked. But, because this might save his life or the lives of other motorists, the sneakiness might be forgiven.
6. Setting up periodic roadblocks. Here drivers are checked for licenses and intoxication, and vehicles are checked for safety.
7. Tough state laws calling for the suspension of driver's licenses, fines, or imprisonment for motorists convicted of drunken driving, speeding, or chronic negligence.[16] These laws can be harsh and often cruel, but careless drivers are cruel, too, often merciless.

The Pedestrian

Just a word about the pedestrian. He deserves a word, because 9,000 to 12,000 get killed by cars each year. The driver, of course, is the central figure in the accident, but he's not always the one at fault. There are jaywalkers who bring on their own demise; there are drunks who stumble in front of cars; there are children who chase balls or pets in front of rolling wheels. Two out of three pedestrians killed are acting in some kind of unsafe way or directly violating traffic regulations. And one in five has the odor of alcohol on his breath. A few rules pertaining to pedestrian conduct are worth reviewing occasionally:

1. Don't try crossing a street or a road unless you're sure traffic is clear on both sides, and don't try to beat an oncoming car. Tripping or stumbling can make you lose.
2. Obey traffic signals and stop signs. You'll get there just as fast if you don't try running against the "walk" sign or dancing between cars that are passing through a green light.
3. Walk on the left-hand side of lighted roads. There's some argument on this. Admittedly, some authorities claim you should move in the direction of the traffic. But most favor moving against it. People have a tendency to daydream and wander when they walk—all of us do. So when you move down a road, you can wander a little into the path of a passing car. If you're facing traffic when you walk, the oncoming car usually alerts you to the danger.
4. Carry a light-colored object when walking on dark roads. It's hard for a motorist to see someone dressed in brown or black, but white or orange or yellow shows up clearly.[17]

Home Accidents

Home is where people fall off chairs and break their legs, burn to death from kitchen fires, get asphyxiated with carbon monoxide. Mom may be a great cook, an expert in love and band-aids, but a winner in the safety department she isn't.

A lot of home accidents result in fatalities. One-fifth of these happen to children under 5, and half strike down people over 65. The most accident-prone person in the home is the 2-year-old boy. This is the age when he's learned to walk, strike matches, turn over electric irons, and fall downstairs. But his behavior isn't unique. There are lots of thoughtless people at 18, 28, 48 who can keep up with him in stumbling over their feet and walking into glass doors.

The most dangerous room in the house is Mom's bailiwick, the kitchen. This is where burns and scalds take place, also explosions, falls, poisonings, and suffocations. Next in order in the home accident department are the stairs, the living room, the porch, the bedroom, the basement, dining room, bathroom, and hallways. But doesn't Dad's castle, the garage, occupy a high place in the accident hierarchy? Surprisingly, no. Except for a few carbon monoxide poisonings, the garage is almost accident free. The yard, though, which is mostly Dad's territory, is just about as dangerous as the kitchen.

Falls are the biggest cause of fatalities in the home, but other common causes of death and serious injury are poor lighting, stairways without railings, unsafe electrical fixtures, scatter rugs that slip, slippery floors, and the kind of housekeeping that lets objects lie in the center of floors and piles of things accumulate near stairways.[18] It takes just a minute to check a home for accident hazards, but it's a worthwhile minute to spend. Everyone should do it on a regular basis.

Recreation Safety

The biggest safety problem in the sports field involves drowning. More than 7,000 people lose their lives in lakes, rivers, and streams each year. Oddly enough, over half of these drownings occur within 20 feet of safety, and they often involve people who are considered fine swimmers.

Fine swimmers also drown in pools. Pools can provide a lot of fun and exercise, of course. But they can bring on misery. It pays to keep a couple of safety fundamentals in mind when you use one. Walk, don't run around the pool. Sliding on wet tiles is about as easy as sliding on ice. As to horseplay, there shouldn't be any. If you want to dunk a buddy, shove your girl friend into the water, or flick people with towels, resist the temptation. Horseplay has its place, but the place isn't around water. If you're lucky enough to own a pool, be sure there's a fence around it with a gate you can lock. This keeps out neighborhood children and neighborhood drunks and pets. And always keep a lot of rescue equipment like long poles and ring buoys near the pool's edge. In case you have to use this equipment or have to dive in and save somebody, be sure you know the number of the fire department or an ambulance service. Their quick arrival can make the difference between life and death, regret and relief.

Here are some swimming safety rules to think about, whether you're at a pool or lake or ocean:

TABLE 13-5
Home Accident Deaths by Type of Accident, 1950–1971

Year	Total Home	Falls	Fires, Burns*	Suffocation, Ingested Object	Suffocation, Mechanical	Poison (solid, liquid)	Firearms	Poison by Gas	Other
1950	29,000	14,800	5,000	**	1,600	1,300	950	2,250	4,100
1960	28,000	12,300	6,350	1,850	1,500	1,350	1,200	900	2,550
1969	27,000	10,000	5,900	2,100	1,200	2,300	1,200	1,200	3,100
1970	27,000	9,800	5,700	2,300	1,100	2,600	1,200	1,200	3,100
1971	27,500	10,000	5,700	2,400	1,000	3,000	1,200	1,200	3,000

* Includes deaths resulting from conflagration, regardless of nature of injury.
** Included in other.

Source: *Accident Facts 1972*, p. 81.

1. Never swim alone. You've heard this before, of course, but so did the corpse they just carried away in an ambulance. Who can help you if you get a cramp or a spasm, or hit your head when you're by yourself?
2. You're young, vigorous, and manly, can lick tigers and sneer at professors. But don't sneer at the calm-looking lake or try to lick a crashing wave. Even young people have limits on their ability. Don't overestimate it.
3. If you're in a boat, and it overturns, stick with it. Hold on to the side and wait for help. Don't try swimming for shore. It may appear close, but it's often way beyond the distance that you can reach.
4. Diving can be fun. And, in the right location, it can provide excellent recreation and give you a chance to show off. But never dive into unknown waters. A rock or log can be just beneath the surface of what looks like a deep pool.
5. It takes a real man to swim in icy waters, particularly when he's been partying late the night before. Leave it to men. Admit you're a boy. Cramps are much more likely when you're tired or when the water's cold.
6. Swim where a lifeguard is available, but never put too much faith in him. Even the strongest and best trained can't protect a fool from himself.
7. Learn to stay afloat for long periods. Some of the finest swimmers can't do this.
8. There are all kinds of new things to try in the water, but don't experiment without good instruction, and experiment slowly. You're not going to master the half-gainer in a few minutes.

Swimming, of course, is a "mild sport." It doesn't offer the he-man contact that football, wrestling, boxing, and lacrosse do. If swimming is such a deadly pastime, what havoc must the "gladiator contests" wreak? Oddly enough, the "manly games" kill darn few in comparison to pastimes like fishing, hunting, and, of course, swimming. Good supervision of the contact sports is apparently the key. Coaches teach football players how to fall, make sure their hockey players are in top condition, fit boxers with mouthpieces and headgear.[19] There is nobody checking on the fellow who goes out to shoot quail or one who decides to fish for salmon or to surf at Waikiki. People would resent recreational supervision if there were such a thing. After all, they're out to have fun, aren't they? They don't need to have somebody telling them what to do.

Industrial and Occupational Safety

A lot of thought, money, and time go into reducing accidents in industry. Not that stockholders are overly concerned about the welfare of employees. They may be, of course. But the main reason behind these safety programs is the cost of industrial accidents. They're brutal, when you consider the cost of insurance, the cost of training replacement personnel, the cost of paying an employee for nonproductive time, the cost in good will with unions and the public. But, despite a lot of effort to reduce industrial accidents, they still happen. And the human being seems to be the main cause. Safety engi-

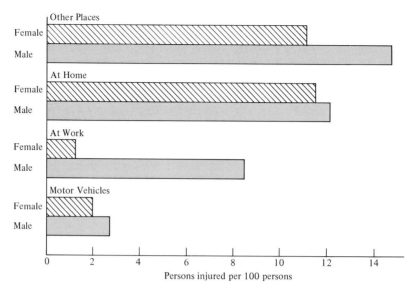

SOURCE: U.S. Public Health Service, National Center for Health Statistics, *Vital and Health Statistics,* Series 10, No. 79.

FIGURE 13-8. *Persons injured, by class of accident and sex, 1971.*

neers have a hard time figuring him out. Horseplay around machinery, poor housekeeping in the shop, and just plain carelessness are the biggest problems. It's not surprising that there are proportionately more people killed in farm work than there are in factories.[20] There are fewer bosses and supervisors on farms and fewer people to keep the human element under control.

Emergency Treatment

There are lots of Americans allergic to penicillin, novocaine, tetanus anti-toxin, sulfa, codeine, and even aspirin. These people can become seriously ill or die if treated with these drugs, yet well-meaning practitioners make this kind of mistake daily. There are 40 million Americans who have hidden conditions that should be made known before they're given emergency medical treatment. Take America's 2 million diabetics. If a diabetic were to go into a diabetic coma, someone might think he was drunk and have him put in jail to sleep it off. The same applies to America's 1.5 million epileptics. There are hemophiliacs, people whose blood doesn't clot properly and who can bleed to death from the slightest cut or bruise. If a hemophiliac is unconscious or can't speak English and someone doesn't see that he gets a transfusion immediately, the outcome can be tragic.

There are millions of people who wear contact lenses. In one who is unconscious for 24 hours or more, unremoved lenses can "chew up" his corneas. This can seriously impair vision or bring on permanent blindness. And then there is the alcoholic trying to kick the habit with Antabuse. He can become violently ill if alcohol enters his system, and a lot of drugs are dissolved in alcohol. So someone trying to help an alcoholic patient can be doing him less than a favor.

Marion C. Collins, a California physician, recognized this problem and formed Medic-Alert in 1963 to deal with it. The organization, working through the American Medical Association, prepares wrist bands, anklets, medallions, and cards for people with medical conditions that first-aid workers should be aware of. Collins feels that more lives can be saved through Medic-Alert than in the operating room.[21]

First Aid

There's a lot of argument about emergency treatment. Some feel it does more harm than good. No matter what the patient's condition might be, he shouldn't be touched until the ambulance arrives. Others feel that any treatment, if done with compassion and reasonable judgment, is better than no treatment at all. Probably the key factors in this controversy involve the type and seriousness of the injury, how long it will take professional care to arrive, the training of the person administering the first aid, and the age and general physical condition of the patient. Supposedly, a top surgeon is one who knows when not to operate. Probably an expert in emergency care is one who knows when to administer the most effective treatment of all—nothing. But we all should know a little about first-aid procedures. We may never use them or intend to use them, but the knowledge gives us a better appreciation of health care delivery.

Promoting Breathing

One of the key first-aid procedures is promoting the breathing process in someone who has ceased to do it. Obviously, a person can't stop breathing for long without making the practice permanent. There are several ways that breathing can theoretically be promoted, but the only reliable method depends on inflating the victim's lungs by blowing into his mouth or nose. This is called "intermittent positive pressure breathing" (IPPB). The rescuer makes a leakproof seal by placing his mouth over the victim's mouth and inflates the victim's lungs approximately 12 times per minute. He keeps his eye on the victim's chest, making sure that it expands with each breath. If it doesn't expand, he can increase the inflation pressure.

A lot of people wonder how breathing "used" oxygen into somebody's lungs can do him any good. Actually, if the mouth-to-mouth resuscitation is done properly, the rescuer's exhaled air is just about as rich in oxygen (18 per cent) as room air. Because he breathes twice as deeply during this procedure as he normally would, he is in effect breathing for two.

Controlling Bleeding

People do bleed to death, and there are ways of preventing this from happening. And there are ways of killing people with these procedures, too.

Probably first aid in this area has done more harm than good, but there are last resort situations when hemorrhaging just has to be stopped. To begin, elevate the wound as much as possible. Then apply direct pressure to the wound. If you have a sterile gauze compress available, which you probably won't, use it. Otherwise, use any cloth that seems reasonably clean, or apply pressure directly with the hands or fingers.

If direct pressure on the wound doesn't stop the blood flow or slow it down appreciably, try putting finger pressure on the main artery that supplies the wounded area. Sometimes you can identify these arteries when they're near the surface. But, if you can't find them, try to identify a pulse close to the wound and apply pressure there.

If bleeding still continues, the last resort is a tourniquet. If somebody really knows what he's doing with a tourniquet, he can save a life. If he doesn't know, and a lot of people really don't, he can kill someone or make him lose a limb. Tourniquets should be placed as close to the wound as possible and should be loosened by a medical attendant only. A lot of first-aid instructors used to teach that a tourniquet should be loosened every 20 minutes. This allowed blood to flow through the wounded limb and prevented the need for amputation later. This is true. But loosening a tourniquet can dislodge a blood clot and bring on enough bleeding to create shock or death. Also, there is a condition known as "tourniquet shock." This is shock that comes from the sudden release of toxins by the injured tissue when the tourniquet is loosened. A few other points to keep in mind when you apply a tourniquet are

1. Attach a note to the victim explaining when and where the tourniquet was applied. A medical attendent who wants to treat the wound at a later time may need this information, and you may not be available to give it.
2. Tighten the tourniquet just enough to control the bleeding. You don't have to twist with all your might.
3. Put the tourniquet as close to the wound as possible, but not right over the wound. It should be between the wound and the heart.
4. Probably a regular tourniquet won't be available. If it is, of course, use it. If not, use any kind of flat article such as a belt, stocking, or bandage. Place a pad over the artery you're trying to compress.

Shock

Shock can be brought on by a loss of blood or serum or the loss of effective blood circulation. It really means any condition in which the key bodily activities become depressed. It can happen when we've had an accident or injury, when we've been hit by a sudden illness, pain, or even extreme stress or a highly emotional situation. Shock can kill and produce brain damage or damage to other vital organs.

Cold and clammy skin almost always is a symptom of shock. Other symptoms are weakness or faintness, sickly pallor, and sweating. The pulse gets rapid and weak, and eye pupils usually enlarge. The patient usually feels restless at first, then gradually slips into stupor and unconsciousness. Here are some things you can do to help a shock patient:

1. Keep him warm, but don't make him too warm. Shock patients burn easily from hot water bottles and heating pads.
2. Loosen belts and ties and any other clothing that restricts circulation.
3. If the victim is conscious, give him plenty of fluid. If he's been burned, give him salt and soda water, but don't give alcoholic beverages or medicine. Alcohol is a depressant, something a shock patient definitely doesn't need.
4. Place the patient on his back or stomach. If he hasn't had a head injury, raise his feet approximately 6 to 12 inches. If he has had a head injury, leave him level.
5. Check the mouth and nose to assure that air passages are open.

Cardiac Resuscitation

If you have a victim whose heart has apparently stopped beating and you want to use cardiac resuscitation, do so only if you've had special training in this technique. If you haven't had special training in this technique, don't try it. It's tricky, and it can cause injury or even death. Seek medical help as quickly as possible, and hope you were wrong in your diagnosis of the non-beating heart.

Childbirth

The birth of a baby can be frightening, not just to the mother, but to anyone giving aid. However, if it's a normal birth there's really nothing to be frightened about. Women and babies have been going through this procedure for millions of years, and the human race is doing just fine. All the helper has to do is make the mother comfortable, or as comfortable as possible under the circumstances. When the baby's head appears, support it so that the mouth and nostrils aren't covered. Wrap the baby when it has completely emerged, and place it on the mother's abdomen. Next will come the placenta. This follows the baby by about 15 minutes. Wrap the placenta and the cord, place them beside the newborn, and your job as the helper is over. Don't cut the cord. Let medical people take care of that. In fact, the cord shouldn't even be touched until the placenta has emerged.

Heat Sickness

Sunburn is the most common of the heat problems. We all get it during the first few days at the lake during the summer, but most of us don't get it so badly that we could really call it a sickness. If it's severe, though, you should see a physician.

Heat stroke is something else. It does call for immediate care, and delay can be fatal. Usually the victim of heat stroke is in a collapsed state, with dry, warm skin. His sweating mechanism has failed, and his body temperature is high. Cool the victim at once. Probably the best method is dunking him in cool water or spraying him with a hose. Then get medical care as fast as possible.

Heat exhaustion is another serious condition. It isn't as potentially fatal as heat stroke. A fellow suffering from heat exhaustion is in a state of shock because the salt and water content of his body has become depleted. He's weak, and he sweats profusely. He should be placed in the shade with his head slightly lower than the rest of his body. Mix some salt water (a teaspoonful of salt to a pint of water) and let him sip it slowly. Then, of course, call a physician.

Burns

For small thermal burns, stick the burned area under cool water or apply ice to relieve the pain. Then apply baking soda with a sterile gauze dressing. Use the same treatment for small chemical burns. If the burns are extensive, cover the burned area with the cleanest cloth available. Have the victim lie down, with his head slightly lower than the rest of his body.

Bones and Joints

If a bone is bruised, and you can never be sure that this is all it is, apply cold cloths or an ice bag. Apply cold cloths to a broken nose, too. If there's a fracture in one of the limbs, and if medical treatment just isn't available, then splint the area where the fracture took place. But don't do anything if the fracture seems to be of the back, the neck, or the skull. Don't let the patient move, and do seek medical aid immediately.

For dislocations—and these are often hard to distinguish from fractures—apply cold cloths or ice bags, and get the patient to a doctor.

Muscles and Ligaments

For a strain or a sprain, apply an ice bag or a wet cloth, and keep the patient from putting weight on the injury. For a cramp, try to contract the opposite muscle forcefully by applying firm hand pressure to the cramped muscle. Also, give the patient sips of salt water. If the cramp persists, seek medical aid.

Wounds

For a mild puncture wound or a cut, place the injured area under cold water, and then cleanse with soap. Use a sterile pad to stop the bleeding and provide protection until the wound heals. If the bleeding is so heavy that you can't stop it, call a physician.

If the victim is bleeding from a punch or some other blow to the nose, keep him sitting or standing. Don't have him lie down. Cover the nose with cold cloths, and use small gauze packs to soak up the blood.

Poisoning

For poisoning, call a poison center or a physician immediately, give water or milk, and try to induce vomiting—assuming the poison center or physician has no objections to this procedure. Don't try to induce vomiting if the patient is unconscious or is having convulsions. Also, leave the vomiting bit alone if the patient swallowed strychnine, a strong acid or alkali, or a petroleum product. If the poison is inhaled, make sure the victim gets to fresh air, and use artificial respiration if necessary.

Foreign Irritations in the Eye

Don't rub an eye that has a foreign body in it. Try to touch the particle with the point of a clean, moist cloth and wash the eye out with cold water. See a physician, of course, if pain persists.

Blisters

Keep blisters clean, and don't irritate them. If they're broken, wash the area well with soap and trim the edges with clean scissors. If they become infected, see a physician.[22]

Notes

1. National Safety Council, *Accident Facts* (Chicago: National Safety Council, 1972).
2. Lynette Shaw and Herbert S. Sichel, *Accident Proneness* (New York: Pergamon Press, 1971), pp. 3–11.
3. Geoffrey T. Mann and Thomas D. Jordan, *Personal Injury Problems* (Springfield, Ill.: Thomas, 1963), pp. 201–211.
4. Roland P. Blake, ed., *Industrial Safety* (Englewood Cliffs, N.J.: Prentice-Hall, 1963), pp. 55–68.
5. Albert P. Iskrant and Paul V. Joliet, *Accidents and Homicide* (Cambridge, Mass.: Harvard University Press, 1968), p. 108.
6. Norman R. Lykes, *A Psychological Approach to Accidents* (New York: Vantage Press, 1954), pp. 1–10.
7. William B. Deichmann and Horace W. Gerarde, *Toxicology of Drugs and Chemicals* (New York: Academic Press, 1969), pp. 1–33.
8. Horatio Bond, ed., *NFPA Inspection Manual* (Boston: NFPA-Fidelity Press, 1970), pp. 11–17.
9. Iskrant and Joliet, *Accidents and Homicide*, pp. 42–48.
10. National Safety Council, *Accident Prevention for Business and Industry* (Chicago: National Safety Council, 1965), pp. 48–63.
11. Ibid., pp. 42–48.
12. National Safety Council, *Accident Facts*, p. 47.
13. J. J. Leeming, *Road Accidents* (London: Cassel, 1969), pp. 33–43.
14. Ralph Nader, *Unsafe at Any Speed* (New York: Grossman, 1972).
15. E. Dahlquist, "Marking Time: Seat Belt Effectiveness," *Motor Trend*, Vol. 24 (1972), 6.
16. Marland K. Strasser et al., *Fundamentals of Safety Education* (New York: Macmillan, 1973), p. 366.
17. Ibid., pp. 364–5.
18. Lykes, *Psychological Approach to Accidents*, pp. 116–129.
19. Iskrant and Joliet, *Accidents and Homicide*, pp. 105–106.
20. Strasser, *Fundamentals of Safety Education*, pp. 296–319.
21. James E. Aaron, Frank Bridges, and Dale O. Ritzel, *First Aid and Emergency Care* (New York: Macmillan, 1972).
22. Ibid., pp. 369–384.

Part Five

Community Health

14 Health Services

No one is sure when the myth started or who originated it. Some say it came from the American Medical Association, others that insurance companies and hospitals fostered it. Still others claim that it blossomed in American medical schools, came to full flower in programs like *Marcus Welby, The Doctors,* and *Medical Center.*

"American medicine is the envy of the world." This is a myth. It's also a myth that American physicians are selfish, irresponsible, sadistic capitalists, more interested in the sounds in their Cadillac engines than those in their patients' chests. The American health care system, if there is such a thing, is far from perfect in the eyes of a Wichita farmer, a London bus driver, a Heidelberg seamstress. Nobody envies us—not even ourselves. Our health care delivery costs, services, and standards really aren't that good. But are they totally inadequate, a disease of incompetency and neglect infecting the entire U.S. citizenry? Not really. If you know a little about America's health services and how they function, you can get excellent medical care in this country.[1] Ignorance of the system, though, can make you sick, can keep you from getting well, even kill you. A less than perfect system calls for individual initiative.

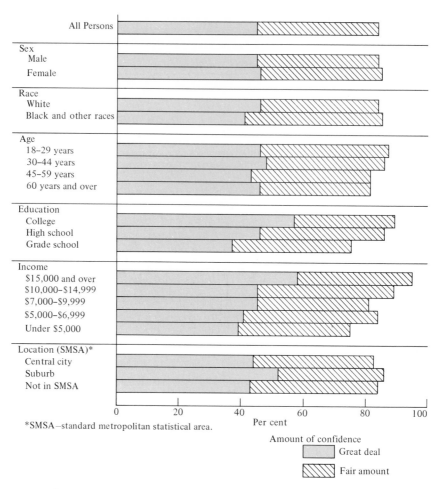

SOURCE: *Social Indicators 1973* (Washington, D.C.: The Social and Economic Statistics Administration, U.S. Department of Commerce), p. 21.

FIGURE 14-1. *Personal confidence in ability to obtain good health care, 1971, by selected characteristics.*

The American Health Care System

If costs were an indication of quality, Americans would be the healthiest people in history. We spend almost 8 per cent of our gross national product on health or about $105 billion a year. This breaks down to about $394 per person, a figure that no other country can, or ever could, match. There are a dozen nations that do a better job than we do in preventing infant deaths, another dozen that have lower maternal mortality rates. There are 17 countries in which men live longer than American males do, ten in which women have a better survival rate.[2] Obviously, our money hasn't bought us longevity, and probably not freedom from sickness while we live.

Of course, our health care system isn't totally to blame. Our personal habits, our life styles, our physical and social environment and genetics enter

354

TABLE 14-1
Where the Health Care Dollar Went, Fiscal Year 1971–1972

Health Care Service	Dollars per Person in the U.S.
Hospitals	153
Doctors	76
Dentists	24
Other professional services	8
Drugs	37
Eyeglasses and appliances	10
Nursing homes	17
Cost of administering insurance and prepayment programs	14
Government public health	10
Other health services	17
Research	10
Construction	19
Total	394

Source: Barbara S. Cooper and Nancy L. Worthington, "National Health Expenditures, 1929–1972," *Social Security Bulletin*, Vol. 36 (January 1973), 12.

the picture, too. Medical care possibly plays a secondary role in our world health rankings. Getting rid of slums and pollution would probably do more for increasing life span than giving everyone a yearly physical examination. Cut down on poverty, and our infant mortality rate would probably look a lot better. And lung cancer and coronary statistics would look better if we cut down on smoking. Our accident statistics would look better if we eliminated alcohol.

But when we're talking about health care, we're really talking about something associated with a doctor, a hospital, or a pill. Other considerations are important, probably more important, to America's health picture. But they're not what we think of as part of the health care delivery system, and they don't come under that $105 billion budget. What is this system? Is it some tightly organized effort directed at eliminating ignorance, sickness, and death; some bureaucratic Washington conglomerate directed by power-hungry politicians with red-tape efficiency? No. The health care system in the United States is very loosely organized, bound together by agreements and cooperation rather than directives and control. Some claim the organization is so loose that you can't say a health care system exists at all. It's really a nonsystem.[3] In any event, there are government agencies, private corporations, volunteer agencies, and professional associations that deal with the health care picture. Whether their combined efforts represent a system or not, you can't have an understanding of America's health care scene without understanding how each of these categories functions.

Federal Government

Health is a privilege available only to those who can financially afford it. This was a concept born with Adam and Eve, nurtured through the Roman Empire, and completely accepted during the Middle Ages. It's only within the last 50 years that the concept has been seriously challenged. It's only

355

within the last 20 or so that the concept has been thrown out. Health care is now looked on as a right the government must assure to all citizens, regardless of financial status, race, or creed. The vehicle the United States uses to carry out such a program is the Department of Health, Education, and Welfare (HEW). This was created in 1953 to assume various responsibilities in the fields of welfare services and education as well as medical care.

The Public Health Service and its programs for Merchant Marines and Indians come under HEW. So do agencies dealing with health planning, the Indian Health Service, the National Medical Library, the Neighborhood Health Center Development, Health Maintenance Organization Development, Assistance for Education in the Health Professions, and the Food and Drug Administration (FDA). The FDA has been involved in some consumer protection and environmental control activities in conjunction with the Environmental Protection Agency. But, in most cases, the government directs its environmental protection activities along other channels.

By and large, HEW is not in the health care delivery business—if you think of health care delivery as taking care of the sick. It does provide advice, assistance, and monetary grants, though, to both governmental and nongovernmental agencies involved in the patient care field.

An exception to this policy came about in 1970, with the establishment of the National Health Service Corps. Here the federal government hires doctors and other health care personnel and sends them to medically deprived areas. Certainly, this active role in health care delivery could be the start of a trend of the government's participation in this area. Also, proposals for national health insurance envision the government's taking a much more active role than it currently does in the delivery system.[4]

There are other parts of the federal government besides HEW involved with health care. The Departments of Commerce and Interior work with the environment. The Office of Economic Opportunity deals with the poverty situation, and the Veterans Administration provides medical care for veterans of the Armed Forces. The Armed Services provide medical care to military personnel and their dependents.[5] The federal government's role in the health care scene depends on your definition of just what health care is.

State Government

Each state has a health department supported by local tax money and grants from HEW. And though their roles vary considerably, each of them normally assumes responsibility for recording vital statistics, such as births and deaths, and maintaining records of diseases, such as tuberculosis and venereal disease. They also establish standards for hospitals and nursing homes, survey them on a regular basis, conduct environmental sanitation programs and various aspects of food and drug control, carry out a public health nursing program, and provide public health laboratory services to identify various types of infectious diseases. Some state health departments run Medicaid programs and operate mental and tuberculosis hospitals. But, whatever their roles, these health departments have come under increasing criticism in recent years. Citizens' groups are looking for them to assume a more active role in planning and delivery of health care.[6]

Local Governments

Most cities, towns, and counties have health departments that treat VD and tuberculosis, inspect restaurants, administer vaccinations, run a hospital for the local poor, check the sewage plants and dairies. Where do they get their money for this operation? Where everyone else gets it, of course—from the federal and state governments. There is local money backing this operation. But our population has shifted from small-town entities to metropolitan areas, which can overlap several counties. So the tax base has shifted from property assessment on a local basis to income assessment on federal and state basis.

It's not just the economic base that has spread. Health problems are no longer confined to a small town or community. Now they transcend paper boundaries and involve several counties, often several states. Water and air pollution that affect people in one part of the state possibly originated in another part, or even a totally different state. And our highly mobile population makes it hard to decide where a TB or VD carrier has gotten his illness and where he's taking it. Local health departments are having a harder and harder time in delineating political jurisdictions and, therefore, in raising local money. So federal and state governments are entering their operations to a greater and greater extent.[7]

Volunteer Groups and Foundations

The American Heart Association, the American Cancer Society, and hundreds of other organizations independent of government support deal with independent health problems or diseases. The larger organizations of this type function at the national level, but some do it on a regional or local basis. Their activities normally involve raising money for research, educating the public, and providing services such as beds and wheelchairs to people afflicted with the illnesses they represent. These volunteer organizations seldom provide any direct patient care.[8]

Foundations are supported by wealthy people and industrial endowments. Their activities involve research, health education programs, and the establishment of health and medical care programs in deprived areas.[9]

Professional Organizations

Professional organizations represent the people in institutions who provide health care, not the people who receive it. There are the American Medical Association, representing physicians, the American Hospital Association, obviously representing hospitals, the American Nurses Association, the American College of Hospital Administrators, the American Public Health Association, and hundreds of others. Their primary purpose, according to their own statements, is to serve the public by protecting it against unqualified practitioners. This is a noble aim and certainly a necessary one. No one would want to be treated by a physician or nurse who hadn't demonstrated some kind of proficiency in the art of healing. And there's more to an effective hospital or nursing home than just giving it that label. But there's been increasing criticism that these organizations are more interested in protecting their own interests than those of the public. Some feel they do their best to impede progress in health care delivery when this progress appears to interfere with the economic well-being of their membership. And, with the lack of any type of accountability for their actions and decisions, they have all the evils of a monopoly. Probably some of this criticism is justified. But, in fairness, members of these organizations probably exhibit no more self-interest than members of any other group who share common backgrounds and goals.[10]

Industrial Organizations

Employers of old looked on health as the responsibility of the individual. If the employee became sick, it was up to him to make himself well so that he could come back to work and make more money for his boss. After all, a day's pay called for a day's work, not a day's sick leave. But the trend in

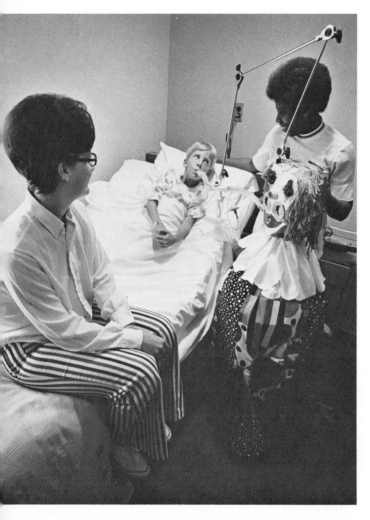

FIGURE 14-2. *You don't have to be a physician to play a leading role in health care.* (*Photograph by* The Wichita Eagle *and* The Wichita Beacon)

recent years has been much more humane. After all, it was just good business to see that an employee received the right kind of care so he could stay on the job and produce as he should. So the employer decided to pay for part of the health care costs. Then unions and employee groups entered the picture. Employers should make this health care benefit package broader, more extensive, and possibly include the employee's family. Industry now provides health benefits to cover everything from injury on the job to complete health maintenance packages. The employee contributes to most of these programs, but the employer, in most cases, foots the majority of the bill. Money is usually paid to insurance companies or groups of doctors, and employees visit health workers in their vicinity when they get sick. Occasionally, an industry operates a small infirmary or outpatient clinic. But, in most cases, employers aren't involved in direct health care delivery.

Some corporations provide excellent health benefit packages. Others provide little or nothing. It's an erratic field, totally dependent on management attitude or strength of unions in a given locality and employees' knowledge about what they can and should receive. Some are fortunate to live in an area or work in a field where corporate health care is comprehensive. And some aren't so fortunate. Lady Luck plays a big role in this aspect of health care delivery.[11]

Health Workers

Lots of organizations with lots of money support the health care system. But be they part of the federal government, an arm of the state government, a private organization, they provide this health care on an indirect basis only. It's the individual worker who takes the temperature, administers the pill, performs the operation. There are hundreds of categories of these people, some with more training than others, some with more authority than others. There's the physician, pretty much the star and quarterback of the health care team; and there are podiatrists, hospital administrators, biomedical engineers, nurses, social workers, and so on.

Physicians often work alone in their own offices and charge their own fees. But not so with the other health care personnel. They work, either directly or indirectly, for physicians. Or, if they maintain their own practices, they get their patients from physician referrals.

Not all people called "doctor" are physicians, of course. Chiropractors, dentists, optometrists, podiatrists, and a few other specialists use this title. These specialists usually aren't licensed to perform any type of surgery or prescribe any medicine you can't buy without prescription in a drugstore. So even though physicians number less than 10 per cent of the health care team, they are the ones who control the key aspects of curing the sick.

This doesn't mean that there aren't outstanding people who perform essential health care services who aren't physicians. Quite often ancillary medical personnel perform tasks that physicians can't or shouldn't because of insufficient experience.[12]

Someone needing treatment should have an idea of the services various members of the health team can provide and what roles they play. Here's a breakdown of some of the more key health delivery personnel.

Physicians

Physicians are the people who have an 8-year span of formal education (usually 4 in college and 4 in a medical school) plus 3 or 4 years' internship and residency. A physician is the highly educated specialist who removes your appendix, gives you a new heart, tells you to lose weight. There are two kinds of physicians. There are M.D.s (Medical Doctors), who constitute the vast majority of all people in this profession. There are also D.O.s (Doctors of Osteopathy). Both require the same educational and training experiences for licensure examination. Both are extremely selective in admitting applicants into their schools of professional education. Actually, the two degrees mean about the same thing. And in California, M.D.s and D.O.s, once licensed, can use either title.

Most people entering medical schools or colleges of osteopathy have bachelor's degrees. Some schools will admit students with only 3 years of undergraduate study, but it's the rare exception whose grades are good enough and who seems to be mature enough to get by without the B.S. or B.A. Then come 2 years of preclinical and clinical science, 2 more years of hospital-based clinical experience, a year of internship, and the state licensure exam.

If a new doctor wants to specialize, and 90 per cent of them do, there's an additional 3 to 5 years of a residency program. This is something like a master–apprentice relationship in a hospital. But the training isn't over at the completion of the residency. There are 2 additional years of full-time specialty practice and finally a written and oral examination in the specialized field. If the doctor passes, and many don't, he receives his diploma. He's then called a "diplomate." Or another way of designating his proficiency is to call him "board-certified" in his specialty.

There are "board-eligible" physicians who have completed their residency training but who have never taken their specialty examinations or have never passed them. This doesn't necessarily mean that the physician is less competent in his area of specialty than one of his board-certified brethren. But if you are interested in whether the person about to treat you is a diplomate or not, you can check in the *Directory of Medical Specialists* available in most libraries. This lists the diplomates in all medical fields.[13]

These specialty fields take in 34 areas. Here are some of the more common:

GENERAL PRACTITIONER

Some don't look on general practice as a specialty. After all, a general practitioner is the doctor who treats the whole person and specializes in nothing. But in this modern age of advanced training and compartmentalization even the general practitioner has his own residency program. It lasts for 3 years, like other residency programs, and begins when he's completed his internship and has been given his license to practice. After the

TABLE 14-2
Physicians, Population, and Physician/Population Ratios for Selected
Years, 1950–1970

Year	Total Physicians*	Total Population†	Physicians per 100,000 Population	Population per One Physician
1950	219,997	156,472,000	141	711
1955	241,711	170,499,000	142	705
1960	260,484	185,370,000	141	712
1963	276,475	194,169,000	142	702
1964	284,224	196,858,000	144	693
1965	292,088	199,278,000	147	682
1966	300,375	201,585,000	149	671
1967	308,630	203,704,000	152	660
1968	317,032	205,758,000	154	649
1969	324,942	207,863,000	156	640
1970	334,028	209,539,000	159	627

* Includes inactive and address unknown.
† Includes Armed Forces in the United States and abroad, civilians in the 50 states, D.C., Puerto Rico, and other U.S. outlying areas; and U.S. government and civilian employees, their dependents, and dependents of Armed Forces personnel abroad.

Source: Reference Data on Socioeconomic Issues of Health AMA: 1971, ed. by K. E. Monroe.

residency, of course, come the board examinations conducted by the American Academy of General Practice.

The majority of general practitioners haven't been exposed to this advanced training, as it's relatively new on the medical scene. But as scientific information and developments continue to grow into some insurmountable mass, there will be more and more demand for physicians to receive training beyond medical school. A human being is highly complex, and to know even a little about the infinite parts that make him up is a great accomplishment.

INTERNAL MEDICINE

Internists are specialists who don't practice surgery, deliver babies, deal with eye and nose problems, or treat children—as a general rule. They're trained primarily in diagnosis. They often coordinate the work of other specialists or become involved with preventive medicine.

The majority of internists practice general medicine, but some confine their work to subspecialties. There are those specializing in heart diseases, lung ailments, digestive tract problems, and allergies. The internist must complete a 5-year residency after his internship and successfully pass the exams prepared by the American Board of Internal Medicine.

PEDIATRICS

Pediatrics is a specialty involving the care of children. Pediatricians administer immunizations, diagnose and sometimes correct congenital deformities, treat diseases that usually occur in childhood, and advise parents on the care of their children. There are subspecialties in pediatrics, such as pediatric allergy and pediatric cardiology.

Community Health

SURGERY

Surgeons, of course, are doctors with knives. They remove gall bladders and cancerous growths, repair malfunctioning hearts, straighten crooked noses. There are general surgeons and those who confine themselves to specific parts of the body, such as neurosurgeons, thoracic surgeons, orthopedic surgeons, and plastic surgeons.

OBSTETRICS AND GYNECOLOGY

Gynecology deals with the treatment of female diseases and disorders, and obstetrics deals with the most female of all physical problems, pregnancy and childbirth. Normally, one physician specializes in both. He counsels mothers during their pregnancy, prescribes any treatment that might be necessary, and handles the delivery.

FIGURE 14-3. *Pediatrician and patient.* (*Photograph by* The Wichita Eagle *and* The Wichita Beacon)

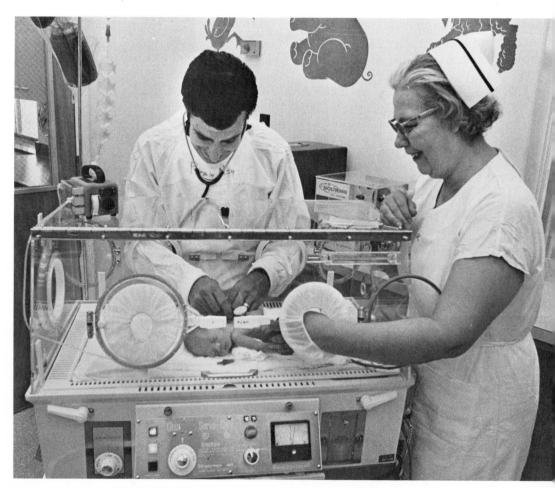

PSYCHIATRY

Sometimes called "headshrinkers," psychiatrists are the people who listen to your problems, counsel, and prescribe shock treatments or drugs to straighten out a confused thinking process. A lot of them work in mental hospitals; some work in private practice; some are also neurologists; some are also psychoanalysts. To be eligible for board examinations in psychiatry only, the candidate has to have had a 3-year residency after completing his internship. But there's more training yet before the psychiatrist can become qualified in any of the subdisciplines.

OTHER SPECIALTIES

Some other key specialties are the following:

Anesthesiology. Anesthesiology involves the administering of anesthesia during operations.

Dermatology. The dermatologist treats skin diseases.

Neurology. The neurologist is sometimes a psychiatrist. He treats diseases of the nerves and the brain.

Ophthalmology. Ophthalmology deals with diseases and malfunctions of the eyes.

Otorhinolaryngology. The otorhinolaryngologist treats nose and throat problems.

Pathology. Pathologists run laboratories, supervise people who look through microscopes to find out what kind of diseases people have and what caused them.

Proctology. The proctologist treats diseases of the rectal and anal area.

Radiology. In radiology diseases are diagnosed and treated by means of the X-ray, radium, and other radioactive substances.

Urology. Urology is concerned with diseases of the urinary tract of the female and male and the genital tract of the male.[14]

Dentists

Dentists have an education almost as lengthy and extensive as that of physicians. Someone can enter one of the 52 dental schools in the country with only 2 or 3 years of predental education, but over 50 per cent of first-year dental students have bachelor's degrees. As in medical school, the first 2 years in dental school are spent on the basic sciences. Sometimes medical and dental students take these basic science courses together. Then come 2 more years of treating patients under the supervision of clinical instructors. Then comes graduation, the award of the D.D.S. (Doctor of Dental Surgery) or D.M.D. (Doctor of Medical Dentistry), and the state licensure examination. There's no internship required as there is in medicine and osteopathy, but a dentist can take additional training and specialize in one of the following areas:

ENDODONTICS

Endodontics involves treating the interior tissues of the teeth. Root canals and pulp capping are two common endodontic procedures.

ORAL PATHOLOGY

Oral pathology is a diagnostic specialty dealing with oral tumors, injuries, and tissue degeneration.

ORAL SURGERY

In oral surgery, oral diseases and injuries are corrected with a knife. Sometimes the oral surgeon corrects defects of the jaw.

ORTHODONTICS

Orthodontics is the specialty dealing with application of braces to teeth or use of some other means of straightening them.

PEDODONTICS

Pedodontics is the counterpart of pediatrics in medicine. It's a dental speciality for children.

PERIODONTICS

Periodontics deals with gum and underlying bone problems.

PROSTHODONTICS

Dentists specializing in prosthodontics make artificial teeth to replace missing ones.

PUBLIC HEALTH DENTISTRY

Public health dentists work with public education programs to teach good dental practices and work on the prevention and control of dental diseases.[15]

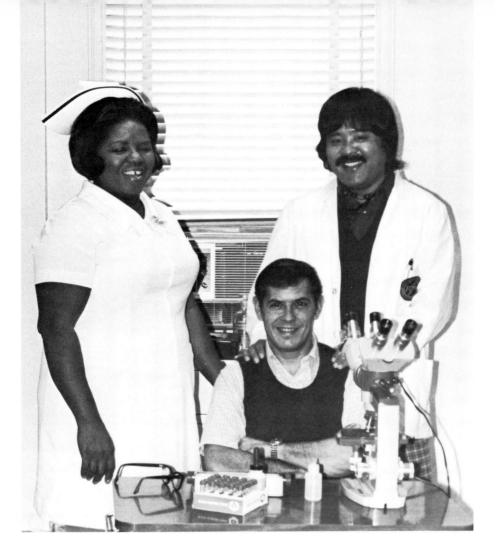

FIGURE 14-4. *Registered nurse and compatriots.*

Registered Nurses

Registered nurses are women, and sometimes men, who carry out patient care activities under the supervision of physicians. They work in hospitals and clinics and public health departments and schools. In addition to being supervised, they supervise the practical nurses who work for them, the nursing aides, orderlies, and attendants.

Because there's quite a bit of responsibility involved in this field, all states require that an R.N. be licensed before he or she can practice. This calls for passing some type of licensure examination after having graduated from a nursing school the state approves of. These schools can take any one of three forms. There are baccalaureate programs, which require 4 or 5 years of study at a college or university. There are diploma programs, which call for 3 years of study in a school affiliated with a hospital. And there are associate's degree programs, usually conducted in community colleges. Here the student can complete his or her nursing academic requirements in only 2 years.

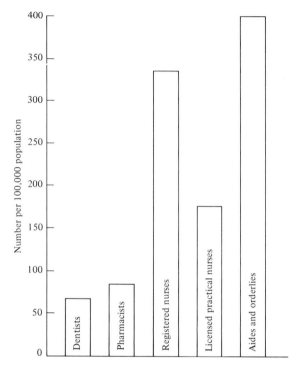

SOURCE: *Socioeconomic Issues of Health,* K. E. Monroe, ed.
(Chicago: Center for Health Services Research and
Development, AMA Publication, 1971).

FIGURE 14-5. *Professional and allied health personnel.*

There are specialties in nursing just as there are in medicine and dentistry. There is the psychiatric nurse, who specializes in caring for the mentally ill; the anesthetist, who administers anesthetics during operations; the nurse-midwife, who cares for pregnant women and manages labor and delivery; the public health nurse; and others.[16]

Allied Medical Practitioners

Allied medical practitioners are a group of people, like dentists, who function independently of physicians. Some undergo extensive training and complex licensure training. Some, in certain sections of the country, just give themselves a title and start to practice.

CLINICAL PSYCHOLOGISTS

Clinical psychologists usually have Ph.D.s. There are people calling themselves clinical psychologists who have master's degrees, some who have no degree at all. But the majority of those accepted in the field have the doctorate of philosophy in clinical psychology. They work in private practice, in clinics, and hospitals. They act as consultants for public schools and community health programs, and do research. It normally takes 3 or 4 years of graduate study beyond the bachelor's degree to qualify for the clinical psychology doctorate, and this includes 1 year of supervised internship in a mental treatment institution.[17]

OPTOMETRISTS

Optometrists don't perform surgery, prescribe drugs, or treat eye diseases the way ophthalmologists do. The latter are physicians specializing in eye problems. Optometrists treat visual defects with corrective lenses and visual training aids only.

Like physicians, they must have a license to practice, and, in order to get it, they have to pass a state board examination. They must be a Doctor of Optometry (O.D.) before they can take the exam, though. This calls for 2 years of preoptometry training plus 4 years at one of 11 accredited optometry colleges in the country. A few states require internship before granting licensure, but most don't.[18]

PODIATRISTS

There are 8,000 podiatrists in the country, who examine feet, perform foot surgery, prescribe physical therapy, prescribe corrective devices for foot problems, administer drugs. A podiatrist carries the title of Doctor of Podiatric Medicine or D.P.M. To get this, he must graduate from one of the five podiatry colleges in the country. To practice, he must pass a state licensure examination.[19]

CHIROPRACTORS AND NATUROPATHS

Chiropractors and naturopaths call themselves doctors (Doctors of Chiropractic, or D.C.; Doctors of Naturopathy, or D.N.). They do undergo a certain amount of advanced training before they can begin to practice in their disciplines. They don't adhere to orthodox medical concepts, though, so they're not permitted to practice in hospitals. If they feel that one of their patients needs hospitalization, they must refer him to an M.D. or a D.O.

Chiropractors, feeling that health problems come from displacements of the spine that irritate peripheral nerves, treat their patients with physical therapy, diet, and counseling. Naturopaths treat their patients the same way, but they emphasize diet to a greater extent. They see human ills as coming from an upset in body balance. Natural forces normally support the body, they feel, but something in the diet can interrupt the way these forces function and bring on illness.[20]

CHRISTIAN SCIENCE PRACTITIONERS

To the Christian Science Practitioner, healing has nothing to do with medication or operations. In fact, orthodox medicine is totally rejected. Healing comes about, according to this philosophy, through prayer, spiritual growth, and moral attunement with God.[21]

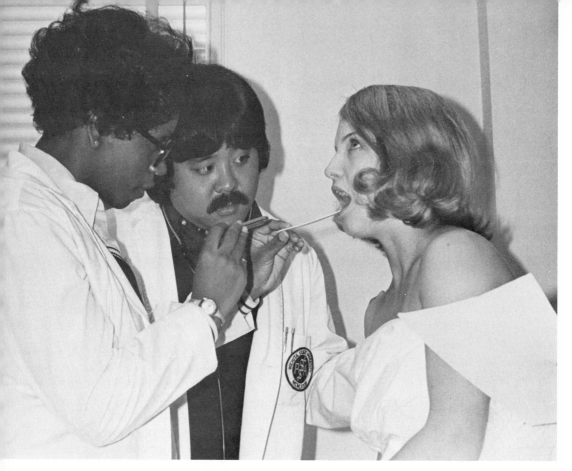

FIGURE 14-6. *A physician's assistant in*
training.

MIDWIVES

Some midwives are registered nurses with advanced training, and some
of them are lay personnel with a limited education. Many are licensed to
practice in poor and rural areas, where the delivery of a baby usually occurs
in the home.[22]

HEALTH-RELATED MANPOWER

Medical. There are two classes of specialists in medical-related fields:
those requiring at least a baccalaureate degree to practice, and ones who
don't need baccalaureate degrees. The former category includes clinical laboratory technicians, dietitians, medical record librarians, speech therapists,
occupational therapists, rehabilitation therapists, health educators, and most
health care administrators. Physicians' assistants, respiratory therapists, and
radiological technicians fall into the category of needing less than a bachelor's degree. Occupational opportunities for both groups are excellent, and
should be so for many years. True, many new educational programs are
developing in this area, and the number of allied health care personnel
should double by 1980. But the demand should still exceed the supply.[23]

368

Dental. The three major dental health–related professions are dental hygienist, dental assistant, and dental laboratory technician. The dental hygienist is the only one who needs a license to practice. The hygienist polishes and scales teeth, processes dental X-rays, instructs patients in toothbrushing techniques and diet, and applies fluoride to teeth. He or she usually gets training in a 2-year college program, which leads to an associate of arts degree or a dental hygiene diploma. There are 4-year programs, though, which lead to a bachelor's degree in this area. People with this educational background often take over a leadership role in dental aspects of public health or education.

There are also 2-year programs in junior colleges to train dental assistants. Sometimes these programs last only 1 year. Sometimes dental assistants are trained on the job in a dental office. Because they don't have to pass a licensure examination or show other qualifications to practice, there's quite a range in their educational backgrounds. But the trend is toward some type of formal training procedure. The assistant prepares patients for treatment, passes instruments, sterilizes instruments, mixes filling materials,

FIGURE 14-7. *He puts teeth in his work.* (*Photograph by* The Wichita Eagle *and* The Wichita Beacon)

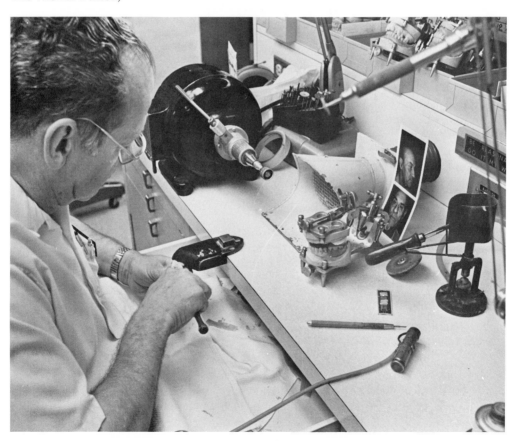

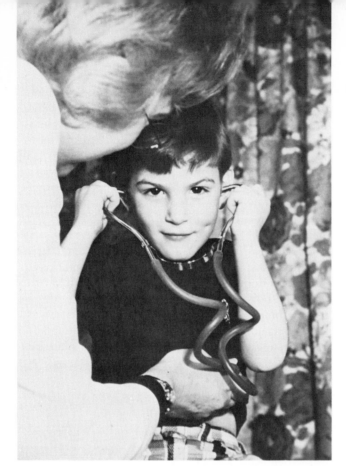

FIGURE 14-8. *Trust.*

and assists with laboratory work. Usually he or she keeps the office records and accounts.

Dental laboratory technicians normally have no patient contact. They're skilled craftsmen who usually work in commercial dental laboratories constructing fixed bridgework, crowns, and other dental appliances. A few of these work directly for a dentist in a dental office, but they still have little or no patient contact. Technicians learn their skills through on-the-job-training only, as there's no formal schooling offered or required in this area.[24]

Nursing. There are licensed practical nurses (L.P.N.), or licensed vocational nurses (L.V.N.) in California or Texas. They have to pass state licensure examinations, but they work under the supervision of registered nurses or physicians when carrying out some of the more direct aspects of patient care, such as taking vital signs and giving baths, injections, and medications. An L.P.N., normally, must have had at least 2 years of high school before beginning his or her training, which usually takes place in a junior college or university setting for 12 to 18 months.

There are also nursing aides, orderlies, and attendants who receive no formal training outside the hospital. Nursing aides assist registered and practical nurses in performing the more routine tasks of patient care. Orderlies and attendants, usually men, perform some of the heavier duties involved with nursing, such as lifting patients, controlling those who are mentally ill, and moving beds and other equipment. Hospitals usually provide classroom instruction for these personnel rather than leaving their total educational experience to on-the-job-training.[25]

Notes

1. Selig Greenberg, *The Quality of Mercy* (New York: Atheneum, 1971).
2. John Fry, *International Medical Care* (Oxford: Medical and Technical Publishing Company, 1972).
3. Edward Yost, *The United States Health Industry* (New York: Praeger, 1969), pp. 3–30.
4. John Upton Terrel, *The U.S. Department of Health, Education and Welfare* (New York: Duel, Sloan, and Pearce, 1965).
5. A. R. Lomers, "Health Care and the Political System," *American Journal of Ophthalmology*, Vol. 73 (April 1972), 600–609.
6. Research Pub. Tax Foundation, *State Programs After Two Years Medicaid* (New York: Research Pub. Tax Foundation, 1968), pp. 6–62.
7. Odin W. Anderson, *Health Care* (New York: Wiley, 1972), pp. 16–51, 206–221, 497–508.
8. Lanthem Willoughby and Anne Newbery, eds., *Community Medicine* (New York: Appleton-Century-Crofts, 1970).
9. Iago Galdston, ed., *Voluntary Action and the State* (New York: International Universities Press, 1961), pp. 83–92.
10. Elton Rayack, *Professional Power in American Medicine* (Cleveland: World, 1967).
11. Margaret F. McKiever, ed., *Friends in Employee Health Services* (Washington, D.C.: Government Printing Office, 1965).
12. Ruth F. Odgers, *Introduction to Health Professions* (St. Louis: Mosby, 1972).
13. Dana W. Atchley, *Physician* (New York: Macmillan, 1961), pp. 17–96.
14. T. M. Richardson, "A Study of Trainee General Practitioners," *British Journal of Medical Education*, Vol. 6 (March 1972), 29–31.
15. Byron S. Hollinshead, *The Survey of Dentistry* (Washington, D.C.: American Council on Education, 1961).
16. Odgers, *Health Professions*, pp. 47–53.
17. D. R. Lipsitt et al., "Psychiatry in Medicine," *Psychiatry in Medicine*, Vol. 1 (January 1970), 1–2.
18. Odgers, *Health Professions*, pp. 29–36.
19. H. K. Koch et al., "Podiatry Manpower U.S. 1970," *Vital and Health Statistics*, Vol. 14 (August 1973), 1–52.
20. M. White et al., "The Chiropractic Physician: A Study of Career Contingencies," *Journal of Health and Social Behavior*, Vol. 12 (December 1971), 300–306.
21. Charles S. Braden, *Christian Science Today* (Dallas: Southern Methodist University Press, 1969), pp. 336–379.
22. Macy Josiah, *The Midwife in the U.S.* (New York: Macy Josiah, 1968), pp. 41–101.
23. M. Murry Lawton and Donald F. Foy, *Medical Assistants* (St. Louis: 1971), pp. 1–45.
24. Odgers, *Health Professions*, pp. 79–85.
25. Ibid., pp. 47–64.

15 Health Care Facilities

The home used to be where most health care took place. Doctors would come and deliver babies, treat tonsillitis, and puncture boils. But then came surgical lights and X-ray machines and cobalt bombs, and the home wouldn't do as a treatment center for more than a splinter or stomachache. This is the day of the thousand-bed medical conglomerate, the health maintenance organization with outreach facilities extending for hundreds of miles, and doctors' group practices of a hundred or more specialists, who can cure anything from a split personality to ugliness. This is the day of scientific medicine, scientific treatment facilities, and planned communities. Here are some of the more typical facilities.

Hospitals

Hospitals used to be places where people went to die. Doctors didn't practice in them, seldom visited them. They were usually operated by religious organizations and catered to the indigent or mentally deranged. They were often cesspools of disease and filth and did more to kill patients than cure them. But with the advent of modern surgery, anesthesia, asepsis, and research, the doctor needed a place to perform the modern medical miracle. The hospital seemed ideal.

372

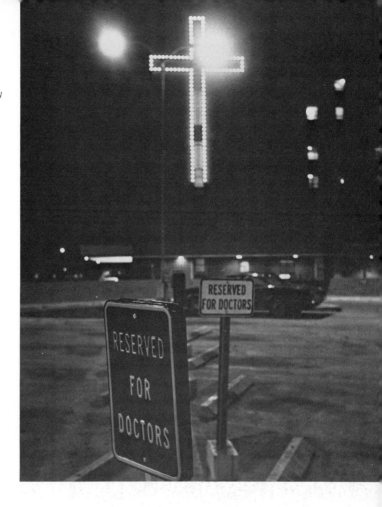

FIGURE 15-1. *A location for today's miracles. (Photograph by* The Wichita Eagle *and* The Wichita Beacon)

So around the turn of the century the marriage between physicians and hospitals took place. There are now over 7,000 hospitals in this country, ranging from 25 beds (they have to be this size before they can be designated a hospital by the American Hospital Association) to over a thousand. There are general hospitals, catering to the diverse ills of the public, and special hospitals, which provide facilities for specific illnesses only. Mental hospitals, tuberculosis hospitals, geriatric hospitals, obstetric hospitals, and various types of surgical hospitals fall into this latter category. Another way of breaking hospitals down is according to their type of ownership. There are government hospitals, voluntary hospitals, and proprietary hospitals.[1]

Government Hospitals

"Government," of course, can refer to federal, state, or local government. The federal government owns hospitals run by the military for their personnel and dependents. And there are U.S. Public Health Service hospitals operated for the American Indians, for veterans, for leprosy patients, for narcotics addicts, and for merchant seamen. Mental hospitals are state operated and owned. The same applies to tuberculosis hospitals. Most medical schools are affiliated with state-owned general hospitals, which provide

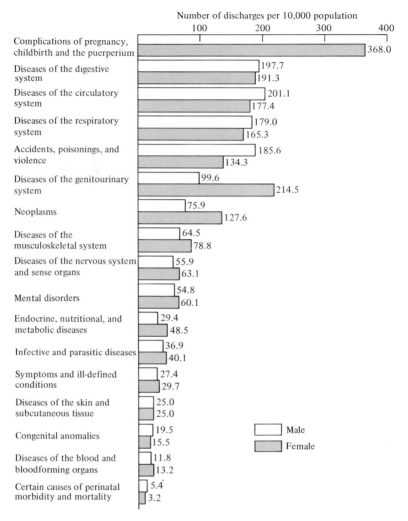

Number of discharges per 10,000 population

100	200	300	400

Complications of pregnancy, childbirth and the puerperium — 368.0

Diseases of the digestive system — 197.7 / 191.3

Diseases of the circulatory system — 201.1 / 177.4

Diseases of the respiratory system — 179.0 / 165.3

Accidents, poisonings, and violence — 185.6 / 134.3

Diseases of the genitourinary system — 99.6 / 214.5

Neoplasms — 75.9 / 127.6

Diseases of the musculoskeletal system — 64.5 / 78.8

Diseases of the nervous system and sense organs — 55.9 / 63.1

Mental disorders — 54.8 / 60.1

Endocrine, nutritional, and metabolic diseases — 29.4 / 48.5

Infective and parasitic diseases — 36.9 / 40.1

Symptoms and ill-defined conditions — 27.4 / 29.7

Diseases of the skin and subcutaneous tissue — 25.0 / 25.0

Congenital anomalies — 19.5 / 15.5

Diseases of the blood and bloodforming organs — 11.8 / 13.2

Certain causes of perinatal morbidity and mortality — 5.4 / 3.2

☐ Male
▨ Female

SOURCE: *Monthly Vital Statistics Report*, Department of Health, Education, and Welfare (Sept. 1973).

FIGURE 15-2. *Annual rate of discharges from short-stay hospitals by diagnostic class of first-listed diagnosis and sex, excluding newborn infants: United States, 1972.*

not only services to the community but complex teaching programs as well. City and county hospitals usually exist for the care of the indigent in their localities.[2]

Voluntary Hospitals

Voluntary hospitals comprise over 70 per cent of all general hospitals in the United States. They're owned by local communities, churches, charitable organizations, and sometimes philanthropic individuals. Although they're organized as corporations, they operate on a nonprofit basis; that is, they

TABLE 15-1
Hospitals—Type of Service and Control: 1950-1971

(Prior to 1960, excludes Alaska and Hawaii. Covers hospitals accepted for registration by the American Hospital Association. Short-term hospitals have an average patient stay of 30 days or less; long-term, an average stay of longer duration.)

Item		1950	1960	1965	1967	1968	1969	1970	1971
Hospitals		6,788	6,876	7,123	7,172	7,137	7,144	7,123	7,097
Beds	(1,000)	1,456	1,658	1,704	1,671	1,663	1,650	1,616	1,556
Rate*		9.6	9.2	8.8	8.5	8.3	8.2	7.9	7.5
Type of Service and Ownership									
Federal hospitals, all types		414	435	443	416	416	415	408	407
Beds	(1,000)	189	177	174	175	175	170	161	148
Nonfederal hospitals		6,374	6,441	6,680	6,756	6,721	6,729	6,715	6,690
Beds	(1,000)	1,266	1,481	1,530	1,496	1,489	1,480	1,455	1,408
Short-term general and special		5,031	5,407	5,736	5,850	5,820	5,853	5,859	5,865
Beds	(1,000)	505	639	741	788	806	826	848	867
Long-term general and special		412	308	283	331	280	260	236	218
Beds	(1,000)	70	67	66	80	67	63	60	54
Psychiatric		533	488	483	470	505	509	519	513
Beds	(1,000)	620	722	685	609	594	570	527	469
Tuberculosis		398	238	178	105	116	107	101	94
Beds	(1,000)	72	52	37	18	22	20	20	18
Nonfederal Ownership or Control									
State hospitals		(†)	556	546	552	559	565	577	580
Beds	(1,000)	(†)	752	708	647	620	598	558	498
Local government hospitals		1,654	1,324	1,495	1,589	1,631	1,665	1,680	1,700
Beds	(1,000)	844	201	216	216	219	220	219	219
Nongovernmental nonprofit hospitals		3,250	3,579	3,670	3,692	3,660	3,650	3,600	3,565
Beds	(1,000)	368	482	552	579	595	607	619	629
For-profit hospitals		1,470	982	969	923	871	849	858	745
Beds	(1,000)	55	46	54	54	55	55	59	61

* Beds per 1,000 population. Based on Bureau of the Census estimated resident population as of July 1, 1972.
† State Hospitals included with "Local."

Source: Hospitals (Chicago: American Hospital Association, Guide Issue, annual).

have no stockholders, and they don't use profits to pay dividends. Boards of trustees appointed by the owners are responsible for their operation, and the boards usually hire administrators to carry out the day-to-day functions of hospital business. These hospitals try to meet their own expenses, but they often can't do it. So the American taxpayer has had to assume part of the burden for building expansion and educational and service programs.[3]

Proprietary Hospitals

Owners of proprietary hospitals are profit-hungry capitalists, bent on getting rich on others' sickness and misfortune—at least, that's the way some look on proprietary institutions. After all, there is something suspicious about a business that makes money out of tragedy. But haven't doctors and undertakers been doing this for years? What about drug firms, medical equipment manufacturing firms? The insurance industry would be in bad shape if we eliminated sickness and death.

But do proprietary hospitals offer the training programs their nonprofit compatriots offer? No, they don't. Proprietary hospitals seldom, if ever, offer internships, residency programs, nurses' training programs, or in-house schooling for auxiliary personnel. After all, education isn't profitable, and owners of proprietary hospitals are out to make a profit.

There are certain hospital services that aren't too profitable, either, so most proprietary hospitals don't offer them. Psychiatric facilities are a good example; another is obstetrical service; and another yet is the emergency room. These facilities are usually provided by nonprofit hospitals in the community, so why should the proprietary hospital owner provide additional facilities of this type? They don't make money.

Proprietary hospitals, then, say their critics, are nothing more than leeches sucking health care delivery blood from the nonprofit system. Voluntary and government hospitals provide services the public needs. Proprietaries provide services that make money and nothing else. Again, we're talking about capitalistic monsters, but the argument isn't too valid. First, there has never been an objective study proving that profitmaking enterprises deliver lower-quality health care than ones working for the public good only. Second, it's hard for an administrator making $50,000 a year and driving a hospital-owned car to justify the nobility of nonprofit sacrifice. Third, although proprietary institutions do provide less comprehensive health care than voluntary types, possibly they should be applauded instead of criticized. Does it make sense to have five psychiatric wings at five general hospitals in a town of 500,000, which also has a mental hospital? This is a fairly typical health care delivery situation. And yet each of these psychiatric wings is often utilized less than 30 per cent of the time; and the same applies to five cobalt bombs in this hypothetical community, which also has multiple facilities for open-heart surgery. Overlapping services are a waste, and waste is something our health care system could do with a lot less of. Possibly, proprietary hospitals limit their services in order to make money only. Possibly, people help others best when they help themselves at the same time.[4]

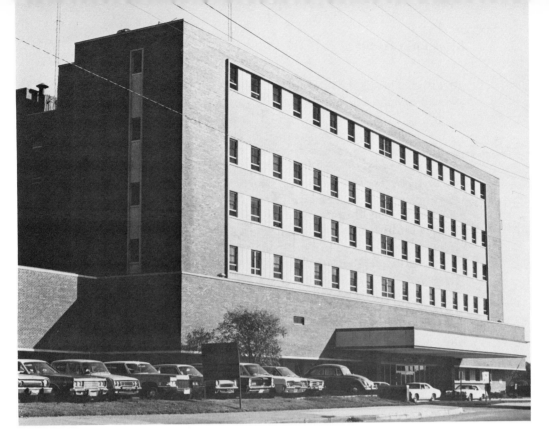

FIGURE 15-3. *Medical center.*

Hospital Accreditation

The Joint Commission on Accreditation of Hospitals (JCAH) is a nonprofit organization, formed in 1952. It's sponsored by the American College of Physicians, the American College of Surgeons, the American Hospital Association, and the American Medical Association. Obviously, it sets standards of hospital care and accredits hospitals that meet the standards established. A hospital has to have been in operation for at least 1 year and have 25 beds before the JCAH will inspect it. Also, it has to be listed with the American Hospital Association.

The evaluation consists of checking the hospital for cleanliness, food handling, records, functioning of the laboratory, fire and safety regulations, emergency plans, and, above all, the practices of the medical staff. Medical records are thoroughly screened; so are records of professional staff meetings. Accreditation is good for 3 years. Then the JCAH checks again to assure that the hospital is meeting acceptable standards.

Accreditation used to be of prestige value only. But now that third-party payees have taken on a bigger role in the health care delivery scene, accreditation has assumed a more meaningful role. Some insurance organizations won't pay money to nonaccredited hospitals, so hospital administrators and medical staffs take the accreditation status quite seriously. Also, accreditation affects the hospital's educational program. A nonaccredited hospital isn't allowed to train interns, residents, or nurses.[5]

Nursing Homes

Nursing homes are for old folks, primarily. Normally they exist for people who are too ill or incapacitated to be cared for by their families. This can be someone in his 20s, of course, as well as someone in his 80s. But most occupants of nursing homes are in the senior citizen status.

Most healthy people ignore these places, and if they think about them at all it's with fear. "God grant that I never have to go to one." Nursing homes are a cross between asylums and the Spanish Inquisition, they believe. Although some nursing homes may be the greatest boon ever given to an ungrateful segment of the population, some of the current-day shacks masquerading as old folks' havens give the fears some credence. Like Caesar's wife, nursing homes should be beyond reproach. But they're certainly not. Here are some of the more common complaints against the establishments:

Unsanitary Conditions

In this day of disinfectant sprays and deodorizers, no health care institution should have an offensive odor. But there are nursing homes that smell of urine, fecal matter, and just plain filth. Some are replete with flies and roaches. Some have dirty floors, and some have dirty mattresses, pillows, and bed linens. Homes of this type shouldn't be licensed, of course. Regrettably, some of them are.

Poor-Quality Health Care

Sometimes it's a shortage of trained personnel, sometimes it's a careless administrator who's responsible for patient injuries. Sometimes the home explains them by saying the patient fell out of bed or climbed over the siderails of the bed. Sometimes, this is true.

Unsafe and Overcrowded Conditions

There are homes with paper drapes (obvious fire hazards), inoperable exit doors and windows, automatic sprinkler systems that don't work, or no sprinkling system at all. Homes with these conditions are tragedies looking for causes and times.

Lack of Therapy Facilities

Some nursing homes aren't rehabilitation oriented. They don't have facilities for physical, speech, occupational, and hearing therapy. They don't have planned programs for recreation. Sometimes indifferent administration brings this about. Sometimes it's lack of finances that causes the problem. In

TABLE 15-2
Long-Term Care Facilities, 1971

Type of Facility	Total	Ownership			Number of Beds			Residents (1,000)	Full-time employees (1,000)
		Government	Profit	Non-profit	Under 25	25–74	75 or more		
All nursing care and related homes	22,558	1,393	17,510	3,655	8,456	8,456	5,646	1,106	584
Nursing care	23,204	890	10,242	2,072	2,073	6,379	4,752	848	493
Personnel care:									
With nursing care	3,645	227	2,366	1,052	1,596	1,271	778	176	68
Without nursing care	5,506	268	4,738	500	4,609	787	110	79	22
Domicillary care homes	203	8	164	31	178	19	6	3	1

Source: Health Resources Statistics (Washington, D.C.: U.S. National Center for Health Statistics, annual).

any event, it's the kind of problem that makes people vegetate rather than adjust.

Poor Menus

Food is an important item to older people. Sometimes meals are the most important events of their days. Yet some nursing homes show little interest in the variety and taste of their menus. Some make no provision for providing special diets for patients who need them. Some don't even feed adequate amounts to maintain good health.

Absence of Social Service Departments

Some of the larger nursing homes have social service departments, but most of the smaller ones don't. Older people do need personal counseling and group work programs. And they need somebody who takes an interest in just them, too.

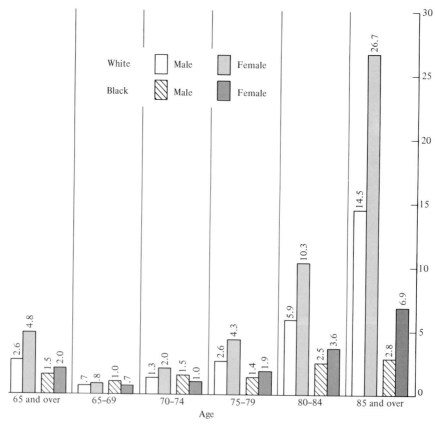

SOURCE: Public Health Service, National Center for Health Statistics, unpublished data; Bureau of the Census, *Current Population Reports,* Series, No. 441, p. 25.

FIGURE 15-4. *Persons in nursing and personal care homes, by age, race, and sex, 1969.*

Finances

There are two classes of people who can afford nursing home care—the wealthy and those on welfare. Patients from middle-class circumstances and their families can go bankrupt meeting the soaring costs of these institutions. And people on welfare have their problems, too. Although most homes have to conform to established welfare rates, they've been known to ask the patients' families for "under-the-table payments," hinting that the welfare rate isn't adequate. And it's suspected that some homes increase their income by getting "kickbacks" from providers of services.

Other Complaints

There are other complaints about nursing homes, lots of them. They have poor color schemes; their atmosphere is drab and cheerless; in some cases, there's lack of central air conditioning as well as inadequate lighting and heat and electrical fixtures. Sometimes there's almost no effort to get the patient out of bed on a daily basis. But, in fairness, there are fine nursing homes as well as poor ones, those that perform as worthwhile a service as any community or country could expect. And though most of them are organized as profitmaking corporations, the profits in this industry aren't all that great. Certainly, the standards of nursing homes can improve, should improve, and have been improving. And, certainly, the people who work in these institutions earn their money by caring for people who are often helpless, often cantankerous, sometimes childish, sometimes uncooperative, usually difficult to deal with. But the nursing home scene, like the rest of America's health care delivery system, isn't some idealistic model the rest of the world envies. We've got a long way to grow.[6]

Group Practice

A group practice is an organization of physicians, often affiliated with clinics and medical centers, which, in turn, are usually associated with hospitals or other types of charitable institutions. The physicians act as a team. They share their skills, their knowledge; they use the same building, laboratory equipment, and ancillary personnel. The physicians' income is divided according to a prearranged plan, based on fee-for-service or a salary. Some call this cooperative medicine rather than competitive medicine.

Certainly, there are several advantages to this type of health care delivery over the single physician's treating patients in his home or office. One of these is having a doctor perform under the scrutiny of his colleagues rather than make decisions and perform services checked by no one other than the patient. Another advantage is that most of the services a patient might need are provided under one roof, and these services are available on a 24-hour basis, 365 days a year. Solo physicians are sometimes hard to find when they're needed. Also, there's an advantage of having a doctor from the same team treat a patient whose personal physician is temporarily unavailable. When a solo physician isn't available, his patients often have to seek

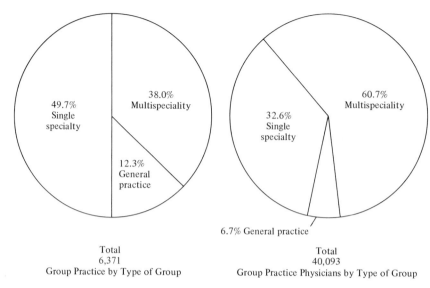

Total
6,371
Group Practice by Type of Group

Total
40,093
Group Practice Physicians by Type of Group

SOURCE: *Socioeconomic Issues of Health,* K. E. Monroe, ed. (Chicago: Center for Health Services Research and Development, AMA Publication, 1971).

FIGURE 15-5. *Per cent distribution of group practices and group practice physicians by type of group, 1969.*

treatment at nearby emergency rooms or with doctors who don't have direct access to the patients' medical records and knowledge of treatment history.[7]

Health Maintenance Organization

About 20 per cent of the American population live within health maintenance organization (HMO) service areas, and about 7 million of us get our health care through this kind of delivery system. Some look on the HMO as a new organization on the health delivery scene, but it's really not. HMOs have been around for over 40 years. But they are becoming more and more visible. Politicians have heralded HMOs as a panacea, a complete answer to America's health care dilemma. Physicians have screamed that they're socialized medicine under another name, monsters that will destroy doctors' initiative, medical standards, and, of course, free enterprise. Some legal experts have looked on them as a trend toward the corporate delivery of health care rather than the individual physician's delivery of the service. What in the world is this thing that people so violently love and hate?

The HMO is really nothing more than an organized system of delivering comprehensive health care to a voluntarily enrolled population. The population pays for this care according to what are called "fixed contract costs." In other words, individuals or families pay for their health care on an annual basis. The HMO cares for these people when they need care or performs some kind of preventive service when they need that. People pay a fixed amount whether they're treated or not, and the HMO gets this money whether it performs a service or doesn't. Obviously, the HMO gets a reward by keeping people well rather than treating them because they're sick. Under the current fee-for-service system, the opposite, of course, is true. Doctors and hospitals don't get paid unless someone needs an operation or needs a pill or cobalt treatment. So HMOs put their emphasis on preventive services, on rehabilitative services and diagnostic services. Ambulatory treatment is given whenever possible, rather than hospitalization.

Critics have claimed that this lowers the quality of health care, that people needing hospitalization may not get it because the HMO is trying to save money. This hasn't proven to be true. A good index of the efficiency of health care delivery is infant mortality. Here the HMO shines. There have been 27.3 infant deaths per thousand births when traditional health delivery systems have been used, but only 22.7 in HMOs. Another statistic involves mortality of the elderly. The index number is 8.8 when they're cared for by the traditional system, only 7.8 when cared for by HMOs. How about operations? Apparently, patients seem to need more of them when someone is paid to do them. In a fee-for-service system, 69 operations per thousand patients per year are performed. Under the HMO, it's 49 operations. For tonsillectomies, the figure is 94 per thousand patients per year under fee-for-service. There are 47 per thousand per year under HMOs.

Another criticism of HMOs is that they're costly. Health care insurance and fee-for-service, supposedly, can deliver just as fine health care service at a much lower price. Not so. When all benefits are taken into account, it costs less to provide health care through health maintenance organizations than any other method of health delivery around.

Another problem of HMOs, critics claim, is that they don't address themselves to critical health care delivery problems in rural areas and ghettos. This is true. HMOs are usually built where doctors like to practice and where there are lots of well-to-do and healthy people to buy the prepayment plans. They're not built in Harlem and Watts and in the small communities in Kansas that can't find a doctor. They have improved the health care delivery picture of a certain segment of our population, though, and possibly they'll serve a more diverse group in the future.[8]

Health Care Corporation

No health care corporations exist yet. But there are many people on the political and medical scenes who think they should and will exist. The health care corporation would be a lot like the health maintenance organization, its only difference being that it would be a franchised operation rather than one that's allowed to grow like Topsy. The franchise would be granted by either the states or the federal government, depending on which health care bill gets passed by Congress. The critics of this type of delivery system claim that we're talking about socialized medicine, and the critics are absolutely right. The HMO, being nothing more than a corporation delivering a health care service in the form and place that it chooses, is still somewhat of a free-enterprise model. The health care corporation would represent almost total government ownership and regulation, the characteristics of any socialistic system. Is this bad? To critics of our current health care delivery system, it most certainly is not. Health care is a right, not some privilege given only to those who can pay for it or those living in the right section of the country. Without the government's forcing health care personnel to practice in certain locations or at least rewarding them heavily for doing it, without the government's putting health care delivery mechanisms in rural areas and ghettos, without the government's forcing health care costs to come into line with the rest of the American economy, these events just won't transpire. The health care corporation is a drastic move. But America's health care, according to its critics, is in a state of crisis. This calls for drastic moves, expensive moves, socialistic trends, and unhappy physicians.[9]

Paying the Health Care Bill

There are several ways of meeting an individual's health care costs. One is by the pay-as-you-go plan. If you or your dependents aren't sick, you don't get treated, and you don't pay a thing. If you do get sick, you dip into your savings or borrow a little and pay the doctor or the hospital and go on from there. This plan works just fine for someone who never gets seriously ill or for Howard Hughes. For others, it may not work out. Major illnesses can cost thousands of dollars that a family doesn't have, possibly bringing on bankruptcy or total poverty.

So there's health insurance. Here a person can pay a predictable amount from month to month and budget for sickness like he does for food, rent, and his automobile. Nearly 80 per cent of our population is covered by some insurance of this type. However, it's not complete coverage. Insurance benefits cover about one-third of the potential medical expenses of the average American family. And insurance companies are raising the premiums and reducing the benefits covered daily. They have to. Doctors' fees and hospital costs go up daily, and insurance companies like to balance their books.

And then there's a group of people who can't afford to or don't want to carry any form of health insurance, no matter what the costs or coverage. The public pays for their medical services with tax dollars. Essentially, then, collective health care financing falls into one of two categories—voluntary health insurance or tax-supported medical services.

Health Insurance

Health insurance is based on the assumption that individuals can't successfully budget against illness costs, that they're better off to pool their risks with those of lots of other individuals so they can spread their costs. Insurance companies issue policies against these pooled chances of getting sick and sell them to individuals, employee groups, and professional organizations.

The group plans are the ones that are most reasonable. They're usually purchased by an employer, who pays a given premium for each subscriber in his organization for a fixed amount of coverage. The costs are higher for

TABLE 15-3
National Health Expenditures, by Object: 1950–1971
(For Calendar Years)

Object of Expenditure	Amount (millions of dollars)							Per Cent		
	1950	1955	1960	1965	1969	1970	1971	1960	1970	1971
Total	12,662	17,745	26,895	40,468	64,142	71,573	79,795	100.0	100.0	100.0
Spent by										
Consumers	8,425	12,282	18,831	28,050	36,615	40,943	45,023	70.0	57.2	56.4
Government	3,440	4,555	6,637	10,066	24,095	26,887	30,646	24.7	37.6	38.4
Philanthropy and other	797	908	1,428	2,348	3,432	3,742	4,125	5.3	5.2	5.2
Spent for										
Hospitals	3,851	5,900	9,092	13,605	24,093	27,597	31,119	33.8	38.5	39.0
Physicians' services	2,747	3,689	5,684	8,745	12,654	14,294	15,725	21.1	20.0	19.7
Dentists' services	961	1,508	1,977	2,808	4,047	4,419	4,860	7.4	6.2	6.1
Drugs and sundries	1,726	2,384	3,657	4,850	6,812	7,297	7,712	13.6	10.2	9.7
Eyeglasses and appliances*	491	604	776	1,230	1,765	1,866	1,984	2.9	2.6	2.5
Nursing-home care	187	312	526	1,328	2,650	3,070	3,495	2.0	4.3	4.4
Research	117	210	662	1,469	1,818	1,842	1,933	2.5	2.6	2.4
Medical facilities construction	843	651	1,048	1,912	2,973	3,366	3,845	3.9	4.7	4.8
Other†	1,739	2,487	3,473	4,521	7,330	7,822	9,122	12.9	10.9	11.4

* Includes fees of optometrists and expenditures for hearing aids, orthopedic appliances, artificial limbs, crutches, wheelchairs, etc.
† Includes the services of registered and practical nurses in private duty, visiting nurses, podiatrists, physical therapists, clinical psychologists, chiropractors, naturopaths, and Christian Science practitioners, and the net cost of insurance and administrative expenses of federally financed health programs.

Source: Research and Statistics Note (Note No. 3) (Washington, D.C.: U.S. Social Security Administration, 1973), and unpublished data.

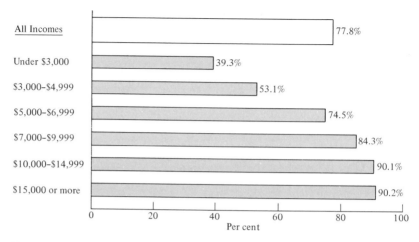

Note: Data are for persons under 65 years old.

SOURCE: Public Health Service, National Center for Health Statistics, unpublished data.

FIGURE 15-6. *Hospital insurance coverage by family income, 1970.*

plans providing the same benefits when they're purchased by individuals. So most people covered by health insurance belong to group plans. The benefits these plans offer are usually one of two types: cash indemnity or service; or sometimes there's a combination of the two. Cash indemnity plans pay what their label implies—money. Someone gets sick and goes to a hospital and then pays the hospital and the doctors who treat him. He then sends the insurance company receipts for what he's paid and gets part or all of his money back. Service plans are contracts between policyholders and physicians and hospitals. If the policyholder gets sick, he sees the physician or hospital concerned and receives the treatment due him. It's then up to the physician or hospital to file a claim for reimbursement from the insurance company.

Most commercial insurance companies use cash indemnity plans. The plans sometimes have deductibles and coinsurance features that are quite flexible and can be shaped to fit the needs of an unlimited number of groups or individuals.[10] Commercial companies don't enter into contracts with hospitals or physicians, though. This is a role carried on by Blue Cross and Blue Shield, the nonprofit sector of the business.

BLUE CROSS

Blue Cross, officially endorsed by the American Hospital Association, offers 75 plans in the United States, insuring against costs for physicians' services, hospital care, laboratory tests, and drugs. This nonprofit mammoth has enrolled 68 million members, one-third of the U.S. population. Six per cent of these people come under group rather than individual subscriptions.

There's no such thing as a typical Blue Cross plan. Each is drawn up by an autonomous regional organization using the Blue Cross name. These

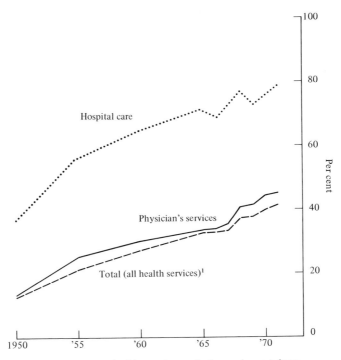

[1] Includes hospital care, physician services, and other services not shown
separately.

SOURCE: Social Security Administration, *Research and Statistics Note,*
No. 3–1973.

FIGURE 15-7. *Consumer expenditures for personal health care covered by private insurance, 1950–1971.*

organizations set their own rates and benefits, make their own contracts with the hospitals in their territories. If a hospital doesn't meet regional organization standards, then no contract is drawn up. So Blue Cross, to a certain degree, controls the quality of hospital care delivery.

The most common type of Blue Cross policy involves coverage, partial or complete, for 30 days of hospital care. The coverage can range to a full year, though, and some plans provide for physicians' services, X-rays, laboratory tests, and drugs. Most of the plans include what is called "extended coverage," providing benefits in the event of a long siege of illness.[11]

BLUE SHIELD

Blue Shield is organized along the same general lines as Blue Cross and serves 60 million subscribers with 72 different plans. Like Blue Cross, it's endorsed by the American Hospital Association and is organized on a nonprofit basis. Blue Shield provides coverage for physicians' services, based on family income. Members are completely covered for physicians' payments if their annual family income is below a given level, provided the physicians involved are willing to accept the Blue Shield rates. When the income is over a given level, the Shield pays a given percentage of the physicians' charges.[12]

MAJOR MEDICAL PLANS

"Major medical" is a form of insurance that a lot of people prefer. Commercial carriers offer it on the assumption that the insured can pay a certain amount of his hospital and medical expenses out of his own pocket. This lets the insurance company provide large amounts of coverage for major expenses at a reasonable cost. The typical major medical plan calls for the insured to pay the first $100 to $500 of the cost of his illness before the company pays anything. Then the company pays only 75 to 80 per cent of the expenses from that point forward. The insured pays the remaining 20 to 25 per cent. Although this may seem a little tough on the fellow who has a serious, long-term illness, it's a financial arrangement that lets carriers issue a lot of coverage at a relatively low cost.[13]

HAPHAZARD COVERAGE

Despite the complexity and comprehensiveness of the plans offered, the health insurance industry is a pretty haphazard approach to health care financing. There are 20 to 30 million Americans without any type of health insurance coverage whatsoever, and most of the policies have severe limitations. Most of them cover hospital care only and make no provisions for care by a physician in his office. The biggest variable concerning the type of insurance a family carries is, of course, the family income. Just about all people in families with incomes of $10,000 or more per year have some type of health care policy. But only 53 per cent of those in families in the $3,000 to $5,000 bracket have health insurance. And with families below $3,000 per year the percentage drops to 39 per cent. Insurance pays for about a third of our health care expenditures. And when you add government programs like Medicare, 50 per cent of the costs are covered. The consumer pays for the rest out of his pocket.

And the health insurance field can be pretty confusing. Seventeen-hundred carriers offer an array of packages that most subscribers don't understand. So lots of people, probably the majority, who think that they have excellent health protection have some pretty serious gaps that they're not aware of. Others have overlapping coverage. Around 22 million have more than one type of coverage for hospital expenses, and 20 million have overlapping insurance for surgical costs. There are 11 million with an overlap for medical expenses.

Medicare, which is supposed to help people 65 and over, covers only 45 per cent of their health care costs. Medicaid, a health program for the poor, has been seriously underfinanced. This has placed a burden on our health delivery system that has forced a cutback in services and brought on cumbersome delivery of the entire health care package. Health insurance, whether provided by the government or nonprofit and profit corporations, isn't fulfilling America's health care needs, and there's nothing to indicate that it ever will.[14]

Tax-Supported Health Services

So public medical care enters the picture. Here citizens' tax dollars are used to deliver health care service to people in various categories of need. There

TABLE 15-4
Personal Health Care—Third-Party Payments and Private Consumer Expenditures: 1950–1971

[In millions of dollars, except per cent. Prior to 1960, excludes Alaska and Hawaii. Third-party payments include private health insurance benefit payments, government expenditures (including those for health insurance for the aged), and philanthropy and the expenditures of employers to maintain industrial in-plant health facilities.]

Item	1950	1955	1960	1965	1969	1970	1971
Personal health care expenditures*	10,885	15,708	23,680	34,821	55,541	62,282	69,027
Third-Party Payments							
Total	3,752	6,576	10,690	16,768	33,583	38,523	43,823
Per cent of total health care	34.5	41.9	45.1	48.2	60.5	61.9	63.5
Private health insurance	992	2,536	4,996	8,729	13,068	15,744	17,891
Per cent of total health care	9.1	16.1	21.1	25.1	23.5	25.3	25.9
Government†	2,440	3,608	5,157	7,342	19,660	21,851	24,933
Per cent of total health care	22.4	23.0	21.8	21.1	35.4	35.1	36.1
Philanthropy and others	320	432	537	697	855	928	999
Per cent of total health care	3.0	2.8	2.3	2.0	1.5	1.5	1.4
Private Consumer Expenditures							
Total‡	8,125	11,668	17,986	26,778	35,026	39,502	43,094
Per cent met by private health insurance	12.2	21.7	27.8	32.6	37.3	40.0	41.5
Hospital care	1,832	2,997	5,119	8,135	11,407	13,495	14,456
Per cent met by private health insurance	37.1	56.0	64.7	71.2	73.3	75.8	78.6
Physicians' services§	2,597	3,433	5,309	8,181	9,689	11,044	12,178
Per cent met by private health insurance	12.0	25.0	30.0	32.8	41.6	44.4	45.2

* All expenditures for health services and supplies except expenses for prepayment and administration, government public health activities, and expenditures of private voluntary agencies for other health services.
† Beginning 1969, includes benefit payments under the health insurance for the aged program.
‡ Includes other expenditures not shown separately. Excludes expenses for prepayment.
§ Includes small amounts for other types of professional services.

Source: Research and Statistics Note (Note No. 3) (Washington, D.C.: U.S. Social Security Administration, 1973), and unpublished data.

TABLE 15-5
Indexes of Medical Care Prices, 1950–1972

(1967 = 100. Prior to 1965, excludes Alaska and Hawaii. These indexes are components of the consumer price index, which was revised beginning 1964.)

Year	Total Medical Care	Drugs and Prescriptions	Physicians' Fees	Obstetrical Case	Professional Services — Tonsillectomy and Adenoidectomy	Dentists' Fees	Optometric Examination and Eyeglasses	Hospital Daily Service Charges
1950	53.7	88.5	55.2	51.2	60.7	63.9	73.5	28.9
1955	64.8	94.7	65.4	68.6	69.0	73.0	77.0	41.5
1960	79.1	104.5	77.0	79.4	80.3	82.1	85.1	56.3
1965	89.5	100.2	88.3	89.0	91.0	92.2	92.8	76.6
1969	113.4	101.3	112.9	113.5	110.3	112.9	107.6	127.9
1970	120.6	103.6	121.4	121.8	117.1	119.4	113.5	143.9
1971	128.4	105.4	129.8	129.0	125.2	127.0	120.3	160.8
1972	132.5	105.6	133.8	133.8	129.9	132.3	124.9	(NA)

NA, Not available.

Source: Consumer Price Indexes for Selected Items and Groups, Monthly and Annual Averages (Washington, D.C.: U.S. Bureau of Labor Statistics).

are federal programs of this type, state programs, county programs, and certain city programs.

Health care for the indigent or the poor dates back to 1935, when the Federal Social Security Act authorized medical services for the aged (65 years of age and older), the blind, and dependent children of families incapable of providing adequate support. A fourth category was added to this indigent list in the mid-1950s, that of the permanently and totally disabled. Later came a fifth category of general welfare cases.[15]

MEDICARE

Medicare is a health insurance program under Social Security that helps people 65 years of age and older to meet their medical expenses. There are two parts to Medicare: hospital insurance and medical insurance.

Hospital Insurance. Hospital insurance helps pay for hospital inpatient services and certain follow-up services, such as:

1. During any benefit period, a patient can receive up to 90 days of inpatient care in a participating hospital. New benefit periods can begin when participants haven't been hospitalized for 60 days or more.
2. On leaving the hospital, the patient can enter any participating extended-care facility for up to 100 days.
3. If the participant needs more inpatient care yet, he has a "lifetime reserve" of 60 more hospital days.
4. If the person doesn't have to or want to enter a hospital or nursing home, he can be treated in his home, by nurses, physical therapists, or other types of health care workers. He's entitled to 100 of these home health "visits."

The government doesn't pay for this entire package. It will pay for room costs in a hospital or nursing home, though, as long as the accomoda-

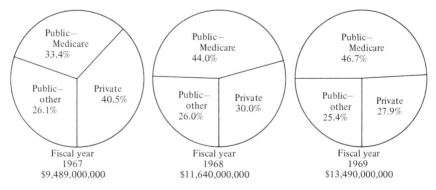

SOURCE: *Socioeconomic Issues of Health,* K. E. Monroe, ed. (Chicago: Center for Health Services Research and Development, AMA Publication, 1971).

FIGURE 15-8. *Personal health care expenditures for the aged by source of funds, fiscal years 1967–1969.*

tions are semiprivate (two to four beds). And it will pay for the meals, standard nursing services, and the costs of drugs, supplies, and any equipment the hospital or nursing home needs for the treatment. The government won't pay for convenience items, private-duty nurses, or the costs of the first 3 pints of blood the patient might need. And this portion of Medicare doesn't cover physicians' fees.

Medical Insurance. Medical insurance is voluntary, and people don't get it unless they sign up for it. This calls for monthly premiums, which help cover the costs of physicians' bills and several other health care items not covered under hospital insurance. The benefits include:

1. Physicians' services.
2. One-hundred yearly home health visits, in addition to the hundred covered under hospital insurance. This second set of visits must be arranged by a physician with the home health agency that takes part in Medicare.
3. Sundry health services a physician might prescribe, such as surgical dressings, artificial limbs, splints, X-rays and radiation therapy, and rental or purchase of various kinds of medical equipment.
4. Ambulance services under certain circumstances, outpatient physical therapy services, and X-ray and clinical laboratory services during hospitalization.

This medical insurance doesn't cover prescription drugs, eyeglasses, examinations for eyeglasses, hearing aids, dental care and dentures, orthopedic shoes, and immunizations. And the monthly premiums aren't the full costs. The participant has to pay the first $50 of his medical expenses each year plus 20 per cent of any additional balance.[16]

VETERANS

People who once served in the Armed Forces and have conditions that were inflicted or aggravated during service can get treated at no cost through the Veterans Administration. The main requirement is that the service-connected disabilities be noted on the military service records. Veterans can also get non-service-connected conditions treated through the Veterans Administration, but they have to show that they're not capable of paying for treatment. And they have to show that they didn't receive a bad conduct, dishonorable, or "undesirable" discharge.[17]

MILITARY PERSONNEL

While they're on active duty, Armed Forces personnel get complete medical and dental care at no cost through military hospitals and clinics. Their wives and their children who are 18 years old or younger usually receive this care as well. Retired military personnel and their families often get the same benefits.[18]

AMERICAN INDIANS

There are more than half a million American Indians who get free medical care through clinics and hospitals operated by the United States Public Health Service.[19]

UNITED STATES MERCHANT MARINE

The government-financed health care that merchant seamen receive dates back to 1798. This was the first tax-supported medical program in the United States.

MENTAL DISEASES

The vast majority of people hospitalized for mental illness get placed in a state hospital. It's been accepted for over 85 years that care of the emotionally ill is predominantly a public function. States also maintain alcohol- and drug-abuse clinics, and so do some local and federal agencies.[20]

DISABLED PERSONS

States also play a major role in caring for and educating people living in their territory who are crippled. For children, there is the Crippled Children's Program, administered by state health departments. Standards for care here are very high, with children receiving treatment only by specialists board-certified in their field.

For adults with physical disabilities, such as amputation, blindness, or paralysis, the states conduct programs in conjunction with the federal government for job training as well as providing various kinds of therapy and treatment. They also administer medical care programs for adults injured during employment. The employer pays for this care by footing the bill for Workmen's Compensation Insurance.[21]

GENERAL HOSPITALS

City or county governments often run general hospitals to take care of the indigent or people with chronic illnesses. The stay of many of these patients is much longer than for those in voluntary general hospitals.[22]

COUNTY HEALTH DEPARTMENTS

The tax-supported services local health departments provide vary from county to county. These are some of the more common ones:

1. Venereal disease control.
2. Communicable disease control.
3. Public health nursing.
4. Public health nutrition.
5. Public health social services.

6. General and child health consultations.
7. Public health dentistry.
8. Sanitation inspection and supervision.
9. Records of births and deaths.
10. School health services.
11. Air pollution control.
12. Industrial health services.
13. Public health education.[23]

Notes

1. William R. Rosengren and Mark Lefton, *Hospitals and Patients* (New York: Atherton Press, 1969), pp. 3–49.
2. C. L. Anderson, *Community Health* (St. Louis: Mosby, 1969), pp. 312–321.
3. Gladys A. Harrison, *Government Controls and Voluntary Non-profit Plan* (Chicago: American Hospital Association, 1961), pp. 1–33.
4. John H. Holmgren, "The Quasi-Public Characteristics of the Private Hospital" (Unpublished M.A. thesis, Wichita State University, 1962).
5. American Hospital Association, *Hospital Accreditation References* (Chicago: American Hospital Association, 1961).
6. Jordan Braverman, *Nursing Home Standards* (Washington, D.C.: American Pharmaceutical Association, 1970).
7. E. Freidson et al., "Organizational Dimensions of Large-Scale Group Medical Practice," *American Journal of Public Health*, Vol. 61 (April 1971), 786–795.
8. Stephen Wilson, *Health Maintenance Organizations*, Report to the Pharmacy Seminar, Detroit, February 1972 (Detroit: Pharmacy Seminar, 1972).
9. William R. Roy, *The Proposed Health Maintenance Organization Act of 1972* (Washington, D.C.: Science and Health Commission Group, 1972).
10. John E. Gregg, *The Health Insurance Market and How to Beat It* (Chicago: Regnery, 1973).
11. AMA Blue Cross Commission, *Blue Cross Report to the Nation* (Chicago: AMA Blue Cross Commission, 1973).
12. Blue Cross Association, *Blue Cross and Blue Shield Fact Book* (Chicago: Blue Cross Association, 1973).
13. Margaret Greenfield, *Meeting the Cost of Health Care* (Berkeley, Calif.: Institute of Government Studies, 1972), pp. 37–67.
14. New York Health Insurance Council, *The Extent of Voluntary Health Insurance Coverage in the United States as of December 1973* (New York: Health Insurance Council, 1973).
15. Mark V. Pauly, *Medical Care at Public Expense* (New York: Praeger, 1971).
16. Herman M. Somers, *Medicare and Hospitals* (Washington, D.C.: Brookings Institution, 1967), pp. 1–56.
17. M. J. Musser et al., "The Veterans Administration as a Health Care System," *Current Psychiatric Therapies*, Vol. 12 (1972), 219–223.
18. U.S. Government, *Military Medical Benefits*, HR 8374, HR 14088, U.S. Government Documents.
19. U.S. Public Health Service, *To the First Americans*, 5th Report on the Indian Health Program of the U.S. Public Health Service (Washington, D.C.: Public Health Service, Department of Health, Education, and Welfare, 1972).

20. Joseph F. Follmann, *Insurance Coverage for Mental Illness* (New York: American Management Association, 1970).

21. Richard T. Smith, *The Social Security Disability Program* (Washington, D.C.: Government Printing Office, 1971).

22. Alan Sheldon, Frank Baker, and Curtis P. McLaughlin, eds., *Systems and Medical Care* (Cambridge, Mass.: MIT Press, 1970), pp. 182–207.

23. C. L. Anderson, *Community Health* (St. Louis: Mosby, 1969), pp. 285–295.

16 Man's Crisis: His Environment

The battle was in doubt at first. Many thought the odds were in favor of the fish and the deer and the ants and the trees. After all, they were hardier than the two-legged predators. They blended more naturally with their environment, they were less hostile, less demanding. But it was this hostility that the oddsmakers really hadn't understood. Man had a need to dominate, a need to indulge, possibly a need to destroy. It was this twisted hunger that would make him the victor. The land, the sea, the air, and all that lived in it didn't really have a chance.

There were some men who respected nature, considered themselves part of it. They killed, of course, and polluted somewhat. But the killing involved a need for survival only; the pollution was minimal, part of the natural scheme of things. But these were red-faced "heathen," savages to be destroyed, swept aside like the beaver and the antelope. Christian soldiers were moving onward; their mighty army would have victory.

Like the red man, the quail, the grouse, the duck, and the woodchuck were the enemy. They provided feasts for fat men in the East, for fat wives and fat daughters. The carrier pigeon was once so plentiful it blotted out the sun. But gunnysacks were filled with them so they could be shipped to markets throughout the world. The species no longer exists. The same is al-

FIGURE 16-1.

396

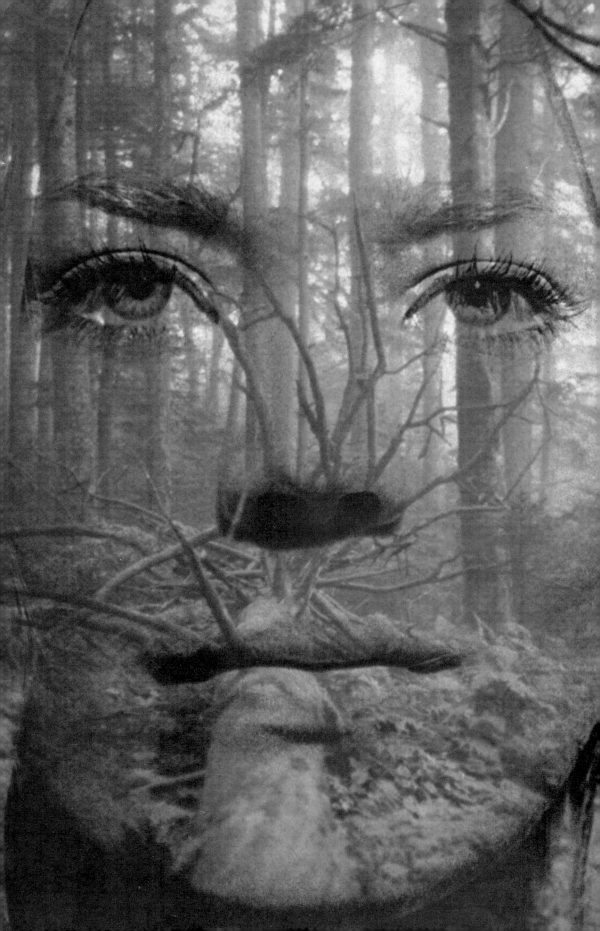

most true of the bald eagle. DDT just about eradicated him, but man took a little pity on this fellow. After all, he was the emblem of the Great Seal of the United States. So there are 750 breeding pairs still living.

The buffalo was almost obliterated. So were the alligator and the crocodile. But these were mean beasts; not too many mourned them. Their hides made excellent purses and shoes and luggage for the Japanese, who imported 127,000 of them during the late 1960s.

But with the whale it was different. It didn't have the viciousness of the crocodile, the slithering creep of the alligator. The mightiest and among the most noble of nature's creatures, man respected him, often romanticized him. It looked for a time as though the whale would survive man's onslaught. Kerosene replaced whaling oil as fuel for lamps. The early whaling industry collapsed, and the thinning schools of these creatures began to grow. But then organization, mechanization, and man's ingenuity entered the picture. There were commercial uses for whale oil—cosmetics, transmission fluids, cat foods. And there were radar equipment and heli-

FIGURE 16-2. *Who cast the first stone?*

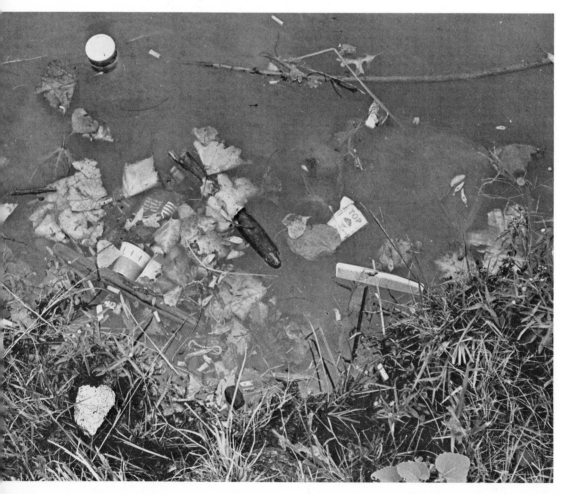

copters and 150-pound harpoons shot from cannons. There are now over 40,000 whales killed each year. The killing since 1920 exceeded all whale killing for the prior 400 years.

Of course, there's the Wild West, where the deer and the antelope and the he-men play. Or does that exist in a Marlboro commercial or a Max Brand novel only? Isn't that a heavy smog washing against the cliffs of the Cascade Mountains? Can you hear the roar of the jeeps and the "tote goats" on the roads? Surely those waters where the salmon and steelhead used to spawn aren't garbage dumps, are they? What about those strip mines cutting an ugly scar across the Ozarks? Indians and cowboys ride no more.[1]

The Science of Ecology

No man is an island. Neither is a bird, a fish, a tree, or a buzzard—not if it wants to stay alive. Insects eat flowers, birds eat insects, and all kinds of species eat the birds. Also, flowers need bees for pollination. All of us need the green plants to capture energy for the sun. Ecologists call communities of this type ecosystems. Elements of these systems depend on other elements for their survival. There are simple systems, such as a one- or two-crop farm, which can be pretty well destroyed by insects or disease. And there are complex systems, like massive forests, which can compensate for blights and pestilence and invasion by new species. If you look at the world as an ecosystem, the relationships are overwhelmingly complex, and the ability to adjust to change seems infinite. But then there's man. His imagination, his creativity, and his greed seem infinite, too.

Some organisms eat plants only; some eat animals only; and some eat both. Plant-eaters are called herbivores and the animal-eaters are called carnivores; the ones who go for either variety are omnivores. These organisms belong to various trophic levels in any given ecosystem (a "trophic level" consists of all living matter that obtains its food in a given way). Green plants comprise the first trophic level; herbivores are on the second; carnivores are on the third or fourth level, depending on their type of prey; and omnivores, like man, are on the third and fourth trophic levels also.[2]

Biomagnification

Although it may seem that everything we eat turns to fat, that calories invade our bodies like germs, it's really not all that easy to gain weight. To gain 1 pound, you have to consume about 10 pounds of something from the trophic level beneath you. This is true for any creature in any trophic level. So, in order to get 1 pound fatter, you have to eat about 10 pounds of perch or trout, which in turn have eaten about 100 pounds of minnows, which in turn have eaten about 1,000 pounds of plankton. And if the plankton has a little DDT in it, the degree of concentration increases as you move from one trophic level to another. This is called biomagnification.

DDT biomagnification has almost extinguished some bird species. Birds eat certain bugs that have absorbed the insecticide, and the DDT works its way into the birds' fatty tissue. This doesn't kill the birds, but it does inter-

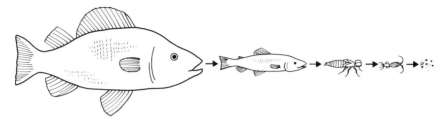

Feeding from the lower trophic level. It's a never-ending cycle.

FIGURE 16-3. *Biomagnification.*

fere with calcium metabolism. Birds with excessive amounts of this chemical in their systems produce fragile egg shells, which break before the young are ready to hatch. So with the increased use of DDT there's been a decrease in feathered friends as well as bugs.[3]

The Rate of Nature's Change

Not that DDT, or any other insecticide, is all bad. It has lowered disease rates, increased food supply, eliminated pests. Man can alter nature, certainly, without destroying it. Frogs do the same when they eat flies, lions when they kill deer. There's no ecosystem that remains constant. And, if the change is gradual, the ecosystem maintains balance and survives. Over the years the forest gets a little denser; a certain type of bug becomes more prominent; another type moves on to another environment; a species of mammal becomes extinct. Orderly change of this type is called succession. It implies that nature's balance is dynamic, not static. But gross interference with this balance or rate of change can affect some basic things in nature itself, like food and water and air.

And it's not just numbers of certain types of life forms that change. The structure and character of these life forms change as well over very long periods of time. If the environment changes, then beings that better adapt to the new ecosystem will replace those that survived in the old. This is the "natural selection" process of evolution. This is what keeps environmental change from eliminating life. But evolution, or Mother Nature herself, has limits. The change can't be so rapid or drastic that the scheme of things doesn't have time to adjust. Without this time, life itself pays the penalty, regardless of the form it takes. Birds could become extinct; so could fish; so could man.[4]

Air Pollution

You don't have to see air pollution to know it's there. You might see it, of course. It can be misty, dirty looking, something that doesn't seem to belong with the sunlight and the air. Sometimes you know it's there by the sting in your eyes, by the wheeze in your cough. You can't see it, or you've gotten so used to it that it doesn't look unnatural. But it makes its presence known in ways that are hard to ignore. It's made women's nylons deteriorate; it's eaten away at granite; it's killed off hundreds of types of plant life—possibly thousands.

Polluted air seems to be the normal kind you get in the 1970s. It was normal for the 1950s and 1960s, too, of course, but the industrial revolution has taken on a faster pace in the past few years. And the faster the pace, the greater the gas fumes, the coal dust, and the oil smoke. There are over 10,000 U.S. communities with some kind of air problem. Despite federal and local government regulations, the number seems to be growing.[5]

Effects of Bad Air

Because we breathe in about 15,000 quarts of air per day, this kind of pollution obviously isn't the best for health. And there are several studies that confirm the obvious. Air pollution has been linked with lung cancer, emphysema, bronchitis, and most other respiratory ailments. Also, it irritates the eyes, irritates the sinuses, and can contribute to acne. To check this out, postmortem examinations were conducted on 300 people who had lived in St. Louis, Missouri, between 1960 and 1966. The subjects were then matched with people who had lived in Winnipeg, Canada, according to smoking habits, sex, age at death, occupation, and length of residence. It was assumed that because St. Louis is highly industrialized and Winnipeg isn't, the Americans would have a significantly higher incidence and severity of emphysema than their Canadian counterparts. The assumption held true, regardless of age. Severe emphysema was three times as common in the St. Louis group. Moderate emphysema was about five times as common. Because this disease is the third leading cause of death for Englishmen over 45 and the fourth leading cause for American males in the same age category, these findings were significant. A belching smokestack was once a sign of prosperity. Although it still may be, there's a question as to just what price even prosperity carries.

Most of us, of course, have pretty healthy respiratory systems, so we look on air pollution as kind of a long-range threat. It's not something that will do away with us this afternoon, put us in the hospital before the month is out. There are those, though, who can't afford this long-range viewpoint. They're usually the older people, those who have chronic respiratory problems or heart disease. If the pollution gets intense enough, this sensitive group can die immediately. This happened in London in 1952. A heavy fog settled over the city, and a lot of smoke and other pollutants were mixed in. The fog stayed much longer than it normally does; the smoke intensified and lingered with the fog. By the time the air cleared, 3,000 people had died. A similar tragedy took place in the Meuse Valley in Belgium in 1930. Air pollution killed only 63 in this instance, but there's no record of how many became pulmonary cripples, how many developed serious lung conditions, how many became just plain sick. And disasters of this type aren't confined to Europe. The United States has smokestacks, automobile fumes, smog, ignorance, and indifference of its own. Combine them in the right amounts, at specific times, and you've got tragedy. An example is the 20 deaths from air pollution that took place in Donora, Pennsylvania, in 1948.[6]

There have been other American tragedies like it, and more will probably come, unless we expect them. And we really don't expect them.

Types of Air Pollution

Chemical pollutants get a lot of publicity from Ralph Nader and his followers. And rightly so. Automotive, industrial, and domestic wastes have assumed a major place in modern society. They kill trees and fish, make a sunny day seem dingy. But there are radioactive and biological pollutants that people often forget about.

The radioactive type got a lot of attention 10 to 20 years ago. This was when nuclear power was new, when each atomic test was in the headlines, when terms like "fallout," "mutation," and "ground zero" were common. Today fear of the hydrogen bomb, nuclear reactors, and radiation might have faded a bit. But radioactive pollutants are with us, and they're not going to get blown away by winds of public opinion. They're destructive, often lethal, and could eliminate every living thing on this earth if they got out of hand.

Biological dusts and pollens aren't nearly as harmful as the other two types of air pollution. But for the poor fellow suffering from asthma or hay fever, they make life miserable. The chemical and radiation type, though, can make life impossible.[7]

Industrial Pollutants

Without the machine, the furnace, the turbine, and the piston, most of chemical air pollution wouldn't exist. It's the price we pay for driving automobiles, turning on electric lights, enjoying hot baths, watching television. We have a standard of living Louis XVI or Beau Brummel wouldn't have dreamed of, but this standard isn't all blessing. There are hydrocarbons from automobiles and petroleum refineries. There are nitrogen oxides coming from all types of oil and gas burners, again including the automobile. There are sulfur oxides that chemical processes emit. There is smoke from incinerators, dust and fumes coming out of the earth where natural resources are mined. In some respects, man never had it so good. In some respects, he's a perennial loser.

One measure of air pollution is monthly dust fall. The Illinois Institute of Technology used this measure in Chicago recently and found the average ranged between 52.9 and 71 tons per square mile. If this sounds like a lot of grime and filth, it is. Louisville, Kentucky, has a little filth of its own. About 440 tons of man-made pollutants get thrown in this city's air each day. And 100 tons of hydrocarbons, up to 80 tons of nitrogen dioxides, and 4 tons of sulfur dioxide enter Seattle's atmosphere on a daily basis from automobiles alone.[8]

Meteorological Conditions

It was a foggy day in London town. Or was it Los Angeles, Las Vegas, Chicago, or Tokyo? A lot of pollution problems are brought on by atmo-

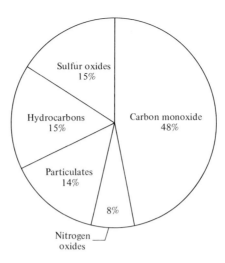

FIGURE 16-4. *Elements of air pollution.*

spheric conditions that corporations can't really control. True, the factories and the cars and the insecticides create the atmospheric muck. But the atmosphere itself helps to spread it around, concentrate it, churn it into a destructive gas. There's a condition known as thermal inversion. Warm air gets trapped by mountains, high buildings, or sometimes wind currents and hangs over a city. When this air is warmer than the atmosphere at ground level, it forms a blanket that keeps the other air from rising and the contaminants along with it. Then warm and radiant sunlight enters the scene to "cook" the hydrocarbons, which turns them into the kinds of gases we call air pollution. The city smells foul and looks dirty, breathing gets difficult, and eyes sting. The atmosphere has contributed to a condition known as

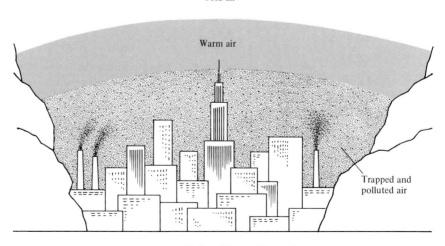

FIGURE 16-5. *Thermal inversion.*

403

photochemical smog, a plague on many of the great industrial centers of twentieth-century mankind.[9]

Rural Contaminants

There was a time when only honeysuckle, new-mown hay, Mom's fresh baked apple pie could be smelled by the barefoot boy with cheeks of tan. Then came smoke, cement plant dust, insecticide aerosols, sawdust, smudge pot fumes, and odors from industrial and organic wastes. It's the kind of air pollution you don't find in the city. It's a unique type of pollution, varying from town to farm to county. It is noxious, though, and definitely destructive. The sweet country air, like the trolley cars of the big city, largely belongs to an earlier time.[10]

Preventing Air Pollution

There's been some talk about new techniques of making smog harmless, eliminating the harmful fumes that come from smokestacks and automobile exhausts, keeping dusts and pollens in a location not inhabited by asthma and hay fever sufferers. Most of this talk is pure nonsense or refers to some type of research project, not some viable program for air pollution control. The main method of keeping the atmosphere somewhat clean is limiting the type and number of contaminants that enter it. To do this, you have to start by gathering data. How much air is available at a given location, and what's the composition of this air? What kind of pollutants is the community producing, and in what quantity? Are there any meteorological factors that work on this pollution?

There are several groups gathering these data for communities planning air pollution control programs. But the National Air Sampling Network of the Public Health Service is the one most commonly used. It has a network of several hundred substations located in every state, plus Puerto Rico and the District of Columbia. It gathers data on all types of chemicals, dust, and smoke contaminants and makes them available to any community, town, or industry that's interested.[11]

LEGISLATION

Obviously, government was going to enter the atmospheric picture. Voters demanded it, Ralph Nader demanded it, and General Motors couldn't stop it. So the Clean Air Act of 1970 was born. This federal law requires that all new light-duty vehicles reduce carbon monoxide, nitrogen oxide, and hydrocarbon emissions by 90 per cent by 1975. As to used cars, the law grants states the authority to control emissions. And the act doesn't deal with automobiles alone. Industrial and municipal smokestacks come under its authority, with the entire United States being divided into "ambient" areas.

An ambient area can be larger than a given state or smaller than one. It's a territory without political boundaries whose atmosphere can be averaged out for air pollution. In some spots the air might be chokingly dirty, in some refreshingly clean. Public health needs and protection of public welfare dictate air-quality standards these areas have to meet. The standards pertaining to health are "primary" ones; "secondary" standards pertain to public welfare.

States have to comply with the federal standards, and they have to develop and carry out some of their own. Theoretically, they can make these standards as stringent as they like, but some companies have challenged this principle in the courts, claiming that the federal standards should take precedence. In any event, the states and the Environmental Protection Agency, the federal government's pollution control arm, are working together to maintain the kind of air that man likes to breathe.[12]

Cost of Air Pollution

There is no way to calculate the cost of corrosion, crop losses, medical bills, cleaning bills, and property damage brought on by smog. The damage is so extensive and often so subtle that it's hard to identify, let alone evaluate. What is the cost of a case of asthma, a dirty building, some gritty artichokes? Damage is in the billions, of course, but how many billions depends on who's making the estimate. The cost of cleaning dirty air, though, is a little more definite. Manufacturing and utility plants are spending about $600 million per year to reduce the hydrocarbon and nitrogen oxide emissions coming out of their smokestacks. The overall pollution control cost is over $1 billion yearly for private industry, and it promises to get much higher.[13]

Water Pollution

It's in our faucets, in our showers, in lakes, oceans, bathtubs, and mud puddles. It even rains water. And the cost is infinitesimal, so the supply seems limitless. But like the buffalo, the bald eagle, and the redwood, the supply isn't limitless. And America, like many other countries, can experience a water shortage. By 1980, we'll need 600 billion gallons a day. By the year 2000, it'll be 1,000 billion gallons. But no matter how we juggle our current resources, there's no way we can have more than 650 billion gallons per day, even by using the most modern processing methods.

And any amount of water won't be enough unless it's pollution free. Water pollution is probably a greater threat to health than air pollution is. There are detergents, pesticides, radioactive wastes, and the like in thousands of rivers and streams. There are septic tanks that drain into underground streams. And though this water can be made safe for drinking and cooking, the problem gets greater as the American industrial giant continues to grow. And there's food we need that has to have reasonably clean water to live. Millions of fish die each year because their habitat has become poisoned by a gross, air-breathing creature with two legs.

Just about all water comes from rainfall. Without this destroyer of baseball games, Sunday picnics, and political rallies, the world would be a desert, a lifeless ball of sand. Before the days of suburbia, paved streets, and parking lots, this priceless commodity would pour to earth and percolate

405

through soil and rocks to underground lakes and streams. Now, of course, it evaporates from cement or falls directly into surface reservoirs. Urbanization has given us two-car garages and patios with barbecue pits. But it's reduced our water supply and interfered with natural purification of the water we get.[14]

Types of Water Pollution

You can contaminate water in an unlimited number of ways, of course. But the pollutants that usually make it unfit for human use fall into one of the following categories:

1. Infectious agents in sewage. These transmit disease for man, animal, fish, and plant.
2. Organic wastes in sewage. These can be industrial wastes as well as human and animal. Both types remove oxygen from the water when they decompose.
3. Sediment. This can build up in harbors, reservoirs, stream channels. It can erode hydroelectric equipment, blanket fish nests, and increase the cost of water treatment.
4. Certain types of plant nutrients that bring on the growth of nuisance aquatic plants such as algae and water weeds.
5. Inorganic chemicals and minerals. These come from industry and agriculture to destroy life in the sea, harden the water, produce corrosion, and make drinking water expensive to purify.
6. Synthetic-organic chemicals. Detergents and pesticides are typical of this category. The miracle of modern technology constantly produces new ones, and each is a new threat to aquatic life and life that isn't aquatic.
7. Radioactive pollution. This can come from nuclear fallout, of course. And it can come from the processing of radioactive ores. It's one of the most destructive forms of pollution. But, fortunately, there's not too much of it.
8. Excessive heat. Water is used a lot for cooling purposes, so it absorbs the heat of what it's supposed to cool. Dumping hot water into a bay or lake or reservoir is hard on aquatic life. If it doesn't kill fish outright, it can change their metabolism so that they die slowly. And it can lower the water's ability to hold oxygen, which can bring on slow death, too.[15]

Sewage Treatment

About one-fourth of all American municipalities discharge untreated wastes into the nearest streams. There's another third that put this waste through primary treatment before discharging it. This involves screening it to get rid of large objects, then putting it in settling tanks to let the sediment work its way to the bottom. The solids, called "sludge," get collected and sent to a "digestion tank," where anaerobic bacteria go to work on it. This brings on the first stages of biochemical oxidation. The final residue is dried in the open air and gets sold as fertilizer or buried or burned. Obviously, munici-

TABLE 16-1
Pollution-Caused Fish Kill, by Source of Pollution and
Type of Water: 1965–1972
(Fish in thousands. Estimates based on reports from state agencies responsible for fisheries management.)

Item	1965	1970	1971	1972
Number of reports	446	560	860*	760
Fish reported killed	11,393	22,286	73,625	17,717
Source of pollution				
Agricultural operations	1,390	1,810	1,023	1,807
Insecticides, poisons,				
etc.	771	1,410	265	1,500
Fertilizers	3	4	66	31
Manure-silage				
drainage	617	396	693	276
Industrial operations	3,764	9,589	4,644	4,694
Chemicals	219	429	2,400	826
Food and kindred				
products	537	2,708	72	328
Mining	295	622	221	310
Paper and allied				
products	495	609	46	721
Petroleum	1,516	40	233	345
Metals	73	135	284	129
Combinations	492	3,620	1,120	1,256
Other	138	1,426	268	779
Municipal operations	5,912	6,602	24,799	8,361
Refuse disposal	17	9	81	38
Sewerage systems	5,211	6,513	21,353	3,697
Water systems	604	20	86	3
Other	79	60†	3,279	4,623
Transportation operations	307	465	664	456
Pipeline	197	50	5	118
Truck	106	85	441	300
Other	3	330	218	38
Other operations	21	3,820	7,245	1,029
Unknown	—	—	35,249	1,369
Type of water				
Fresh	11,256	11,991	15,206*	10,666
Salt	102	536	2,015*	38
Estuary	36	9,759	56,404*	7,010
Average duration of				
kill (days)	2.6	3.3	3.4	3.4

* Includes unknown.
† Includes 58,100 in 1970 killed by power operations.

Source: Pollution-Caused Fish Kills (Washington, D.C.: U.S. Environmental Protection Agency, Water Quality Office, annual).

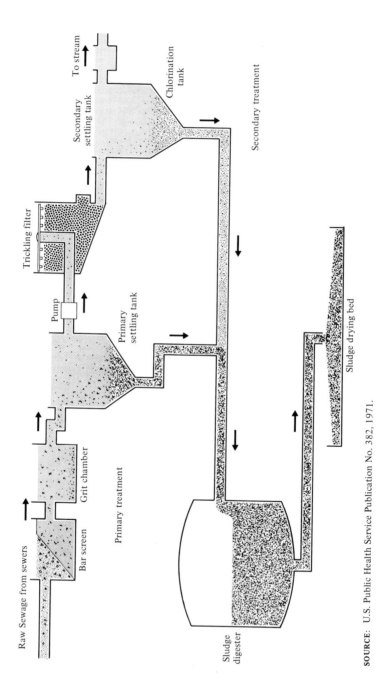

FIGURE 16-6. *Sewage plant.*

SOURCE: U.S. Public Health Service Publication No. 382, 1971.

palities that dump their wastes in the water without putting it through primary treatment dump unfiltered residue as well.

About half of American municipalities use secondary treatment as well as primary treatment. Here the liquid part of the waste in the settling tank goes through another filtering process. The common way to do it is spray it onto a bed of coarse stones, where the droplets trickle to the bottom of the bed and flow into an underground drainage system. The cycle is repeated several times, making the maximum use of sunlight and aerobic bacteria for oxidation and purification. Then comes chlorination to kill the odor and remaining bacteria before the liquid gets dumped back into the river or bay.

If primary and secondary treatments sound effective, the sound doesn't ring true. Only about a third of all organic wastes, be they from animals or vegetables, get removed by primary treatment. Secondary treatment removes about 90 per cent, but we're talking about organic waste only. Neither process removes a significant amount of the inorganic variety. So in today's cities, with their appalling industrial parks, churning automobiles, trucks, airplanes, and gas stations, a tremendous amount of pollution gets poured into rivers and streams, whether the sewage is treated or not.

Around the turn of the century, the streams were getting about 15 per cent of the pollutants they get today. But that was before America's great surge of progress, the two-car garage, the television set, and automatic data processing. Also, waste treatment plants rely heavily on bacterial action. This works fine on wastes that come from people or other organisms. But bacteria can't do much with leftovers from the nylon industry and the detergent and plastic industries, or with pesticides, herbicides, and medicines. The same applies to acids draining from mines, radioactive material, and salt.

And the picture probably won't improve in the near future. There's likely to be an increased urban growth rate, which is going to increase the sewage discharge, which will require additional primary and secondary treatment plants. These are being built, of course. But if the building rate continues at its current pace, municipal sewage discharge will be 52 per cent greater in 1980 than it was in 1960. Possibly there will be a surge in treatment plant construction. The federal government might panic; state and local governments might become a little upset, too. With a massive effort, we might be able to keep the 1980 sewage discharge rate just about the same as it is today.[16]

Recycling Used Water

We don't use water just once. Water in most streams gets at least two exposures to the living world. Water in major rivers, like the Ohio and Mississippi, can be used three or four times. Of course, each time water gets used it gets polluted. And this calls for a cleaning process before it can be used again. This may not sound too aesthetic, but there's really nothing wrong with the procedure if the water is properly cleaned. The better and more economically this can be done, the more often the water can be used.

There's been a lot of research on this recycling process. Scientists have experimented with distillation, foaming, ion exchange, freezing, adsorption by carbon and other filters, electrodialysis, electrolysis, and solvent extrac-

TABLE 16-2
Federal Funds for Pollution Control and Abatement—Summary: 1970, 1972, and 1973

(In millions of dollars. For years ending June 30. Obligations refer to liabilities, contracts, and other commitments entered into requiring the payment of money by the government. Outlays refer to the issuance of checks or disbursements of cash by the government to liquidate obligations. Outlays during any fiscal year may be payments of obligations incurred in prior years or in the same year.)

Media or Pollutants	Obligations		
	1970	1972	1973 (est.)
Total	1,071	1,868	5,336
Water	677	1,167	4,344
Air	189	373	535
Land	35	55	57
Living things, materials, etc.	100	200	314
Multimedia*	69	73	86
Selected pollutants†			
Radiation	116	141	174
Noise	36	77	103
Pesticides	30	40	45
Solid wastes	20	91	116

Agency	Outlays		
	1970	1972	1973 (est.)
Total	751	1,314	1,917
Environmental Protection Agency‡	388	763	1,147
Atomic Energy Commission	116	138	162
Department of Defense	42	142	213
Department of Agriculture	91	77	110
Department of Interior	37	73	103
Department of Commerce	22	12	16
Department of Transportation	11	40	73
National Aero and Space Administration	15	16	36
National Science Foundation	7	15	15
Other	23	38	42

* More than one of media shown above.
† Funds for "Selected pollutants" included in "media" breakdown above.
‡ Includes funds for activities carried out by U.S. Departments of Health, Education, and Welfare; Agriculture; and Interior; and by the Atomic Energy Commission and the Federal Radiation Council prior to December 2, 1970.

Source: *Special Analyses, Budget of the United States Government* (Washington, D.C.: U.S. Office of Management and Budget).

tion. And they've met with a certain amount of success. It's possible that the recycling and treatment methods we know today can become obsolete in the future, possibly archaic. And it's possible that new treatment methods won't be economically feasible or feasible in any other way. Technological progress has conquered some diseases, some famine, and a certain amount of filth. It might conquer the dirty water problem, too. But don't count on it. Like any other approach, technology meets with more failure than it does success.[17]

Food Pollutants

You have to have food to live. It's like air and water. If you get the wrong kind of it or a poisoned version of it, it'll kill you. If you don't get any, you'll die, too. So man takes a chance every time he bites into a steak, slurps on an ice cream soda, swallows a vitamin pill. This chance he has to take, but there's no reason why the odds can't be as highly in his favor as possible. Certainly, the odds are much better than they were in Abe Lincoln's day, even in Teddy Roosevelt's day. There probably weren't a hundred major food items sold in general stores before the twentieth century. And most of these were produce and dry staples from local farms. Perishable foods got consumed before they perished. And though there were home canning and other ways of preserving certain items, it wasn't done on a broad commercial scale. Vinegar and sugar were the key preservative agents. They didn't keep the food from spoiling for long, but no one worried about it too much. No one had much of an idea about foodborne diseases.

Then Pasteur's germ theory caught on, railroads provided transportation for manufacturing plants, farm machinery replaced the plow and mule, and mechanical refrigeration was perfected. By 1900, the commercial food industry came into its own, and the number of items on grocery store shelves began to increase rapidly.

What also increased rapidly were foods saturated with formaldehyde, boric acid, and other misery-producing preservatives; candy colored with poisonous dyes; canned goods with misleading and fraudulent labels; and filth. It was time for the government to enter the picture, which it did in 1906 by passing the Pure Food and Drug Law. But this law was vaguely worded and didn't provide much enforcement authority. It wasn't until 1958 that the Food and Drug Administration got the power to approve food additives before they were put on the market. By this time, there were hundreds of additives already in use. So the new legislation had a grandfather clause that exempted substances "generally recognized as safe" (GRAS).

There are hundreds of GRAS additives. There are sequestrants, which keep soft drinks from turning cloudy and fats and oils from becoming rancid. There are emulsifying agents, which force substances that normally don't mix to do so. Without these, you wouldn't have homogenized milk. And there are anticaking agents, which keep salt and sugar from becoming crystalline lumps. Without additives food would spoil, sometimes be less nutritious, probably be more expensive. But most of the GRAS items have never been completely tested for long-term harmful effects. Can one or more of them produce cancer over a 30-year period? How about birth defects, glandular deficiency, stomach ulcers? True, these items probably cause no more harm than pure drinking water and fresh air, but we know the difference between dirty and clean water and polluted and clean air. We ought to be sure of the difference between contaminated and uncontaminated food as well.[18]

Food Contamination by Microbes

There are about a million cases of food poisoning in the United States each year. This may not seem surprising, because everyone gets an occasional stomachache or case of diarrhea. But the million involve the serious cases, the ones that call for doctors and hospitals. Shigella organisms, staphylococci, and salmonellae are usually what bring the sicknesses on. And usually it's dirty kitchens, careless cooks, and sick waitresses who spread this kind of disease rather than the food industry. Some will protest this, claiming that sanitary practices in food packaging plants are less than perfect. Without a doubt, this is true. The Food and Drug Administration initiates about 3,500 legal actions each year against various commercial segments in the food and drug industries. There are prosecutions, citations, seizures, and about 7,500 detentions. Industry itself sometimes voluntarily recalls food from the marketplace that could kill people or make them wish they were dead. But, despite managerial inefficiency, worker indifference, union selfishness, and capitalistic self-indulgence, the corporate world of food isn't what brings on most of the diarrhea or gas pain. It's carelessness, sometimes a little ignorance, sometimes total indifference to sanitary practices. Washing hands after using the latrine is too much trouble; covering foods so flies can't light on it is "nonsense." Who worries about a little potato salad left in the sun? It tastes better when it's warm.[19] Here are a few cases of misery that could have been avoided with a little thought:

    1. The roast beef and gravy tasted great. It was tender, yet firm, flavored with just the right amount of salt, and good and hot. True, it had been reheated after having been prepared the day before and allowed to cool in the open air. But this way no one had to wait to be served. Having meals prepared just when people are ready to eat can be a big problem at a banquet. Preparing the food early and then reheating it got rid of all the worries. There were a few worries that developed later, though. Of the 170 people who attended the dinner, 155 came down with severe diarrhea.

    Clostridium perfringens organisms were the culprits. They worked their way into the beef and gravy. But the fellow preparing the beef and gravy paved the way for them. If he had followed the rule of keeping cooked food at 140° Fahrenheit or above until serving it, or cooling it below 45°F, probably the guests would have felt fine.

    2. A similar incident took place at sea. There were 17 persons who came down with diarrhea, vomiting, cramps, and the like a few hours after eating their noon meal. It was the salad that did them in. There were chopped pimientos, boiled eggs, mayonnaise, lettuce, mustard, and macaroni hand-mixed by two cooks. The salad tasted great, despite the *Staphylococcus aureus* that poured out of one of the cook's cut fingers. No one tasted the bacteria, but eventually their presence became known.

This wouldn't have happened, of course, if the cook had used utensils to mix the salad instead of his cut fingers. In fact, even if fingers aren't cut, it's better to keep them out of food. Utensils can be sanitized a lot more thoroughly than hands can.

3. In this case there were vomiting and nausea, too. And there were also problems with speaking and breathing, and the victims' vision got blurred. Some even became temporarily paralyzed. The sickness here was botulism, which affected four people, killing one. Home-canned chili had caused the problem. The temperature and pressure hadn't been high enough during the canning process to keep toxin from forming.

Despite Safeway, Krogers, and A&P, a lot of people still do canning. It can save money, and it can provide a variety of things hard to find in stores. But it's a dangerous process when people don't use pressure cookers. Without them, they often don't get the high temperatures and pressures necessary to destroy toxin-producing spores. And even a touch of this toxin can kill or bring on serious illness. Also, toxin strikes without warning. You can't taste it or smell it, so you never know it's there until it's too late.

4. Eleven people in a small community came down with trichinosis. They had stomach cramps, chills, muscle pain, ran very high fevers, and became extremely weak. They were lucky. Trichinosis can and often does kill. *Trichinella sprialis* is the parasite that brings the disease on. It is sometimes present in uncooked pork. In the case of the 11 victims we're referring to, all had eaten raw, smoked sausage that had come from a particular hog.

These people could have enjoyed their sausage and felt fine if they'd cooked it. Before being served, pork should always be brought to 150°F, which destroys the parasite. However, the 150°F has to be the internal temperature of the meat, not just the temperature on the surface. So the cook should always use a thermometer.

5. Two people became dizzy and numb and vomited profusely after eating some mushrooms. They couldn't understand it; the mushrooms were fresh, they'd picked them themselves. And they had cleaned them thoroughly before preparing them for supper. The problem lay with the mushrooms themselves, which were poisonous.

It's best to leave the picking of mushrooms and other "wild foods" to Euell Gibbons. He knows the difference between those that will hurt you and those that won't. Most people don't.

6. No one was quite sure what caused the people who attended a church dinner to become sick after eating the barbecued chicken. It was the barbecued chicken, of course, that caused the problem. But there was a lot of argument about which phase of the preparation had brought on the upset. Maybe it was the lack of refrigeration. The chickens had been cooked the day before the dinner, refrigerated, then reheated, cut into quarters, then allowed to stand in the open air between 10 A.M. and 5 P.M. No doubt about it, this might not have had the best effect on people who ate the poultry. And maybe this wasn't the problem at all. The hands of one of the cooks had several abrasions and small cuts. The chicken had traveled from these hands to people's mouths. Or maybe the meat saw that cut the chicken into quarters was at fault. This wasn't the cleanest meat saw that had ever graced a church social.

There could have been any number of things that contaminated the chicken. Possibly it was a combination of factors that brought on the trouble. Everyone who had worked on the preparation of the dinner realized that sanitation wasn't quite up to par. But, after all, these were just minor details. You shouldn't get bogged down in details.[20]

Radiation

There were the blinding light, the mushroom cloud, the rumbling shock wave, and the sickening wind. Hiroshima was leveled, and the radiation age was born. Now man could worry about isotopes and fallout, gamma rays and radioactive wastes. But, in fairness, the radiation hazard was with us long before man smashed his first atom. It comes from the sun, from certain elements, from meteorites, from the universe. Many feel that evolution wouldn't take place without natural radiation. This is what brings on mutation of the genes. But the man-made variety can be a lot more intense and harmful than the type Mother Nature comes up with. Some of the more common types of man-made radiation are the following:

RADIOTHERAPY

Radiotherapy is the major source of man-made radiation in the 1970s. We use it to make X-rays of various shapes and sizes. We treat certain illnesses with it, too.

INDUSTRIAL X-RAYS

Manufacturers use X-rays to discover flaws in castings and welds and other products that might have structural defects.

RADIOACTIVE ISOTOPES

Radioactive isotopes are atoms of radioactive elements. They're used a lot in medical diagnosis and treatment. And sometimes they're used in industry.

RADIOACTIVE FALLOUT

Radioactive fallout comes from the explosion of nuclear devices. It usually affects just a limited number of people but can contaminate cities, nations, the world.[21]

Bodily Effects of Radiation

Radiation can kill cells. Only relatively large doses of it kill, but recovery isn't always complete from the damage smaller doses bring on. A lot depends on the types of cells and tissues involved. Tissues that constantly regenerate through cell division and multiplication are the most vulnerable. Gonadal

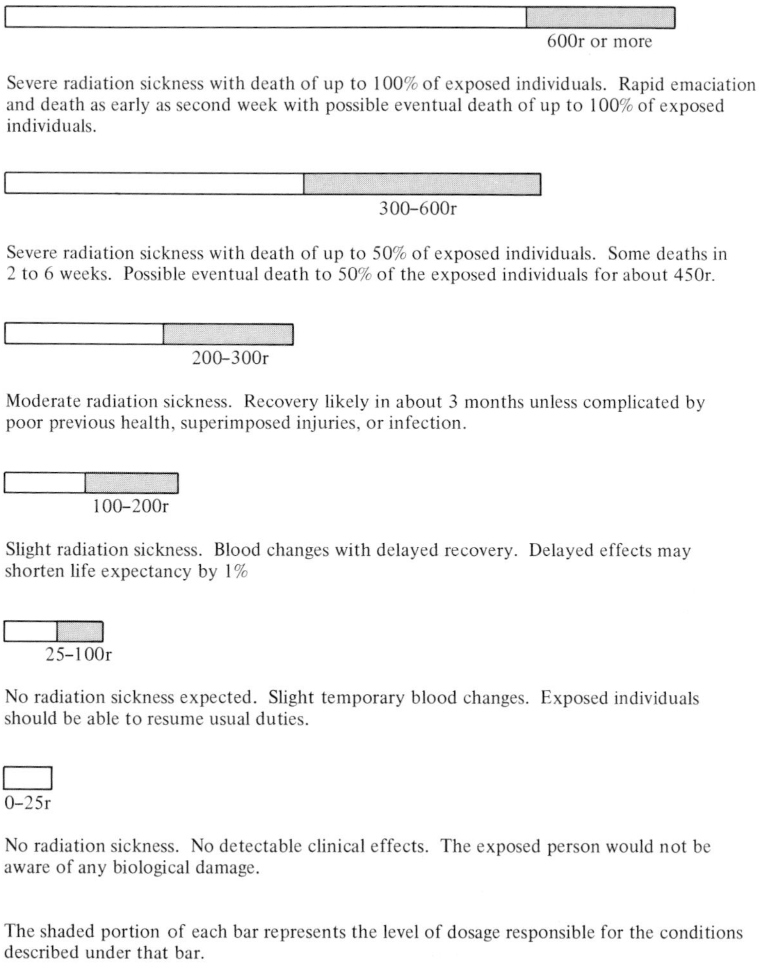

```
┌─────────────────────────────────────────────┬──────────┐
│                                             │░░░░░░░░░░│
└─────────────────────────────────────────────┴──────────┘
```
600r or more

Severe radiation sickness with death of up to 100% of exposed individuals. Rapid emaciation and death as early as second week with possible eventual death of up to 100% of exposed individuals.

```
┌─────────────────────────┬──────────────────┐
│                         │░░░░░░░░░░░░░░░░░░│
└─────────────────────────┴──────────────────┘
```
300–600r

Severe radiation sickness with death of up to 50% of exposed individuals. Some deaths in 2 to 6 weeks. Possible eventual death to 50% of the exposed individuals for about 450r.

```
┌──────────┬──────────────┐
│          │░░░░░░░░░░░░░░│
└──────────┴──────────────┘
```
200–300r

Moderate radiation sickness. Recovery likely in about 3 months unless complicated by poor previous health, superimposed injuries, or infection.

```
┌─────┬─────────┐
│     │░░░░░░░░░│
└─────┴─────────┘
```
100–200r

Slight radiation sickness. Blood changes with delayed recovery. Delayed effects may shorten life expectancy by 1%

```
┌────┬──────┐
│    │░░░░░░│
└────┴──────┘
```
25–100r

No radiation sickness expected. Slight temporary blood changes. Exposed individuals should be able to resume usual duties.

```
┌──────────┐
│          │
└──────────┘
```
0–25r

No radiation sickness. No detectable clinical effects. The exposed person would not be aware of any biological damage.

The shaded portion of each bar represents the level of dosage responsible for the conditions described under that bar.

SOURCE: *Peacetime Radiation Hazards in the Fire Service*, U.S. Department of Health, Education, and Welfare and U.S. Atomic Energy Commission, 1961, p. 15.

FIGURE 16-7. *External radiation doses.*

germ cells are a good example. The skin is another. This type of tissue damage usually falls into two classes:

SOMATIC TISSUE DAMAGE

"Somatic" is used to describe the general tissue throughout the body. A lot of damage to it, of course, can bring on lesions and abnormalities and localized destruction. Sometimes the effects of radiation don't show immediately, but they can slowly alter cell functions, possibly bring on leukemia or other forms of cancer.

415

GENETIC DAMAGE

Genetic damage doesn't show in the individual who received the radiation. His offspring and their offspring are the ones who pay with malformed bodies and sensory impairments. The radiation damages the original victim's reproductive cells, so his ability to pass on healthy characteristics to his children gets damaged, too. There's no need for massive radiation doses to bring this tragedy about. Minor amounts of it can produce all the heartbreak people can stand.[22]

Radioactive Fallout

When nuclear devices are exploded, radioactive material spreads throughout the atmosphere. Fallout is the return of this material to earth. Sometimes people use the term to describe radiation contamination of soil, air, food, and water.

No two fallout patterns are the same. The height of the burst, the yield, and the meteorological conditions determine the size, amount, and shape of these contaminants. Also, there are ionization effects to consider. These affect the radiation dosage as much as the quantity of radioactive material does.

There's about 110 pounds of highly radioactive substance for every megaton of fission. Luckily, most of this material has a very short radioactive life. In a little over 2 days, the radioactivity of the fallout material is less than 1/100 of what it was within an hour after the explosion. In 2 weeks, the radioactivity is 1/1,000; in 3 months, 1/10,000. So most fallout, except in the area where the bomb exploded, has lost most of its destructive potential by the time it gets back to earth. This doesn't mean, of course, that we should ignore it. In technically advanced countries, fallout accounts for a sizable percentage of the radiation dosage found in human bone marrow. It may not be a large enough dose to kill, but no one can be sure of just what the long-range effects of this condition are.[23]

Radioactive Waste Disposal

Potentially, disposal of radioactive wastes is a much bigger problem than fallout. There are so many different types of radioactive wastes coming out of industry that there's no single or simple solution as to how to get rid of them. You can't destroy the radioactivity. Only time, which allows for radioactive decay, can deal with the problem. The waste eventually has a very low radioactivity level and becomes almost harmless. How long this takes depends on the type of radioactive material being treated, the amount of this material involved, and the conditions of the area where it's being disposed of. But no matter how carefully the problem has been studied or approached, no completely satisfactory disposal method exists.

Processing sites of the United States Atomic Energy Commission receive most radioactive waste coming out of reactors. It gets shipped to the sites, where it "cools" for 90 days, which lets radioactive isotopes with short lives decay. Then the residue is classified according to energy level and disposed of as follows:

1. The high-level radioactive wastes get placed in storage tanks for long-term decay.
2. Medium-level wastes sometimes go into storage tanks, too. And sometimes they're held in trenches or put in artificial ponds until they decay to a level where it's safe to discharge them into the environment. Sometimes the medium-level wastes get mixed with concrete in steel drums and get dumped at sea or buried.
3. The low-level variety, which has a radioactive concentration of less than 1 microcurie per gallon, usually is diluted with water and released to the sea, the air, or the land.[24]

There's been a lot of research into ways of disposing of these wastes more quickly, safely, and cheaply. Chemical processing seemed to offer a certain amount of promise a few years ago. But it, like other methods, didn't meet with much success. Possibly there is a more efficient method in the offing. But, until it's found, radioactive wastes will be a public hazard and a major public expense.[25]

Noise Pollution

They put a plug in the guinea pig's left ear. Then they exposed it to 122 decibels of cacophonous screeching, yelling, blasting, blowing, snorting,

FIGURE 16-8. *Tomorrow's child inherits tomorrow's world.*

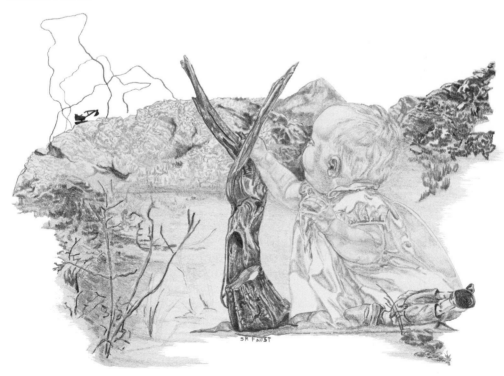

growling called rock 'n' roll music. The 122 decibels was selected because that's about the sound level most teenagers face at discotheques, dance halls, and rock concerts. Incidentally, a whisper is about 30 decibels loud, ordinary conversation around 60, a motorcycle around 110, a jet plane 140, a close-range cannon 160. The guinea pig's plugged ear turned out just fine. There was no damage to the hair cells in the cochlea, none to the tympanic membrane, none to the ability to hear. Not so for the ear exposed to the pulsating sounds of youth's ritualistic vibrations. There was irreparable damage, and never again would the guinea pig's world sound quite the same. Of course, you can't apply the findings in an animal experiment to humans. But research on two-legged animals has pointed to similar conclusions. Modern society, with shotgun blasts, riveters, power mowers, city traffic, and trumpet solos, is turning the old into Sonotone users, the young into the turned-off society having trouble turning back on.[26]

Noise's Effect on Health

Sound is a physical force. It comes from waves traveling through the atmosphere, which create energy and heat. If you focus sound vibrations at 179 decibels, the heat released by the energy can start a fire, kill a small animal. If you focus 130 decibels on someone's eardrum, you can do permanent damage to his hearing. And if someone faces 100 decibels or so, over an extended period, he can have permanent damage, too. So modern society faces a modern health problem—noise.

It's something like air pollution. It's with you every day; it seems like a natural part of your environment. Surely it can't be producing harm. Something you can hardly notice can't really harm you. Unfortunately, people lose their hearing without being aware that they're losing it. You don't need much acuity to hear an ordinary 60-decibel conversation. And the pressure of loud sound destroys peripheral hearing long before it affects the ability to hear speech. Someone who has a 40 per cent hearing impairment according to an audiometer test may not even be aware that he's going deaf.

Also, loud noise may cause high blood pressure. Granted, this has never been absolutely proven. But many authorities feel that the constriction of blood vessels and reduced output from the heart come from noise as well as from smoking, overeating, and lack of exercise. Continuous noise may even bring on peptic ulcers. And what about sleep? Do we really sleep through train whistles, sirens, sonic boom explosions, parties and loud TV sets in the next apartment? If we do sleep, do we really rest? According to brain wave studies, we really don't. When you wake up exhausted in the morning, when you need three cups of coffee before you can face your family and job, when you doze in your classes, stumble exhausted through the day oblivious to happenings and friends, possibly you're not undernourished, don't have a cold, don't have iron deficiency anemia. The jet planes that soared overhead, the drag racers that went by your window at 2 o'clock in the morning, and the blaring radio down the hall might really be at fault, even though you weren't aware of them.[27]

Cost of Noise

And, unlike the best things in life, noise isn't free. American industry's bill is about $4 billion annually for noise-produced accidents and lost production time. One company reduced its typing errors by 29 per cent, employee turnover by 37 per cent, absenteeism by 47 per cent, and errors by machine operators by 52 per cent by soundproofing the office. A noisy New York bank plagued with high employee turnover finally resorted to hiring deaf people. And there was a factory manager who made a major reduction in costly worker errors by moving the assembly line out of hearing distance of the boiler room.[28]

Control of Noise

Of course, we can control the problem. Other countries do. Paris garbage cans have to be covered by rubber or plastic lids. And Paris doesn't permit transistor radios in public places. West Germany has a similar type of law pertaining to radios and extends it to TV as well. And, despite the West Germans' desperate need for housing, construction noise is limited. Britain has antinoise legislation. So do Russia and many of the countries behind the Iron Curtain; many of the countries we send aid to for industrial growth.

America deals with the noise problem on a local basis, which often isn't too effective. There are thousands of cities, towns, and counties jealous of their own prerogatives, and rightly so. But quite often their governments don't think noise pollution is a serious problem, aren't even aware of it as a problem, or fail to enforce legislation dealing with the problem. This legislation, also, can be pretty inadequate. There's a California law that lets a 50-horsepower motorcycle make as much noise as a 300-horsepower Cadillac.[29]

Modern home construction often contributes to the situation. This is the day of lots of glass and open floor plans, which bring on acoustical bedlam. But many people are willing to tolerate noise, thinking they'll get used to it, just so their homes or apartments comply with the standards of American suburbia.[30]

But can't you have a home, an office, a club that's too quiet? You certainly can. This is a form of pollution in its own right. Someone's whisper seems like a shout, human footsteps like rhinoceros footsteps, drumming on a table like drums in a band. But this problem isn't hard to deal with. There's "white noise" or "acoustical perfume" that can change the environment from vacuum-like silence to the relaxing hum of country spring. There are soft music, the taped sound of running brooks and chirping birds, even whispered poetry. Silence is a pollution modern technology can deal with. Noise isn't. And the problem will get worse without public awareness, public indignation, public demands for solutions.[31]

Notes

1. Sterling Brubaker, *To Live on Earth* (Baltimore: Johns Hopkins Press, 1972), pp. 11–47.

2. Arthur S. Boughey, *Contemporary Readings in Ecology* (Belmont, Calif.: Dickenson, 1969).
3. World Health Organization, *Health Hazards of the Human Environment* (Geneva: World Health Organization, 1972), pp. 205–210.
4. Ibid., pp. 78–89.
5. W. L. Faith and Arthur A. Atkinson, Jr., *Air Pollution* (New York: Interscience, 1972).
6. Arthur C. Stern, ed., *Air Pollution,* Vol. 1, 2nd. ed. (New York: Academic Press, 1968).
7. Morris B. Jacobs, *The Chemical Analysis of Air Pollutants* (New York: Interscience, 1960).
8. Joe O. Ledbetter, *Air Pollution* (New York: Dekker, 1972), pp. 40–81.
9. Louis J. Bottan, *The Unclean Sky* (Garden City, N.Y.: Doubleday, 1966).
10. Jacobs, *Chemical Analysis,* pp. 252–276.
11. Wesley E. Brittin, Ronald West, and Robert Williams, eds., *Air and Water Pollution* (Boulder, Colo.: Colorado Associated University Press, 1970), pp. 425–459.
12. George H. Hagevik, *Decision Making in Air Pollution Control* (New York: Praeger, 1970), pp. 128–165.
13. Howard E. Hesketh, *Understanding and Controlling Air Pollution* (Ann Arbor, Mich.: Ann Arbor Science Publishers, 1972), pp. 356–365.
14. Brittin et al., *Air and Water Pollution,* pp. 1–113.
15. R. Michael Stevens, *Green Land—Clean Streams* (Philadelphia: Temple University Press, 1972), pp. 1–15.
16. R. L. Bolton and L. Klein, *Sewage Treatment* (Ann Arbor, Mich.: Ann Arbor Science Publishers, 1971).
17. Russel L. Culp and Gordon L. Culp, *Advanced Wastewater Treatment* (New York: Van Nostrand Reinhold, 1971).
18. Beatrice Trum Hunter, *Consumer Beware!* (New York: Simon and Schuster, 1971), pp. 79–109.
19. Fred W. Tanner, *Food–Borne Infections and Intoxications* (Champaign, Ill.: Garrard Press, 1953).
20. (Staff) Review of Minnesota Extension Bulletin 339, *Food Poisoning: Salmonellosis and Staphylococcus Poisoning,* Consumer Bulletin No. 53 (August 1970), 15–17.
21. Lawrence H. Lanzl, John H. Pringel, and John H. Rust, eds., *Radiation Accidents and Emergencies in Medicine, Research, and Industry* (Springfield, Ill.: Thomas, 1965), pp. 13–27.
22. Richie Calder, *Living With the Atom* (Chicago: University of Chicago Press, 1962), pp. 100–122.
23. International Atomic Energy Agency, *Environmental Contamination by Radioactive Materials* (Vienna: International Atomic Energy Agency, 1959).
24. C. W. Shillings, ed., *Atomic Energy Encyclopedia in the Sciences* (Philadelphia: Saunders, 1964).
25. C. W. Easley, *Basic Radiation Protection* (New York: Gordon and Breach, 1969), pp. 99–105.
26. David M. Lipscomb, "High Intensity Sounds in the Recreational Environment: Hazard to Young Ears," *Clinical Pediatrics,* Vol. 8, No. 2 (February 1969), 63–68.
27. Donald F. Anthrop, "Environmental Noise Pollution: A New Threat to Sanity," *Bulletin of the Atomic Scientists,* Vol. 25, No. 5 (May 1969), 13.
28. Robert A. Baron, "Let Quiet Be Public Policy," *Saturday Review,* No. 53 (November 7, 1970), 66–67.
29. Ibid.
30. Leo L. Beranek, ed., *Noise Reduction* (New York: McGraw-Hill, 1960).
31. American Public Health Association, Inc., *Principles for Healthful Rural Housing* (New York: American Public Health Association, 1957), p. 26.

Index